ANTI-INFLAMMATORY COOKBOOK
FOR
BEGINNERS

The Ultimate Guide to Reducing Inflammation

And Supporting the Immune System.

2001 Days Plus 8-Week Meal Plan with Delicious Recipes

by

Abbie Bates

Table of Contents

Welcome to the world of the anti-inflammatory diet!

In these pages I will take you on a journey of discovery in search of well-being through conscious nutrition. The anti-inflammatory diet is much more than just a simple diet: it's an opportunity to transform your life, to put your health and wellbeing at the center, to take care of your body and mind in ways you may never have considered before.

Inflammation is a natural response of the body to stressful situations or external aggressions, but when it becomes chronic, it can have a significant impact on our health. This book is dedicated to providing you with the knowledge, tools and recipes you need to fight inflammation and improve your overall health.

Together we will explore the power of anti-inflammatory foods, you will learn to recognize foods that can promote inflammation and those that can fight it, and you will discover how to prepare delicious and nutritious meals that will be good for your body and your spirit.

This knowledge could lead to a positive change in your life. I invite you to be open and willing to change, to explore new flavors, new eating habits and, above all, to put your health first. Every small step you take toward an anti-inflammatory diet will be an investment in your future well-being.

I'm excited to share this journey with you, and I believe you will find inspiration and motivation to start or continue your journey to a healthier, more fulfilling life.

Without further ado, let's dive into the wonderful adventure of the anti-inflammatory diet together!

With love,

Abbie Bates

Introduction

ANTI INFLAMMATORY COOKBOOK for BEGINNERS lays the foundation for a journey to wellness and health through an anti-inflammatory diet. In a world increasingly plagued by chronic diseases and busy lifestyles, chronic inflammation has become a widespread problem that threatens our vitality and longevity.

In the first chapter, we explore the fundamental concept of inflammation and discover how it is a natural response of our body to injury and infection, but becomes harmful when it becomes chronic and uncontrolled. This chronic inflammation is often the root of numerous diseases, including obesity, diabetes, heart disease, and even some forms of cancer. The good news is that we can influence inflammation through our food choices. In chapter two, we look in detail at the multiple benefits of an anti-inflammatory diet. From reducing the risk of chronic disease to potentially reducing the painful symptoms of existing inflammatory conditions, the benefits are extraordinary. An anti-inflammatory diet can also increase our energy, improve skin quality, and even positively impact our mood.

This book was written by experts in the fields of nutrition and health, and was created to guide you step-by-step in adopting an anti-inflammatory approach to your diet and lifestyle. Through a vast collection of recipes curated by experts, we will help you discover the pleasure of eating healthily and deliciously, without compromising your health. We are confident that after reading this book and following our advice, you will be able to experience a positive transformation in your overall health and well-being. It's time to embrace the Anti-Inflammatory Diet and begin your journey to a more vibrant, healthy life. Welcome to this extraordinary journey of healing and well-being!

The concept of an anti-inflammatory food pyramid

The anti-inflammatory food pyramid is a nutritional guide designed to promote overall health by emphasizing foods with known anti-inflammatory properties. At its foundation are whole, nutrient-dense foods such as fruits, vegetables, and whole grains, which form the basis of a well-balanced diet. The pyramid encourages the consumption of lean proteins, healthy fats, and specific herbs and spices known for their anti-inflammatory benefits. By minimizing processed foods and unhealthy fats, and incorporating lifestyle factors like regular exercise and stress management, this dietary approach aims to reduce inflammation in the body, contributing to improved well-being and a lowered risk of chronic diseases.

Top Tier (Consume Sparingly):
- Saturated and trans fats (limit as much as possible): red meat, fried foods, highly processed foods with trans fats.

Middle Tier (Consume in Moderation):
- Lean animal proteins: chicken, turkey, fish.
- Healthy fats: extra virgin olive oil, avocado, nuts, flaxseeds.
- Low-fat dairy: yogurt, low-fat cheese.

Moderate Tier (Consume in Moderate Amounts):
- Fruits: berries, cherries, apples, oranges.
- Leafy green vegetables: spinach, kale, broccoli, cauliflower.
- Legumes: beans, lentils, chickpeas.
- Whole grains: quinoa, farro, whole oats.

Base Tier (Consume Freely):
- Herbs and spices: turmeric, ginger, garlic, parsley.
- Green tea and herbal teas.
- Water: maintain adequate hydration.

Healthy Lifestyle Practices:
- Regular physical activity.
- Stress management through practices like yoga and meditation.
- Sufficient and quality sleep.

ANTI-INFLAMMATORY PYRAMID

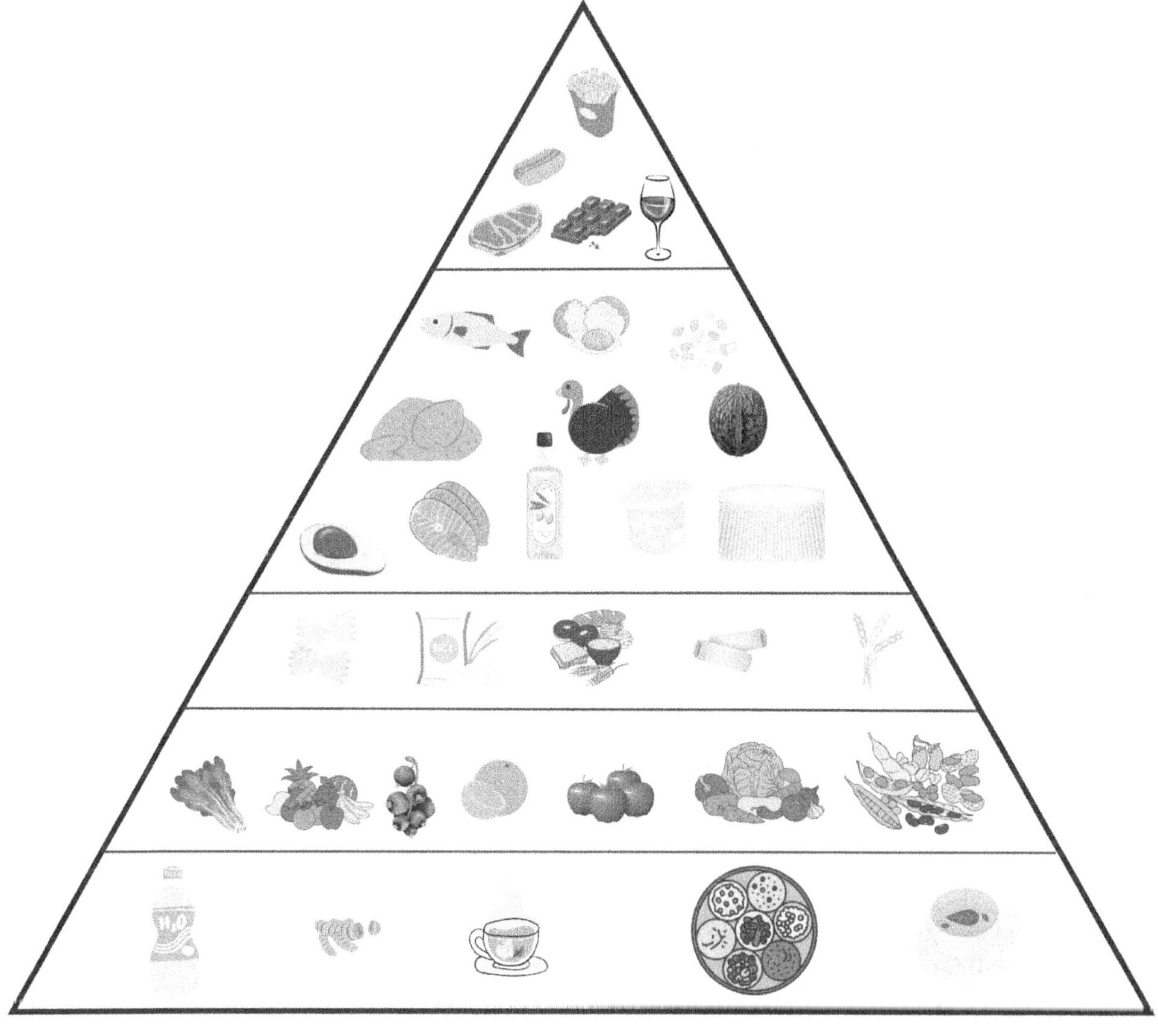

Healthy lifestyle practices: Regular physical activity, Stress management through practices such as yoga and meditation. Sufficient and quality sleep.

Chapter 1: Understanding Inflammation

Definition of inflammation

Inflammation: A Natural Response of the Body

Inflammation is a natural and fundamental biological process in our body. It is the immediate and complex response of the immune system to damage or infection. This chapter explores in detail this extraordinary defense mechanism that lies at the heart of our biological system.

Inflammation as a Defense Response

Inflammation is, first and foremost, a defense response. When the body detects a threat, such as a wound or bacterial infection, it activates a series of reactions to protect itself. This response is intended to limit damage and repair damaged tissue. For example, if you cut your hand, you will notice that the area will swell and become red. These are signs of inflammation that indicate your body is trying to heal.

Role of Immune Cells

Immune cells play a critical role in inflammation. When an injury or infection occurs, immune system cells, such as white blood cells, travel to the affected site. These cells work in a coordinated manner to fight pathogens and remove damaged cell debris. Inflammation helps concentrate these cells in the affected area to maximize the effectiveness of the immune response.

Phases of Inflammation

Inflammation is commonly divided into different stages. The first phase is called the vascular phase, in which blood vessels temporarily narrow to reduce blood flow to the damaged area, thus preventing excessive blood loss. Subsequently, the blood vessels dilate, allowing the flow of blood, which brings with it the cells of the immune system to fight the infection. This phase is accompanied by symptoms such as swelling and redness. The second phase, called the cellular phase, involves the action of immune cells. White blood cells, for example, engulf and destroy pathogens, playing a critical role in clearing the infection.

Acute Inflammation vs. Chronic

It is important to note that inflammation can be divided into two main types: acute inflammation and chronic inflammation. Acute inflammation is a temporary response and usually goes away when the threat is eliminated and the damaged tissue is repaired. It is a beneficial process that promotes healing. On the other hand, chronic inflammation is a problem. This form of inflammation persists for a long time term and is often triggered by factors such as obesity, insulin resistance or an unhealthy lifestyle. Chronic inflammation can contribute to the development of chronic diseases, including type 2 diabetes, heart disease, rheumatoid arthritis and even some forms of cancer. Therefore, understand the difference between these two types of inflammation It is essential for health management.

Acute Inflammation vs. Chronic

Acute Inflammation: A Protective Response

Acute inflammation is the most common form of inflammation and is a protective, well-regulated response of the body to injury or infection. This form of inflammation is usually transient and aims to repair damage and eliminate the underlying cause. When you get hurt, for example, your body immediately activates acute inflammation to limit the damage and begin the healing process. One of the hallmarks of acute inflammation is swelling, which is the result of increased blood flow to the affected area. This extra blood flow brings with it immune cells that fight the infection and remove damaged cell debris. Pain, another common symptom, is an important response that warns you to avoid further damage.

Chronic Inflammation: A Harmful Process

On the other hand, chronic inflammation is a form of long-term inflammation that persists even when there is no obvious threat. This type of inflammation is often caused by factors such as obesity, insulin resistance, chronic stress, or an unhealthy lifestyle. Unlike acute inflammation, chronic inflammation is dysfunctional and is linked to numerous chronic diseases. A crucial aspect of chronic inflammation is that it can be silent and underreported, as visible symptoms such as swelling and pain are often missed. This makes it difficult to recognize it without a specific medical evaluation. However, in the long term, chronic inflammation can contribute to the development of conditions such as type 2 diabetes, heart disease, rheumatoid arthritis and many others.

The Health Implications

Understanding the difference between acute and chronic inflammation is critical because it guides our health decisions. Acute inflammation is a necessary and beneficial response of our body, while chronic inflammation is harmful and can compromise our well-being. An essential part of health management is preventing or treating chronic inflammation through conscious lifestyle and nutrition choices. An anti-inflammatory diet, which will be discussed in detail in later sections of the book, is an effective tool for mitigating chronic inflammation and reducing the risk of associated chronic diseases.

The Classic Signs of Inflammation

Redness

One of the most obvious signs of inflammation is redness in the affected area. This color change is the result of increased blood flow to the affected area. During inflammation, blood vessels dilate to allow immune system cells to reach the site of inflammation more easily. The accumulation of blood leads to visible redness, which is often accompanied by an increase in local temperature.

Swelling

Swelling is another hallmark of inflammation. During inflammation, blood vessels become more permeable, allowing fluids, proteins, and immune system cells to leak out of the vessels and accumulate in the affected area. This fluid buildup causes swelling, which can vary in intensity depending on the severity of the inflammation.

Heat

Heat is often associated with inflammation and is the result of increased blood flow and metabolic activity in the affected area. When the immune system activates, there is an increase in blood flow, which can cause a warm sensation in the area. This sensation of heat is particularly evident when we touch the inflamed area.

Ache

Pain is a universal sign of inflammation. During inflammation, the nerve endings in the affected area are sensitized, making the area more sensitive to external stimuli. This makes pain a protective response that limits movement or contact with the inflamed area, thus contributing to the repair of damaged tissue.

Loss of Function

In some cases, inflammation can lead to a temporary loss of function in the affected area. For example, if a joint is inflamed due to infection or trauma, mobility may be limited due to pain and swelling. This loss of function is a protective mechanism that prevents further damage to the area. Importantly, these classic signs of inflammation are manifestations of acute inflammation, which is a normal and beneficial physiological response. However, when inflammation becomes chronic, these signs may not be as obvious or pronounced, which can make it more difficult to recognize without a thorough medical evaluation. Understanding these classic signs of inflammation is critical to recognizing when inflammation is present in our bodies and taking appropriate steps to manage it. The next step in our journey to health and wellness through an anti-inflammatory diet is to understand how we can positively influence inflammation through our food choices and lifestyle, a theme we will explore further in later sections of the book

Key Molecules: Cytokines and Inflammatory Mediators

Cytokines: Messengers of the Immune System

Cytokines are signaling molecules produced by cells of the immune system to communicate with each other. They function as messengers, transmitting important information that regulates the inflammatory response. During inflammation, cytokines are released in response to a danger signal. Some cytokines, called pro-inflammatory cytokines, promote inflammation. For example, tumor necrosis factor alpha (TNF-α) and interleukin-1 (IL-1) are cytokines that stimulate immune cells to react against a threat. This response is important for fighting infections and injuries. On the other hand, there are anti-inflammatory cytokines that limit inflammation and promote resolution. For example, interleukin-10 (IL-10) plays a key role in mitigating inflammation and preventing excessive tissue damage. This balance between pro-inflammatory and anti-inflammatory cytokines is essential for an adequate inflammatory response.

Inflammatory Mediators: Amplifiers of Inflammation

Inflammatory mediators are molecules that amplify inflammation, facilitating communication between cells immune system and increasing the effectiveness of the inflammatory response. A known inflammatory mediator is histamine, which is released during allergic inflammation and causes symptoms such as itching and swelling. Another important inflammatory mediator is prostaglandin, which is involved in many inflammatory reactions. Prostaglandins regulate the dilation of blood vessels and sensitivity to pain. Prostaglandin inhibitors, such as aspirin and nonsteroidal anti-inflammatory drugs (NSAIDs), are often used to reduce inflammation and pain.

Inflammatory Cascade

Inflammation is the result of a complex cascade of events in which cytokines and inflammatory mediators play central roles. The typical sequence begins with a warning sign, such as a wound or infection. This signal activates cells of the immune system, which in turn release pro-inflammatory cytokines. Pro-inflammatory cytokines coordinate the arrival of immune cells to the site of inflammation and promote inflammation. Inflammatory mediators, such as prostaglandins, further amplify inflammation and can cause symptoms such as pain. The ultimate goal of this cascade is to eliminate the threat, repair damaged tissue, and restore homeostasis. Once this task is completed, anti-inflammatory cytokines step in to limit inflammation and promote resolution.

Implications for Diet and Lifestyle

Understanding cytokines and inflammatory mediators is critical to understanding how our diet and lifestyle can influence inflammation. Some foods, such as those rich in omega-3 fatty acids, can reduce the production of pro-inflammatory cytokines, while others, such as refined sugars, can promote inflammation.

Chronic Inflammation and Related Diseases

Chronic Inflammation as a Risk Factor

Chronic inflammation has been identified as an important risk factor for numerous chronic diseases. These conditions include type 2 diabetes, heart disease, rheumatoid arthritis, neurodegenerative diseases such as Alzheimer's, some forms of cancer, and many others. This connection has been widely studied by the scientific community and has led to a deeper understanding of the underlying causes of these diseases.

Type 2 diabetes

Chronic inflammation is closely related to insulin resistance, a key factor in type 2 diabetes. Inflammation can interfere with the ability of cells to respond to insulin, which regulates blood sugar levels. This can lead to the buildup of blood sugar and the progression of type 2 diabetes.

Heart Diseases

Heart disease, including atherosclerosis (hardening of the arteries), is often associated with chronic inflammation. Inflammation can contribute to the buildup of plaque in the arteries, increasing the risk of vascular occlusions and cardiovascular events such as myocardial infarction. Additionally, inflammation can affect the function of the heart tissue itself.

Rheumatoid arthritis

Rheumatoid arthritis is an autoimmune disease in which the immune system attacks the joints, causing inflammation and chronic pain. Persistent inflammation is a key feature of this condition and can lead to permanent joint damage.

Neurodegenerative diseases

Recent studies have highlighted the role of inflammation chronic in neurodegenerative diseases such as Alzheimer's and Parkinson's disease. Inflammation in the brain can contribute to the death of nerve cells and the worsening of symptoms.

Cancer

Chronic inflammation has been associated with an increased risk of some forms of cancer. Inflammation can influence the tumor microenvironment, promoting the growth of tumor cells and the formation of new blood vessels that feed the tumor.

Obesity and Inflammation

Obesity is a significant risk factor for chronic inflammation. Adipose tissue (adipose tissue) can release pro-inflammatory cytokines, thus contributing to systemic inflammation. This inflammation can further worsen obesity and increase the risk of related diseases.

A Vicious Circle

What makes chronic inflammation especially problematic is that it can become a vicious cycle. For example, obesity can trigger chronic inflammation, which in turn can worsen obesity, creating a continuous cycle of inflammation and health deterioration.

The Promising Way of Prevention

Understanding the connection between chronic inflammation and these diseases offers a promising avenue for prevention and treatment. This awareness has prompted the search for strategies to mitigate chronic inflammation through lifestyle and dietary changes. An anti-inflammatory diet, rich in foods that reduce inflammation and low in those that promote it, has emerged as an effective approach to preventing or managing these diseases.

Inflammation and Nutrition

The Power of Nutrition in Inflammation

Inflammation is a natural and necessary biological process, but when it becomes chronic, it can lead to serious health problems. One of the major influences on chronic inflammation is our diet. The foods we choose to consume can trigger or reduce inflammation in our bodies, and this knowledge gives us the power to shape our health through our food choices. Pro-inflammatory foods vs. Anti-inflammatories. In the context of inflammation, foods can be divided into two main categories: pro-inflammatory and anti-inflammatory.

Pro-inflammatory foods

These foods can increase inflammation in the body. They include refined sugars, high glycemic index carbohydrates, saturated and trans fats, processed meats, sodium-rich foods and sugary drinks. These foods can trigger chronic inflammation when consumed in excess and on a regular basis.

Anti-inflammatory foods

These foods, in contrast, can reduce inflammation or promote resolution of inflammation. They include fruits and vegetables, especially those rich in antioxidants like vitamins C and E, omega-3 fatty acids (found in fatty fish like salmon), nuts, seeds, legumes, whole grains, and spices like turmeric and ginger. These foods contain compounds that can fight inflammation and support overall well-being.

Role of Omega-3 Fatty Acids

Omega-3 fatty acids are especially important in fighting inflammation. These polyunsaturated fats are present in foods such as oily fish (salmon, mackerel, tuna), flax seeds, fish oil and walnuts. Omega-3s have been shown to reduce the production of pro-inflammatory cytokines and promote anti-inflammatory cytokines. This balance helps reduce chronic inflammation.

Fiber and Intestinal Microbiota

Dietary fiber is another ally in the fight against inflammation. A diet rich in fiber, coming from vegetables, fruits and whole grains, supports a healthy intestinal microbiota. The microbiota, or intestinal flora, is made up of trillions of microorganisms that live in our intestines and play a fundamental role in regulating the immune system and inflammation. A high-fiber diet promotes a health-promoting gut environment and can reduce systemic inflammation.

The Harmful Effects of Sugar

Sugar has been linked to chronic inflammation. Excessive consumption of refined sugar and sugary drinks can increase blood sugar levels and promote inflammation. This is especially relevant in the fight against type 2 diabetes and other inflammation-related conditions.

Anti-inflammatory Lifestyle and Nutrition

In addition to considering specific foods, a healthy lifestyle is essential to combat chronic inflammation. Regular exercise, stress management, and quality sleep are all key to keeping inflammation under control. These factors may help reduce oxidative stress and systemic inflammation.

The Path to an Anti-Inflammatory Diet

The heart of the book is dedicated to exploring a wide range of anti-inflammatory foods and recipes. Readers will be guided through selecting nutrient-dense foods and discover how to combine ingredients to create flavorful meals that promote wellness and reduced inflammation. With a thorough understanding of the principles of an anti-inflammatory diet, readers will be able to make informed food choices that promote long-term health.

Causes of inflammation

External Causes

Physical Trauma

Here we examine how physical injuries, such as cuts, bruises, and fractures, trigger an inflammatory response. It discusses how our body immediately sends immune cells to the site of injury to prevent infection and promote healing. The importance of acute inflammation as a protective response and how, in some cases, it can progress to chronic inflammation is emphasized.

Infections

Bacteria, viruses and other pathogens can trigger an inflammatory response to try to neutralize the infectious agent. The concept of "low-grade inflammation" associated with chronic infections such as viral hepatitis or HIV infection, in which the inflammation persists long-term, is discussed.

Exposure to Environmental Toxins

Exposure to environmental toxins, such as air pollutants, pesticides or heavy metals, can trigger inflammatory reactions. The body tries to protect itself from toxic exposure by activating inflammatory defense mechanisms. Additionally, the long-term health risks associated with continued exposure to these substances are addressed.

Chronic Injuries and Inflammation

Let us now address the topic of chronic injuries, such as those caused by repetitive processes or persistent irritants. We see how repeated stress injuries, for example in professional or sporting settings, can lead to chronic inflammation, explaining the importance of correct management of such injuries to prevent ongoing inflammation.

Autoimmune Processes

We cover the role of autoimmune diseases, in which the immune system mistakenly attacks its own tissues and organs. These autoimmune processes can trigger chronic inflammation and irreparably damage target organs. We give examples of autoimmune diseases, such as systemic lupus erythematosus and Crohn's disease, to illustrate how inflammation is central to their manifestations.

Dietary causes

Refined Sugars and Glycemic Index

We examine the effect of refined sugars and high glycemic index foods on promoting inflammation. Excessive consumption of simple sugars, such as glucose and fructose, can increase blood sugar levels and trigger inflammatory responses. There are links between the glycemic index of foods and inflammation, further highlighting the importance of a low glycemic index diet.

Saturated Fats and Trans Fats

What is the role of saturated fats and trans fats in chronic inflammation? Foods high in saturated fat, such as red meat and high-fat dairy products, can contribute to systemic inflammation. Additionally, trans fats, often found in processed and fried foods, can increase inflammation and the risk of chronic disease.

Processed Foods and Food Additives

What are the negative effects of processed foods and food additives on inflammation? Preservatives, artificial colors and flavors found in many processed foods contribute to chronic inflammation. The high salt and sodium content in many food options is also the cause. packaged.

Foods Rich in Omega-6 vs. Omega 3

The balance of omega-6 and omega-3 fatty acids in the diet can influence inflammation. A diet rich in omega-6, often combined with vegetable oils such as corn and soybean oil, promotes inflammation when it is disproportionate to omega-3, which have anti-inflammatory effects. We present strategies to improve the ratio of these fatty acids through the selection of appropriate food sources.

Anti-inflammatory foods

Let's consider an overview of foods with anti-inflammatory properties. Fruit vegetables, nuts, seeds, whole grains and spices like turmeric and lo ginger help reduce inflammation in the body. Let's examine the scientific basis behind these foods and how they can be incorporated into an anti-inflammatory diet.

Role of Hydration and Drinks

Now let's talk about drinks and their role in managing inflammation. Adequate water consumption and the role of green tea, turmeric tea and other beverages can contribute to the reduction of inflammation

Causes Related to Lifestyle

Tobacco Smoke and Inflammation

A harmful and serious aspect is the impact of tobacco smoking on chronic inflammation. The smoke of cigarette contains toxic chemicals that can trigger inflammatory reactions in the body. It is important to emphasize the correlation between smoking and chronic inflammatory diseases, such as chronic obstructive pulmonary disease (COPD) and cancer.

Alcohol Consumption and Inflammation

Alcohol abuse can damage the liver and trigger inflammatory responses. Moderation is important just as responsible alcohol consumption, if at all appropriate, is good.

Quality Sleep and Inflammation

Another crucial factor is sleep in managing inflammation. In fact, poor quality sleep or insufficient quantity of sleep can contribute to chronic inflammation. There are mechanisms by which sleep affects the immune system and inflammation, and practical advice is offered for improving sleep quality.

Stress and Inflammation

Chronic stress also causes cellular inflammation. In fact, a high level can activate inflammatory responses and compromise the immune system. So stress management strategies, including relaxation and mindfulness techniques, are important as they can help reduce inflammation.

Physical Activity and Reduction of Inflammation

The positive role of physical activity in chronic inflammation is known. Regular exercise can have anti-inflammatory effects, improving insulin sensitivity, reducing visceral fat accumulation, and promoting overall well-being.

Social and Community Impact

The last piece of advice I would like to give in terms of the causes that can promote chronic inflammation is to highlight how social support and a sense of community can influence chronic inflammation. Positive interpersonal relationships and belonging to supportive communities can help reduce stress and promote mental health, indirectly contributing to the management of inflammation.

Genetic and Autoimmune Causes

Genetic predisposition to inflammation

Some people may be genetically predisposed to developing exaggerated inflammatory responses. Genetic variants are associated with an increased risk of chronic inflammatory diseases, such as rheumatoid arthritis or Crohn's disease. It is important to understand your family history and genetic predispositions to take preventative measures.

Autoimmune Diseases and Inflammation

Here we will focus on autoimmune diseases and their role in chronic inflammation. These conditions, such as systemic lupus erythematosus, multiple sclerosis and Sjögren's syndrome, can trigger systemic inflammatory responses due to incorrect activation of the immune system against its own tissues. It would be important to manage these diseases to reduce inflammation and prevent tissue damage.

Treatments for Autoimmune Diseases

There are treatments available for autoimmune diseases, with a focus on approaches aimed at reducing inflammation. Immunosuppressive drugs, biologic therapies, and immune system modulating therapies are available. Having information about health management strategies for those living with autoimmune diseases is as important as prevention strategies.

Prevention and Risk Reduction

In the medical field, prevention is an aspect of undeniable importance and usefulness. Perhaps the best advice that can be provided is that risk prevention and reduction of autoimmune diseases and excessive inflammatory responses can be seen as a healthy lifestyle, including conscious food choices and stress reduction. Helping to keep inflammation under control is essential even in the case of genetic predisposition.

Prevention and Risk Reduction

In the medical field, prevention is an aspect of undeniable importance and usefulness. Perhaps the greatest advise is that the prevention and reduction of the risk of autoimmune disorders and excessive inflammatory reactions can be viewed as a healthy lifestyle, which includes conscientious food choices and stress reduction. Helping to keep inflammation under control is essential even in the case of genetic predisposition.

The Importance of Early Diagnosis

The importance of early diagnosis of autoimmune diseases to prevent chronic inflammation and tissue damage cannot be emphasized enough. Recognizing the early symptoms of autoimmune diseases and the need to consult a healthcare professional for an accurate and timely diagnosis should be a routine choice for everyone.

Age-Related Causes

Aging of the Immune System

The immune system undergoes significant changes with age, influencing the inflammatory response. Unfortunately, there is a weakening of the immune defenses over time, which can make the body more susceptible to infections and chronic inflammation. Alterations in immune cell activity, with a focus on cells called "silent inflammatory," can promote chronically active inflammation.

Chronic Inflammation and Aging

There is a link between chronic inflammation and aging. Chronic inflammation can be considered a characteristic of aging itself and contributes to the onset of age-related chronic diseases. Inflammation can accelerate the cellular and tissue aging process.

Age-Related Diseases and Inflammation

We examine some of the most common age-related chronic diseases, such as atherosclerosis, dementia, and osteoporosis, and the central role of inflammation in their pathogenesis. Chronic inflammation may contribute to the onset and progression of these diseases, underscoring the importance of managing inflammation in healthy aging.

Lifestyle and Aging Factors

Lifestyle choices can also influence age-related inflammation. A balanced diet, regular exercise, quality sleep and stress management help mitigate inflammation in aging.

Strategies for Healthy Aging

Let's look at practical strategies to promote healthy aging and manage chronic inflammation in adulthood. Tips on how to incorporate an anti-inflammatory diet into your daily routine, how to maintain adequate physical activity, and how to manage specific age-related challenges, such as bone health and brain health.

Causes Related to Obesity and Body Composition

Adiposity and Inflammation

Excess adipose tissue, particularly visceral fat, may be an important mediator of chronic inflammation. In fact, adipose cells release pro-inflammatory cytokines, such as TNF-alpha and IL-6, which can trigger and maintain systemic inflammation. Obesity is often associated with chronic inflammation and increased risk of chronic disease.

Insulin Resistance and Inflammation

Let's examine the link between insulin resistance and inflammation. Accumulation of body fat, especially around the abdomen, could lead to decreased insulin sensitivity. This can trigger a series of events that contribute to chronic inflammation and type 2 diabetes.

Role of Hormones and Inflammation

We also examine the role of hormones, particularly adiponectin and leptin, in regulating inflammation. It explains how adiponectin, a hormone produced by adipose tissue, has anti-inflammatory effects, while leptin, involved in the regulation of appetite, can promote inflammation when it is present in excess. Hormone imbalance can contribute to chronic inflammation.

Body Composition and Chronic Inflammation

The concept of "healthy metabolism" examines how body composition, including percentage of fat and muscle mass, can influence inflammation. An increase in muscle mass and a decrease in fat mass may be associated with a reduction in chronic inflammation. Exercise and a proper diet can improve body composition.

Role of Diet in Obesity and Inflammation

A diet high in sugar, saturated fat, and highly processed foods contributes to body fat accumulation and inflammation.

Importance of Physical Exercise

Physical activity can play a crucial role in managing obesity and chronic inflammation. Regular exercise promotes weight loss, improves insulin sensitivity and reduces systemic inflammation.

Effects of inflammation on health

Damage to Tissues

Local Inflammatory Reactions

Let's start by exploring local inflammatory reactions. When the body detects damage or infection, it triggers an acute inflammatory response. This response is intended to isolate the affected area and begin the repair process. However, in the presence of chronic inflammation, this response can become harmful. Immune cells and pro-inflammatory cytokines can build up in the tissue, damaging surrounding healthy cells.

Cell Damage

Chronic inflammation can cause direct damage to cells. Oxygen-reactive molecules, called free radicals, are generated as part of the inflammatory process and can damage DNA, proteins and cellular lipids. This damage can lead to genetic mutations, cellular malfunctions and, ultimately, cell death.

Excessive Immune Response

An excessive inflammatory response can cause tissue damage. In an attempt to fight persistent inflammation, the immune system can become overactive and mistarget healthy tissue. This phenomenon is known as autoimmunity and is associated with many autoimmune diseases, such as lupus and multiple sclerosis. Autoimmunity can cause significant tissue damage, leading to debilitating symptoms.

Inflammation and Deterioration of the Endothelium

The endothelium is a layer of cells that lines the insides of blood vessels. Chronic inflammation can damage the endothelium, compromising its function. This can lead to a decrease in vascular dilation, increasing the risk of hypertension and atherosclerosis. Inflammation in the endothelium can also promote the formation of blood clots, increasing the risk of cardiovascular events.

Damage to Organ Tissues

Organ tissues can be severely damaged by chronic inflammation. Long-term liver inflammation, for example, might result in cirrhosis, a condition in which normal liver tissue is replaced by tissue that is scarred. In the digestive system, chronic inflammation can damage the intestinal lining, contributing to disorders such as Crohn's disease and ulcerative colitis. Additionally, inflammation can damage the connective tissue in the joints, leading to rheumatic diseases such as rheumatoid arthritis.

Effects on the Nervous System

Chronic inflammation can also affect the nervous system. Inflammation in the brain can cause damage to neurons and contribute to neurodegenerative disorders such as Alzheimer's and Parkinson's disease. Additionally, inflammation can increase the permeability of the blood-brain barrier, allowing harmful substances to enter the brain.

Damage to Muscle Tissues

Chronic inflammation can also affect muscle tissue. This phenomenon is evident in conditions such as myositis, where the immune system attacks the muscles. Muscle inflammation can cause weakness, pain, and decreased physical function.

Management of Inflammation for Tissue Health

The importance of managing inflammation to maintain tissue health is very important. Adopting an anti-inflammatory diet and promoting a healthy and conscious lifestyle can mitigate chronic inflammation. It is also possible to resort to medical therapies to control inflammation in chronic diseases.

Cardiovascular diseases

Atherosclerosis and Inflammation

One of the major cardiovascular diseases related to inflammation is atherosclerosis. Inflammation is involved in the formation of atherosclerotic plaques within the arteries, it can damage the arterial wall, triggering an immune response that leads to the accumulation of immune cells and lipids in the arteries. This process can restrict blood flow and increase the risk of cardiovascular events such as heart attack and stroke.

Inflammation and Hypertension

Inflammatory cytokines negatively influence the regulation of blood pressure, contributing to high values. In fact, chronic inflammation can damage blood vessels and promote hypertension, further increasing the risk of cardiovascular disease.

Role of Lipoproteins and Inflammation

We look at the role of lipoproteins, particularly low-density lipoproteins (LDL) often called "bad cholesterol," in the context of cardiovascular inflammation. LDL can undergo oxidative changes due to inflammation, becoming particularly harmful to arterial walls. These modified lipoproteins can contribute to the formation of atherosclerotic plaques and local inflammation.

Chronic Inflammation and Risk of Thrombosis

The risk of thrombosis (blood clots) is associated with chronic inflammation. Inflammation contributes to the blood's tendency to clot, increasing the risk of vascular occlusions and interrupting blood flow. There is a link between inflammation and thrombotic events, such as myocardial infarctions and strokes.

Management of Inflammation for Cardiovascular Health

Preserving cardiovascular health is done by managing inflammation which should be reduced. The elements to do this are conscious lifestyle choices and the adoption of an anti-inflammatory diet.

Autoimmune Diseases

Introduction to Autoimmune Diseases

We now provide an overview of autoimmune diseases, such as systemic lupus erythematosus, rheumatoid arthritis, multiple sclerosis and others. These conditions involve the immune system which, instead of protecting the body, mistakenly attacks healthy tissue. Inflammation is often a central element in this autoimmune process.

Role of Inflammation in Autoimmunity

Chronic inflammation can trigger or exacerbate autoimmune diseases. It is the pro-inflammatory cytokines that can contribute to the abnormal activation of the immune system and the production of autoantibodies, which attack the body's tissues.

Effects of Inflammation on the Symptoms of Autoimmune Diseases

Inflammation directly influences the symptoms of autoimmune diseases. Inflammatory processes in the affected tissues cause pain, swelling and tissue damage. These symptoms often characterize autoimmune diseases and can vary in intensity depending on the degree of inflammation present.

Inflammation and Progression of Autoimmune Diseases

Inflammation may contribute to the course of autoimmune illnesses; in fact, if not controlled, it causes irreparable damage in the affected tissues, with long-term implications for organ function and patient quality of life.

Impact on Obesity

Inflammation in Adipose Tissue

The accumulation of excess body fat, particularly visceral fat (fat around internal organs), may be an important mediator of inflammation. Fat cells produce pro-inflammatory cytokines, such as TNF-alpha and IL-6, which can trigger and maintain inflammation systemic.

Insulin Resistance and Inflammation

Body fat increase, particularly around the abdomen, can contribute to a loss in insulin sensitivity, which means the body has difficulties using insulin properly to manage blood sugar levels. This state of insulin resistance can trigger a series of events that contribute to chronic inflammation.

Role of Hormones in Obesity and Inflammation

Adiponectin, a hormone produced by fat cells, has anti-inflammatory effects, while leptin, involved in appetite regulation, could promote inflammation when present in excess. Hormone imbalance may contribute to chronic inflammation in obesity.

Body Composition and Inflammation

We look at the concept of "healthy metabolism" and how body composition, including percentage of fat and muscle mass, influences inflammation in obesity. An increase in muscle mass and a decrease in fat mass may be associated with a reduction in chronic inflammation.

Role of Diet in Obesity and Inflammation

The role of diet in obesity and chronic inflammation is critical. In fact, a diet high in added sugars, saturated fats and highly processed foods can contribute to the accumulation of body fat and inflammation.

Importance of Physical Exercise

Finally, the role of physical activity in the management of obesity and chronic inflammation is crucial. In fact, regular exercise promotes weight loss, improves insulin sensitivity and reduces systemic inflammation.

Mental health

Inflammation and the Central Nervous System

Inflammation in the body can have direct effects on the central nervous system. Inflammatory cytokines can cross the blood-brain barrier and activate inflammatory processes in the brain. These brain inflammatory processes can affect cognitive and emotional functions.

Excess adipose tissue, particularly visceral fat, may be an important mediator of chronic inflammation. In fact, adipose cells release pro-inflammatory cytokines, such as TNF-alpha and IL-6, which can trigger and maintain systemic inflammation. Obesity is often associated with chronic inflammation and increased risk of chronic disease.

Insulin Resistance and Inflammation

Let's examine the link between insulin resistance and inflammation. Accumulation of body fat, especially around the abdomen, could lead to decreased insulin sensitivity. This can trigger a series of events that contribute to chronic inflammation and type 2 diabetes.

Role of Hormones and Inflammation

We also examine the role of hormones, particularly adiponectin and leptin, in regulating inflammation. It explains how adiponectin, a hormone produced by adipose tissue, has anti-inflammatory effects, while leptin, involved in the regulation of appetite, can promote inflammation when it is present in excess. Hormone imbalance can contribute to chronic inflammation.

Body Composition and Chronic Inflammation

The concept of "healthy metabolism" examines how body composition, including percentage of fat and muscle mass, can influence inflammation. An increase in muscle mass and a decrease in fat mass may be associated with a reduction in chronic inflammation. Exercise and a proper diet can improve body composition.

Role of Diet in Obesity and Inflammation

A diet high in sugar, saturated fat, and highly processed foods contributes to body fat accumulation and inflammation.

Importance of Physical Exercise

Physical activity can play a crucial role in managing obesity and chronic inflammation. Regular exercise promotes weight loss, improves insulin sensitivity and reduces systemic inflammation.

Effects of inflammation on health

Damage to Tissues

Local Inflammatory Reactions

Let's start by exploring local inflammatory reactions. When the body detects damage or infection, it triggers an acute inflammatory response. This response is intended to isolate the affected area and begin the repair process. However, in the presence of chronic inflammation, this response can become harmful. Immune cells and pro-inflammatory cytokines can build up in the tissue, damaging surrounding healthy cells.

Cell Damage

Chronic inflammation can cause direct damage to cells. Oxygen-reactive molecules, called free radicals, are generated as part of the inflammatory process and can damage DNA, proteins and cellular lipids. This damage can lead to genetic mutations, cellular malfunctions and, ultimately, cell death.

Excessive Immune Response

An excessive inflammatory response can cause tissue damage. In an attempt to fight persistent inflammation, the immune system can become overactive and mistarget healthy tissue. This phenomenon is known as autoimmunity and is associated with many autoimmune diseases, such as lupus and multiple sclerosis. Autoimmunity can cause significant tissue damage, leading to debilitating symptoms.

Inflammation and Deterioration of the Endothelium

The endothelium is a layer of cells that lines the insides of blood vessels. Chronic inflammation can damage the endothelium, compromising its function. This can lead to a decrease in vascular dilation, increasing the risk of hypertension and atherosclerosis. Inflammation in the endothelium can also promote the formation of blood clots, increasing the risk of cardiovascular events.

Damage to Organ Tissues

Organ tissues can be severely damaged by chronic inflammation. Long-term liver inflammation, for example, might result in cirrhosis, a condition in which normal liver tissue is replaced by tissue that is scarred. In the digestive system, chronic inflammation can damage the intestinal lining, contributing to disorders such as Crohn's disease and ulcerative colitis. Additionally, inflammation can damage the connective tissue in the joints, leading to rheumatic diseases such as rheumatoid arthritis.

Effects on the Nervous System

Chronic inflammation can also affect the nervous system. Inflammation in the brain can cause damage to neurons and contribute to neurodegenerative disorders such as Alzheimer's and Parkinson's disease. Additionally, inflammation can increase the permeability of the blood-brain barrier, allowing harmful substances to enter the brain.

Damage to Muscle Tissues

Chronic inflammation can also affect muscle tissue. This phenomenon is evident in conditions such as myositis, where the immune system attacks the muscles. Muscle inflammation can cause weakness, pain, and decreased physical function.

Management of Inflammation for Tissue Health

The importance of managing inflammation to maintain tissue health is very important. Adopting an anti-inflammatory diet and promoting a healthy and conscious lifestyle can mitigate chronic inflammation. It is also possible to resort to medical therapies to control inflammation in chronic diseases.

Cardiovascular diseases

Atherosclerosis and Inflammation

Chapter 3: Foods to Avoid

Pro-inflammatory foods

Foods High in Added Sugars

Types of Added Sugars

Added sugars are simple carbohydrates, such as glucose and fructose, that are deliberately added to foods during the manufacturing process. A distinction is made between natural sugars, such as those found in fruit, and added sugars, such as high fructose corn syrup and table sugar, which are often incorporated into foods and drinks to improve their flavor.

Inflammation and Glycemic Spikes

Consuming added sugars can lead to rapid and significant blood sugar spikes after meals. These blood sugar spikes trigger an inflammatory response in the body, with an increase in pro-inflammatory cytokines.

Role in Obesity

Now let's highlight the role of added sugars in obesity. High consumption of added sugars leads to an excess of calories in the diet, contributing to weight gain. Additionally, chronic inflammation caused by added sugars alters satiety signals in the brain, leading to higher overall calorie consumption.

Negative effects on metabolic health

The negative effects of added sugars on metabolic health are also examined. It explains how high sugar consumption can increase the risk of developing insulin resistance, a key factor in type 2 diabetes. It also addresses the importance of reducing sugar consumption to keep blood sugar levels stable. blood and promote metabolic health.

Strategies for Reducing Added Sugar Consumption

We conclude by providing practical suggestions for reducing the consumption of added sugars in the diet. Reading food labels to identify hidden sugars in packaged foods is encouraged, as well as suggest the adoption of healthier alternatives such as coconut sugar, honey or moderate use of sweeteners natural.

List of foods that often contain added sugar

- **Sugary drinks:** Carbonated drinks, fruit juices with added sugar, sweetened iced teas, sports drinks.
- **Sweets and desserts:** Cakes, biscuits, donuts, ice cream, sweets, milk chocolate, puddings.
- **Baked goods:** White bread, muffins, sugary breakfast cereals, pastries, packaged pancakes.
- **Sauces and condiments:** Ketchup, salad dressings, barbecue sauces, sweet soy sauce.
- **Packaged foods:** Breakfast cereals, protein bars, flavored yogurts, jellies, puddings.
- **Canned or jarred foods:** Fruit in syrup, fruit preserves, ready-made spaghetti sauces, canned soups.
- **Salty foods:** Some salad dressings, snacks such as chips and sweet popcorn, sauces for seasoning meat and chicken.
- **Drinking alcohol:** Sugary cocktails, flavored liqueurs, some low-alcohol beers.
- **Fast Food:** Many fast food chains use added sugars in their menus, including sandwiches, sauces and drinks.
- **Children's foods:** Children's cereals, children's fruit juices, children's cereal bars, children's canned fruit.
- **"Light" or "low-fat" foods:** Often, to compensate for the lack of fat, these products contain more sugar to improve the flavor.
- **"Sugar-Free" Foods:** Some foods labeled "sugar-free" may contain artificial sweeteners that can be equally problematic for your health.

Remember that reading food labels carefully is essential to spot added sugars, as they can appear under different names such as high fructose corn syrup, cane sugar, rice syrup, barley malt and many others. Reducing your consumption of these foods can contribute to healthier eating and better management of inflammation. Trans and Saturated Fats' Harmful Effects.

The Harmful Effects of Trans and Saturated Fats

Saturated Fats: Sources and Impact

Saturated fats are predominantly present in foods of animal origin such as fatty meat, butter, lard and cheese. Excessive consumption of saturated fats increases levels of LDL cholesterol (known as "bad cholesterol") in the blood, thus increasing the risk of cardiovascular disease. It is important to limit the consumption of these sources of saturated fat to promote heart health.

Trans Fats: Hydrogenation Process

Let's now address the issue of trans fats, which are often the result of an industrial process called partial hydrogenation. Vegetable oils are transformed into solid trans fats through this process and as such fats are often used in the food industry to improve the shelf life of products. These trans fats are harmful because they can increase LDL cholesterol levels and lower HDL cholesterol levels (known as "good cholesterol"), increasing the risk of heart disease.

Cardiovascular risks

Cardiovascular risks are associated with the consumption of trans and saturated fats. In fact inflammation, can be a result direct of high levels of trans fats in the blood, which can damage the walls of the arteries and contribute to formation of atherosclerotic plaques.

Chronic Inflammation and Autoimmune Diseases

Trans and saturated fats play a role in triggering or worsening autoimmune diseases. When inflammation causes an excessive immune response, it contributes to autoimmune conditions such as rheumatoid arthritis and lupus. It would be important to avoid these fats for those suffering from autoimmune diseases.

Strategies to Reduce Trans and Saturated Fat Consumption

We conclude by providing practical suggestions for reducing the consumption of trans and saturated fats in the diet. It would be better to choose healthier alternatives, such as monounsaturated fats (found in olive oil and nuts) or polyunsaturated fats (found in vegetable oils), for cooking and seasoning meals.

Gluten and Dairy in Some Individuals as Pro-Inflammatory Foods

Gluten and dairy can act as pro-inflammatory foods, but with one important consideration: this reaction does not occur in all individuals. This is a food sensitivity that affects only some people.

Gluten and Gluten Sensitivity

Let's analyze gluten, a protein found in wheat, rye and barley. For some people, consuming gluten can trigger an inflammatory response in the immune system. This reaction can occur in individuals with non-celiac gluten sensitivity or the autoimmune condition known as celiac disease. Associated symptoms, which may include gastrointestinal problems, fatigue and inflammation.

Dairy products and lactose intolerance

The section goes on to look at dairy products, including milk, cheese and yogurt, and lactose intolerance. This condition is due to the body's inability to digest lactose, milk sugar, due to a deficiency of lactase, the enzyme responsible for its digestion. Lactose intolerance can cause symptoms gastrointestinal disorders such as bloating, cramps and diarrhea, which may be associated with inflammation.

Identifying Food Sensitivities

It would be a priority to be able to identify gluten sensitivity or lactose intolerance. In this context it is important to keep a food diary and monitor symptoms after consuming these foods. Additionally, you should consult a healthcare professional for an accurate diagnosis.

Management of Food Sensitivities

To manage food sensitivities to gluten or lactose, you should eliminate the offending foods from your diet and research gluten- or lactose-free alternatives. Not all people are sensitive to these foods, but for those who are, reducing or eliminating them can lead to significant improvements in health and reduced inflammation.

Role of Alcohol in Inflammation

Alcohol as an inflammatory product

Let's say right away that alcohol is an inflammatory product. When alcohol is metabolized in the body, yes produce toxic metabolites that can damage cells and tissues. This process of alcohol metabolism can trigger an inflammatory response in the body, with an increase in pro-inflammatory cytokines. This can lead to chronic inflammation, which has been associated with a number of health conditions, including heart disease, liver damage and gastrointestinal disorders.

Liver Damage and Inflammation

Here we explain how alcohol abuse can lead to inflammation of the liver, a condition known as alcoholic hepatitis. This inflammation can progress to liver cirrhosis, a serious and potentially fatal disease. It highlights the importance of moderating or completely avoiding alcohol consumption to prevent liver damage.

Effects on the Cardiovascular System

We also examine the effects of alcohol on the cardiovascular system. While some studies suggest that moderate alcohol consumption may have cardio-protective effects, excessive consumption can trigger inflammation and contribute to the risk of heart disease.

Link between Alcohol and Chronic Inflammation

Let us now highlight the link between chronic alcohol use and persistent systemic inflammation. Excessive alcohol consumption can negatively affect the immune system, compromising the body's ability to respond appropriately to threats. This can increase the risk of infections and chronic inflammatory diseases.

Sodium and High Salt Foods

Excess salt can contribute to high blood pressure and inflammation. Reducing the use of salt in meal preparation and choosing foods with a lower sodium content is highly recommended not only for this type of diet but as general health indications.

Chapter 4: Foods to Include

Key anti-inflammatory foods

Key anti-inflammatory foods

This paragraph is crucial in Chapter 4, as it highlights foods that play an essential role in reducing inflammation in the body and promoting optimal health. The foods mentioned here are rich in nutrients and compounds that have been shown to have anti-inflammatory properties and can contribute to overall well-being.

Colorful Fruits and Vegetables

Let's start by looking at the wide range of colorful fruits and vegetables that should be included in your diet. These foods are rich in antioxidants, vitamins and minerals that help fight inflammation. They mention red fruits like strawberries, orange fruits like carrots, green leafy vegetables like spinach and many other nutritious options.

Healthy Fats

We've already talked about healthy fats, like omega-3 fatty acids. These fatty acids, found in oily fish, walnuts, flaxseed and olive oil, are known for their anti-inflammatory properties. We want to reiterate how important it is to include these fat sources in your diet to balance the inflammatory effects of saturated fats.

Lean Proteins and Vegetable Sources

The paragraph also addresses the role of proteins in the anti-inflammatory diet. We recommend including lean proteins such as chicken, turkey, fish, and plant proteins such as legumes and tofu. These foods provide essential amino acids and nutrients that can help reduce inflammation and promote tissue repair.

Spices and aromatic herbs

In addition to classic foods, it is important to highlight the power of spices and aromatic herbs in anti-inflammatory cuisine. Some spices, such as turmeric and black pepper, contain powerful anti-inflammatory compounds. Regular use of these spices can add flavor to dishes and help fight inflammation.

Whole foods and cereals

Let's now look at the importance of whole foods and cereals in the anti-inflammatory diet. These foods provide fiber, vitamins and minerals that can help keep blood sugar levels stable and reduce inflammation. The use of whole grains such as quinoa, spelled and oats is recommended.

Foods rich in antioxidants

Foods rich in antioxidants

This type of food is essential in this diet because it promotes health and reduction of inflammation. The Antioxidants are natural compounds that help fight free radicals in the body, which are molecules unstable linked to inflammation and cellular damage.

Colorful Fruits and Vegetables

For example, there is a wide range of colorful fruits and vegetables that represent an excellent source of antioxidants. These foods are high in vitamins like C, E, and beta-carotene (a type of vitamin A), which function as antioxidants in the body. Fruits like oranges, strawberries, blueberries, and leafy greens like spinach are mentioned as some of the most antioxidant-rich options.

Nuts

There are also nuts such as walnuts, almonds and hazelnuts, which are rich in antioxidants such as vitamin E and selenium. These foods can be eaten as a healthy snack or added to salads and main dishes for a crunchy, nutritious twist.

Antioxidant drinks

Now let's consider drinks rich in antioxidants, such as green tea and white tea. These drinks contain catechins and polyphenols, which are antioxidant compounds known for their health benefits. Moderate consumption of coffee, which contains antioxidants and may have beneficial effects on health, is also discussed.

Cocoa and Dark Chocolate

We also mention cocoa and dark chocolate as sources of antioxidants. Cocoa is especially rich in flavonoids, which may help protect the heart and improve vascular health. We recommend choosing dark chocolate with a high cocoa content to maximize the benefits.

Spices Antioxidants

Finally, we again highlight the use of spices such as turmeric, which contains curcumin, a powerful natural antioxidant and anti-inflammatory. Including these spices in your cooking can not only add flavor to your dishes, but also help fight inflammation.

List of foods with the greatest levels of antioxidants

- **Berries:** Strawberries, blueberries, raspberries, blackcurrants and wild strawberries are particularly rich in antioxidants, including vitamin C and anthocyanins.
- **Citrus fruits:** Oranges, tangerines, grapefruits and lemons are rich in vitamin C and other antioxidants such as flavonoids.
- **Walnuts:** Walnuts, almonds and hazelnuts contain vitamin E, selenium and other beneficial antioxidants.
- **Leafy Greens:** Spinach, kale, chard, and other leafy greens are rich in antioxidants, including vitamin C, vitamin K, and carotenoids like lutein.
- **Cocoa and dark chocolate:** Cocoa contains flavonoids, while dark chocolate with a high cocoa content offers antioxidant benefits.
- **Green Tea:** Green tea is known to be rich in catechins, a type of flavonoid with antioxidant properties.
- **Spices:** Turmeric, ginger, oregano, rosemary and other spices contain antioxidant compounds.
- **Cherries:** Cherries are rich in antioxidants, especially anthocyanins, which give them their red color.
- **Grapes:** Grapes contain resveratrol, an antioxidant compound associated with health benefits.

- **Legumes:** Beans, lentils and chickpeas are rich in antioxidants such as vitamin C and polyphenols.
- **Seeds:** Flax seeds, chia seeds and sunflower seeds are sources of antioxidants, including omega-3 fatty acids and vitamin E.
- **Dried fruits:** Prunes, dried apricots and raisins are among the dried fruits with a high content of antioxidants.
- **Broccoli:** This cruciferous vegetable is rich in vitamin C, carotenoids and other antioxidants.
- **Peppers:** Red, yellow and green peppers are rich in vitamin C and other antioxidants.
- **Carrots:** Carrots are a good source of carotenoids, including beta-carotene, an antioxidant that the body can convert into vitamin A.

Remember that a balanced diet that includes a variety of these foods can help provide a full range of antioxidants and health benefits.

Foods that support digestive health

Foods that support digestive health

It is important to enjoy good digestive health and which foods can help keep it in balance. Efficient digestion is crucial not only for optimal nutrient absorption, but also for reducing inflammation in the gastrointestinal tract.

Dietary Fiber

Fiber-rich foods, such as fruits, vegetables, legumes and whole grains, play a vital role in promoting digestive health. Fiber helps prevent constipation, promotes bowel regularity and nourishes the beneficial bacteria in the gut, known as the microbiota.

Yogurt and Fermented Foods

Let's continue by examining the role of fermented foods in digestive health. Yogurt, kefir, sauerkraut and kimchi are examples of foods rich in probiotics, beneficial bacteria that can improve body balance intestinal microbiota. These foods can help reduce inflammation in the gastrointestinal tract and improve digestion.

Water and Hydration

Hydration is a key component of digestive health. Drinking enough water is essential for keeping the digestive tract functioning well, preventing constipation and facilitating the passage of food through the intestine.

Foods Rich in Digestive Enzymes

Consider the role of digestive enzymes naturally present in some foods, such as pineapple and papaya. These enzymes can help break down foods and improve digestion.

Easy to Digest Foods

Including easily digestible foods in the diet in case of digestive problems is essential. These foods can include white rice, zucchini, and skinless chicken. They are lighter options on the digestive system and can be helpful during periods of gastrointestinal sensitivity.

Carbon hydrates and resistant starch

Carbonates and resistant starch can have a positive effect on digestive health. These compounds, found in foods such as green bananas and cold potatoes, can promote the growth of beneficial bacteria in the gut and contribute to bowel regularity.

Chapter 5: How to Plan an Anti-Inflammatory Meal

Meal planning guidelines

Macronutrient Balance

Lean Proteins for Satiety and Tissue Repair

We start by examining the role of lean protein in the anti-inflammatory meal. Protein plays a crucial role in promoting satiety and tissue repair. This section outlines how to include lean protein sources such as chicken, turkey, fish, legumes, and tofu in your meals to provide your body with the essential amino acids needed for muscle growth, recovery, and function.

- Complex Carbohydrates for a Sustainable Source of Energy
- Healthy Fats for Cellular Function and Nutrient Absorption
- Colorful Fruits and Vegetables for Powerful Antioxidants
- Healthy Fats to Reduce Inflammation
- Lean Proteins for Muscle Support and Anti-Inflammation
- Foods Rich in Fiber for Intestinal Regularity
- Spices and Aromatic Herbs for Taste and Health

Portion Sizes and Calorie Control

Know your portion sizes

Many people tend to overestimate or underestimate their portion sizes, which can affect their overall calorie intake.

Calorie Calculation and Control

Another fundamental aspect concerns the calculation and control of calories. You should calculate your daily calorie needs based on age, gender, physical activity and other individual factors. Understanding this value helps you plan meals that meet your calorie needs without exceeding.

Balancing Calories in and Calories Out

Here we also highlight the importance of balancing calorie intake with calorie consumption through physical activity. This is crucial for weight control and maintaining a healthy body weight.

Balanced Meal Planning

Another essential aspect concerns planning balanced meals in terms of calories. Balance proteins, carbohydrates and fats so that the meal provides the right calorie intake and supports nutritional needs, and focus on nutritious, antioxidant-rich foods to maximize anti-inflammatory benefits.

Food Variety and Rotation

Benefits of Dietary Variation

Consuming a wide range of foods allows you to get a greater diversity of nutrients, vitamins and minerals. This can help keep the body well-nourished and support optimal function.

Prevention of Food Sensitivities

Another fundamental aspect concerns the prevention of food sensitivities. Constant exposure to the same foods can increase the risk of developing food sensitivities or intolerances. Food rotation, that is, changing food sources, helps avoid this problem.

Experimentation with New Ingredients

Experimentation with new ingredients and recipes is also encouraged. Trying new ones can make cooking more interesting and fun. Additionally, it can lead to the discovery of anti-inflammatory foods that may have been overlooked in the past.

Seasonality and Location

Seasonality and locality of foods are another important aspect. It explains how choosing seasonal and local foods not only reduces the ecological footprint but also provides fresh and nutritious food. This highlights the importance of adapting meal planning to the resources available in your region.

Variety in Protein Sources and Carbohydrates

It is important to vary protein and carbohydrate sources. Including a variety of fish, lean meats, legumes, whole grains and vegetables offers a full range of nutrients and supports well-balanced anti-inflammatory nutrition.

Rotation of Fat Sources

Rotating fat sources is also crucial. Change between oils such as olive oil, oil coconut and flaxseed oil can provide a variety of essential fatty acids that support health.

Weekly Meal Planning

Benefits of Weekly Meal Planning

Among the various advantages are:

- **Saves Time:** Planning meals in advance reduces the time spent in the kitchen during the week, allowing you to prepare and cook more efficiently.
- **Better Nutritional Control:** Planning meals in advance gives you more control over ingredients and portions, helping you maintain a balanced, anti-inflammatory diet.
- **Stress Reduction:** Knowing in advance what to cook eliminates the last-minute stress associated with what to prepare for meals.

- **Money Savings:** Meal planning helps you avoid impulse purchases and food waste, saving money.

Preparing Meals in Advance

Preparing meals in advance is an essential aspect of weekly meal planning. Cooking in larger quantities and saving meals for the following days, this helps you save time and avoid less healthy food choices when you are hungry and in a hurry.

Adaptation to Individual Needs

Individual Dietary Considerations

This may include specific calorie needs, the
food preferences, food allergies or intolerances, and any pre-existing medical conditions. For example, those with a vegetarian or vegan diet may have to make different food choices than those who include meat in their diet.

Planning Meals Suitable for Your Needs

This may involve researching and identifying alternatives to problematic foods, such as choosing plant-based protein sources for vegetarians or selecting gluten-free grains for those with gluten intolerance.

Flexibility and Moderation

Another key point is the importance of flexibility and moderation. While the goal is to follow the anti-inflammatory diet, it is equally important to allow occasional indulgences to satisfy personal desires. This helps prevent feelings of restriction and makes the eating plan more sustainable in the long term.

Listening to the Body

The importance of listening to the body. Each individual has different signals of hunger and satiety, and your meal plan should reflect this. Listening to feelings of hunger and satiety can help you avoid calorie overload and promote a healthy relationship with food.

Recording and Monitoring

Finally, nutrition logging and monitoring are useful tools for tailoring your meal plan to individual needs. Keeping a food diary can help identify eating patterns, any adverse reactions to specific foods, and support the overall goal of anti-inflammatory eating.

Examples of Daily Meal Plans

These are examples in broad terms as we will see later how to better structure food plans

Example Daily Meal Plan 1: Reducing Inflammation

At this point in the book, a daily meal plan aimed at reducing inflammation is presented. It includes a breakfast of low-fat yogurt with fruit and nuts, a lunch of a large salad of spinach, quinoa and baked salmon, and a light dinner of grilled chicken and steamed vegetables. Nutritious snacks such as mixed nuts and baby carrots are also recommended throughout the day.

Example of Daily Meal Plan 2: Energy Support

This second example of a daily meal plan is designed to sustain energy throughout the day. Includes a protein-rich breakfast with eggs, avocado and wholemeal bread, a lunch with a turkey sandwich with coleslaw and a balanced dinner with grilled salmon, quinoa and broccoli. Snacks include fresh fruit and Greek yogurt to keep you energized.

Example of Daily Meal Plan 3: Weight Management

This third example of a daily meal plan focuses on weight management. Breakfast includes a smoothie bowl with fruit, spinach and chia seeds, lunch features a grilled chicken salad with light dressing and dinner features a large portion of grilled vegetables and tofu. Snacks consist of fresh fruit and almonds.

Example of Daily Meal Plan 4: Digestive Health Support

This fourth daily meal plan example is designed to support digestive health. Breakfast includes probiotic yogurt with blueberries, lunch features a fiber- and veggie-rich lentil soup, and dinner includes steamed salmon with brown rice and asparagus. Snacks include kefir and baby carrots.

Part II: The Recipes
Chapter 6: Breakfast Recipes
50 Anti-Inflammatory Breakfast Recipes

In these recipes, the values are expressed like this: Ingredients for 4 servings, Nutritional values per medium portion

1.Greek Yogurt Parfait with Blueberries and Walnuts

Ingredients: 2 cups Greek yogurt,1 cup fresh blueberries, 4 tablespoons chopped walnuts, Honey for drizzling (optional)

Preparation:

- In each of 4 glasses, layer ½ cup of Greek yogurt.
- Add ¼ cup of fresh blueberries over the yogurt in each glass.
- Sprinkle 1 tablespoon of chopped walnuts on top of the blueberries.
- Repeat the layering process, ending with a sprinkle of walnuts on each parfait.
- If wanted, drizzle honey over the surface.
- Serve immediately.

Nutritional Values: Calories: 360 kcal, Protein: 10g, Carbohydrates: 40g, Dietary Fiber: 6g, Sugar: 20g, Fat: 18g, Saturated Fat: 2g, Cholesterol: 10mg, Sodium: 50mg, Potassium: 300mg

2.Buckwheat Porridge with Apples and Cinnamon

Ingredients: 1 cup buckwheat groats, 2 cups water, 1 apple, sliced, 1 teaspoon cinnamon, 1 tablespoon honey

Preparation:

- In a medium saucepan, combine 1 cup of buckwheat groats and 2 cups of water. Bring to a boil.
- Reduce heat, cover, and simmer for 10-12 minutes or until the water is absorbed.
- Add 1 sliced apple, 1 teaspoon of cinnamon, and 1 tablespoon of honey to the cooked buckwheat.
- Continue to cook for another 2-3 minutes, stirring regularly.
- Serve the porridge in bowls with extra apple slices and a sprinkle of cinnamon.

Nutritional Values: Calories: 280 kcal, Protein: 7g, Carbohydrates: 60g, Dietary Fiber: 10g, Sugar: 14g, Fat: 3g, Saturated Fat: 0.5g, Cholesterol: 0mg, Sodium: 5mg, Potassium: 400mg

3.Banana and Oat Pancakes

Ingredients - 2 ripe bananas, 1 cup rolled oats, 1/2 cup Greek yogurt, 2 eggs, 1 teaspoon vanilla extract, 1 teaspoon baking powder, A pinch of salt

Preparation:

- In a blender, combine 2 ripe bananas, 1 cup of rolled oats, 1/2 cup of Greek yogurt, 2 eggs, 1 teaspoon of vanilla extract, 1 teaspoon of baking powder, and a pinch of salt. Blend until smooth.
- Lightly oil a nonstick skillet over a medium-high flame.
- Pour 1/4 cup of the pancake batter onto the skillet for each pancake.
- Cook until surface bubbles appear, then flip and cook until golden brown.
- Garnish with juicy fruit, honey, or maple syrup if preferred.

Nutritional Values: Calories: 290 kcal, Protein: 6g, Carbohydrates: 55g, Dietary Fiber: 6g, Sugar: 18g, Fat: 5g, Saturated Fat: 1g, Cholesterol: 30mg, Sodium: 400mg, Potassium: 430mg

4.Scrambled Eggs with Tomatoes and Spinach

Ingredients - 8 large eggs, 2 tomatoes, diced, 2 cups fresh spinach, Salt and pepper to taste, 2 tablespoons olive oil

Preparation:

- In a bowl, whisk 8 large eggs and season with salt and pepper.
- In a pan over a medium-high flame, heat 2 tablespoons of olive oil.
- Cook for just a few minutes, or until the diced tomatoes mellow.
- Cook until the spinach is wilted, about 2 cups.
- Pour the beaten eggs over the vegetables and cook, stirring, until the eggs are set. Serve hot.

Nutritional Values: Calories: 240 kcal, Protein: 15g, Carbohydrates: 6g, Dietary Fiber: 2g, Sugar: 3g, Fat: 17g, Saturated Fat: 4g
Cholesterol: 370mg, Sodium: 290mg, Potassium: 550mg

5.Green Smoothie with Spinach, Banana, and Avocado

Ingredients: - 2 cups fresh spinach, 2 ripe bananas, 1 ripe avocado, 2 cups water or almond milk, Honey or agave nectar (optional)

Preparation:

- Blend 2 cups of fresh spinach, 2 ripe bananas, 1 ripe avocado, and 2 cups of water (or almond milk) until smooth.
- If you want to sweeten with honey or maple nectar.
- Serve immediately.

Nutritional Values: Calories: 170 kcal, Protein: 3g, Carbohydrates: 23g, Dietary Fiber: 6g, Sugar: 10g, Fat: 9g, Saturated Fat: 1g
Cholesterol: 0mg, Sodium: 20mg, Potassium: 670mg

6.Yogurt with Chia Seeds and Fruit

Ingredients: - 2 cups Greek yogurt, 4 tablespoons chia seeds, 2 cups mixed fruit (e.g., berries, sliced banana), Honey for drizzling (optional)

Preparation:

- In each of 4 serving bowls, add 1/2 cup of Greek yogurt.
- Sprinkle 1 tablespoon of chia seeds over the yogurt in each bowl. Sprinkle with 1/2 cup mixed fruit.
- Drizzle with honey if desired.
- Serve immediately.

Nutritional Values: Calories: 260 kcal, Protein: 12g, Carbohydrates: 28g, Dietary Fiber: 8g, Sugar: 15g, Fat: 11g, Saturated Fat: 2g, Cholesterol: 10mg, Sodium: 70mg, Potassium: 470mg

7.Herb Omelet with Asparagus and Sun-Dried Tomatoes

Ingredients: - 8 large eggs, 1 cup asparagus, trimmed and cut into 1-inch pieces, 1/2 cup sun-dried tomatoes, chopped, 1/4 cup fresh herbs (e.g., parsley, chives), chopped, Salt and pepper to taste, 2 tablespoons olive oil

Preparation:

- In a bowl, whisk 8 large eggs and season with salt, pepper, and chopped fresh herbs.
- In a pan over a medium-high flame, heat 2 tablespoons of olive oil.
- Add the asparagus and cook until tender

- Add the sun-dried tomatoes to the skillet and sauté briefly.
- Pour the beaten eggs over the asparagus and tomatoes. Cook, lifting the edges to let uncooked eggs flow underneath.
- Once the omelet is set, fold it in half and slide it onto a serving plate.
- Garnish with extra fresh herbs.
- Serve hot.

Nutritional Values: Calories: 240 kcal, Protein: 14g, Carbohydrates: 9g, Dietary Fiber: 2g, Sugar: 4g, Fat: 16g, Saturated Fat: 4g
Cholesterol: 370mg, Sodium: 270mg, Potassium: 570mg

8. Avocado Toast with Sunny-Side-Up Eggs

Ingredients: - 4 slices whole-grain bread, 2 ripe avocados, 4 large eggs, Salt and pepper to taste, Olive oil for cooking eggs, Optional toppings: red pepper flakes, cherry tomatoes, arugula
Preparation:
- Toast 4 slices of whole-grain bread until golden brown.
- Cut the ripe avocados in half, remove the pit, and scoop the flesh into a bowl. Using a fork, mash the avocados and sprinkle with both pepper and salt.
- In a pan over a medium-high flame, add a little olive oil. Crack 4 large eggs into the skillet and cook sunny-side-up until the whites are set but the yolks are still runny.
- Carefully spread the mashed avocado across the bread slices.
- Carefully place a sunny-side-up egg on top of each avocado toast.
- Season with more salt, pepper, and any optional toppings you prefer.
- Serve immediately.

Nutritional Values: Calories: 260 kcal, Protein: 10g, Carbohydrates: 22g, Dietary Fiber: 7g, Sugar: 2g, Fat: 16g, Saturated Fat: 3g
Cholesterol: 190mg, Sodium: 260mg, Potassium: 750mg

9. Brown Rice Porridge with Dried Figs

Ingredients: 1 cup brown rice, 4 cups water, 1/2 cup dried figs (chopped), 1 teaspoon ground cinnamon, 2 tablespoons brown sugar, a pinch of salt
Preparation:
- In a pot, combine the brown rice and water. After bringing to a boil, remove off the heat
- Simmer, covered, for about 45 minutes or until the rice is tender and the water is absorbed.
- Add the dried figs, ground cinnamon, brown sugar, and a pinch of salt to the cooked rice. Mix well.
- Continue to cook for another 5 minutes, stirring occasionally, until the figs are soft and the mixture has a porridge-like consistency.
- Serve hot and garnish with additional dried figs if desired.

Nutritional Values: Calories 220, Carbohydrates 49g, Protein 4g, Fat 1g, Fiber 4g

10. Whole Wheat Crepes with Raspberry Sauce

Ingredients: 1 cup whole wheat flour, 2 eggs, 1 1/2 cups milk, 2 tablespoons olive oil, 1 teaspoon sugar, a pinch of salt, 1 cup fresh raspberries, 2 tablespoons powdered sugar
Preparation:
- In a bowl, mix the whole-wheat flour, eggs, milk, olive oil, sugar, and a pinch of salt until you have a smooth batter.
- Heat a non-stick pan and lightly grease it with oil.
- Pour a ladle of batter into the hot pan and cook until the bottom becomes golden. Place it on the opposite side to cook.
- Continue the process until all of the batter has been used.
- To prepare the raspberry sauce, blend the fresh raspberries with powdered sugar.
- Serve the crepes hot with the raspberry sauce drizzled on top.

Nutritional Values: Calories 180, Carbohydrates 26g, Protein 7g, Fat 5g, Fiber 4g

11. Coconut Parfait with Pineapple and Mango

Ingredients: 1 cup shredded coconut, 1 cup Greek yogurt, 1 cup fresh pineapple (diced), 1 cup fresh mango (diced), 2 tablespoons honey, a handful of toasted coconut for garnish
Preparation:
- In a bowl, combine the shredded coconut and Greek yogurt.
- In four dessert glasses, create alternating layers of the coconut yogurt mixture, diced pineapple, and diced mango.
- Drizzle a teaspoon of honey on each glass.
- Garnish with toasted coconut.
- Serve chilled as a refreshing dessert.

Nutritional Values: Calories 330, Carbohydrates 46g, Protein 6g, Fat 14g, Fiber 5g

12. Buckwheat Pancakes with Honey and Fresh Fruit

Ingredients: 1 cup buckwheat flour, 2 eggs, 1 cup milk, 2 tablespoons honey, 1 cup mixed fresh fruit (e.g., berries, banana, or apple), a pinch of salt
Preparation:
- In a bowl, whisk together the buckwheat flour, eggs, milk, honey, and a pinch of salt until you have a smooth batter.
- Heat a non-stick pan and lightly grease it with oil.
- Pour a ladle of batter into the hot pan and cook until the bottom becomes golden. Place it on the opposite side to cook.
- Continue the process until all of the batter has been used.
- Serve the pancakes with the mixed fresh fruit on top.
- Drizzle with additional honey if desired.

Nutritional Values: Calories 280, Carbohydrates 51g, Protein 10g, Fat 4g, Fiber 6g

13. Greek Yogurt with Walnuts and Honey

Ingredients: - 2 cups Greek yogurt, 1/2 cup chopped walnuts, 4 tablespoons honey
Preparation:
- Divide the Greek yogurt among four serving bowls.
- Sprinkle each bowl with chopped walnuts.
- Drizzle 1 tablespoon of honey over each bowl.
- Serve and enjoy!

Nutritional Values: Calories: 290 kcal, Protein: 14g, Carbohydrates: 23g, Dietary Fiber: 2g, Sugar: 18g, Fat: 18g, Saturated Fat: 3g, Cholesterol: 15mg, Sodium: 60mg, Potassium: 270mg

14.Strawberry Chia Seed Smoothie Bowl

Ingredients: - 2 cups strawberries, fresh or frozen, 1 cup Greek yogurt, 2 tablespoons chia seeds, 1 tablespoon honey, Optional toppings: sliced strawberries, chia seeds, nuts, and shredded coconut

Preparation:
- In a blender, combine the strawberries, Greek yogurt, chia seeds, and honey.
- Blend until smooth.
- Split the smoothie mixture among four serving bowls.
- Top with additional sliced strawberries, chia seeds, nuts, and shredded coconut as desired.
- Serve immediately.

Nutritional Values: Calories: 160 kcal, Protein: 9g, Carbohydrates: 20g, Dietary Fiber: 6g, Sugar: 11g, Fat: 6g, Saturated Fat: 1g

Cholesterol: 5mg, Sodium: 30mg, Potassium: 280mg

15.Herb Frittata with Peppers and Onions

Ingredients: - 8 large eggs, 1 cup red bell pepper, diced, 1 cup onion, diced, 1/4 cup fresh herbs (e.g., basil, thyme), chopped, Salt and pepper to taste, 2 tablespoons olive oil

Preparation:
- In a bowl, whisk 8 large eggs and season with salt, pepper, and chopped fresh herbs.
- Heat 2 tablespoons of olive oil in an ovenproof skillet over medium heat.
- Add the diced red bell pepper and onion and sauté until softened.
- Pour the beaten eggs over the peppers and onions. Cook, lifting the edges to let uncooked eggs flow underneath.
- Once the frittata is set around the edges, transfer the skillet to the oven and broil until the top is golden brown.
- Slice into wedges and serve hot.

Nutritional Values: Calories: 190 kcal, Protein: 11g, Carbohydrates: 6g, Dietary Fiber: 1g, Sugar: 2g, Fat: 14g, Saturated Fat: 3g

Cholesterol: 370mg, Sodium: 160mg, Potassium: 190mg

16.Whole Wheat Carrot and Walnut Muffins

Ingredients: 1 1/2 cups whole wheat flour, 1/2 cup rolled oats, 1 1/2 teaspoons baking powder, 1/2 teaspoon baking soda, 1/2 teaspoon ground cinnamon, 1/4 teaspoon salt, 2 large eggs, 1/4 cup honey, 1/4 cup unsweetened applesauce, 1/4 cup Greek yogurt

1 teaspoon vanilla extract, 1 1/2 cups grated carrots, 1/2 cup chopped walnuts

Preparation:
- Preheat the oven to 350°F (175°C) and line a muffin tin with paper liners.
- In a large bowl, whisk together the whole-wheat flour, rolled oats, baking powder, baking soda, ground cinnamon, and salt.
- In another bowl, beat the eggs and mix in the honey, applesauce, Greek yogurt, and vanilla extract.
- Combine the wet and dry ingredients, then fold in the grated carrots and chopped walnuts.
- Spread the batter among the muffin cups in a uniform layer.
- Cook for 18-20 minutes, or until a toothpick put into the center of the cake comes out clear.

- Let the muffins to cool down completely before serving.

Nutritional Values: Calories: 280 kcal, Protein: 9g, Carbohydrates: 42g, Dietary Fiber: 5g, Sugar:18g, Fat: 10g, Saturated Fat: 1g

Cholesterol: 85mg, Sodium: 300mg, Potassium: 350mg

17.Papaya Stuffed with Yogurt and Nuts

Ingredients: - 2 ripe papayas, halved and seeds removed, 2 cups Greek yogurt, 1/4 cup mixed nuts (e.g., almonds, walnuts, pistachios), chopped, 2 tablespoons honey

Preparation:
- Scoop Greek yogurt into the papaya halves.
- Drizzle honey over the yogurt.
- Top with the shredded mixed nuts.
- Serve the papaya halves as a refreshing and nutritious breakfast or snack.

Nutritional Values: Calories: 270 kcal, Protein: 12g, Carbohydrates: 36g, Dietary Fiber: 5g, Sugar: 24g, Fat: 9g, Saturated Fat: 1g, Cholesterol: 10mg, Sodium: 70mg, Potassium: 670mg

18. Buckwheat Crepes with Honey and Nuts

Ingredients: 1 cup buckwheat flour, 2 eggs, 1 1/2 cups milk, 1/4 teaspoon salt, 2 tablespoons melted butter, Honey, to taste, Chopped nuts, to taste

Preparation:
- In a bowl, mix the buckwheat flour with the eggs.
- Add in the milk carefully, stirring carefully to prevent lumps.
- Add the salt and melted butter, continuing to mix until smooth.
- Let the batter to cool down in the refrigerator for a minimum of 30 minutes.
- Heat a slightly oiled nonstick skillet over medium heat.
- Pour a ladle of batter into the pan, tilting it to evenly spread the batter across the surface.
- Cook the crepe for about 2 minutes on each side or until golden brown.
- Repeat the process with the remaining batter.
- Once ready, fold the crepes as desired and serve warm, with a generous drizzle of honey and a handful of chopped nuts.

Nutritional Values: Calories: 220, Protein: 8g, Fat: 10g, Carbohydrates: 25g, Fiber: 3g, Sugar: 6g, Sodium: 180mg

19. Millet Porridge with Apples and Cinnamon

Ingredients: 1 cup millet, 2 cups water, 2 cups milk (dairy or plant-based), 2 apples, peeled, cored, and diced, 2 tablespoons honey or maple syrup, 1 teaspoon ground cinnamon, 1/4 teaspoon salt, Chopped nuts or dried fruits for garnish (optional)

Preparation:
- Rinse the millet under cold water.
- In a medium saucepan, combine millet, water, and a pinch of salt. Bring to a boil, then reduce heat to low, cover, and simmer for 15-20 minutes or until millet is tender.
- Boil the milk in a separate pan until it is hot.
- Once the millet is cooked, stir in the warm milk, diced apples, honey (or maple syrup), cinnamon, and salt. Cook over low heat, stirring occasionally, until the mixture thickens to your desired consistency.

- Remove from heat and let it sit for a few minutes to allow flavors to meld.
- Serve the millet porridge warm, topped with additional diced apples, a sprinkle of cinnamon, and optional chopped nuts or dried fruits.

Nutritional Values: Calories: 280, Protein: 9g, Fat: 5g, Carbohydrates: 52g, Fiber: 6g, Sugar: 16g, Sodium: 220mg

20. Mushroom Omelet with Parsley

Ingredients: 3 large eggs, 1/2 cup mushrooms, sliced, 2 tablespoons butter or olive oil, Salt and pepper, to taste, 2 tablespoons fresh parsley, chopped, 1/4 cup grated cheese (optional)

Preparation:

- Crack the eggs into a mixing dish and whisk until fully mixed. Season with salt and pepper.
- In a non-stick skillet, heat 1 tablespoon of butter or olive oil over medium heat.
- Add the sliced mushrooms to the skillet and sauté until they are golden brown and tender. Remove mushrooms from the skillet and set aside.
- In the same skillet, add the remaining tablespoon of butter or olive oil.
- Pour the beaten eggs into the skillet, swirling them to ensure an even spread.
- As the eggs set at the edges, gently lift them with a spatula, letting the uncooked eggs flow underneath.
- Once the eggs are mostly set but still slightly runny on top, add the sautéed mushrooms evenly over one half of the omelet.
- Sprinkle chopped parsley and grated cheese (if using) over the mushrooms.
- Carefully fold the other half of the omelet over the mushrooms, creating a half-moon shape.
- Cook for an additional minute or until the cheese melts, and the omelet is cooked to your liking.
- Slide the omelet onto a plate, garnish with additional parsley if desired, and serve immediately.

Nutritional Values: Calories: 320, Protein: 17g, Fat: 25g, Carbohydrates: 4g, Fiber: 1g, Sugar: 2g, Sodium: 360mg

21. Peach Smoothie with Flaxseeds

Ingredients: 2 ripe peaches, peeled and sliced, 1/2 cup plain Greek yogurt, 1/2 cup almond milk (or any milk of your choice), 1 tablespoon flaxseeds, 1 tablespoon honey or maple syrup (optional), Ice cubes (optional)

Preparation:

- In a blender, combine the sliced peaches, Greek yogurt, almond milk, and flaxseeds.
- If you prefer a sweeter smoothie, add honey or maple syrup to the blender.
- Process the ingredients at a high speed in a blender until the mixture is creamy and smooth.
- If a thicker consistency is desired, add ice cubes to the blender and blend until smooth.
- Modify the level of sweetness and consistency of the smoothie as desired.
- Quickly put the peach smoothies into glasses and serve.

Nutritional Values: Calories: 180, Protein: 8g, Fat: 6g, Carbohydrates: 25g, Fiber: 5g, Sugar: 18g, Sodium: 90mg

22. Sweet Potato Pancakes with Maple Syrup

Ingredients: 1 cup cooked and mashed sweet potatoes, 1 cup all-purpose flour, 1 tablespoon baking powder, 1/2 teaspoon cinnamon, 1/4 teaspoon nutmeg, 1/4 teaspoon salt, 1 cup milk (dairy or plant-based), 1 large egg, 2 tablespoons melted butter or oil, Maple syrup, for serving

Preparation:

- In a large bowl, combine the mashed sweet potatoes, flour, baking powder, cinnamon, nutmeg, and salt.
- Mix together the milk, egg, and the melted butter or oil in an independent basin.
- Mix the wet components into the dry ingredients until they are barely mixed. Do not mix too much; a few lumps are acceptable.
- Lightly butter a grill or nonstick pan over a medium-high flame.
- Scoop 1/4 cup portions of batter onto the griddle, spreading them slightly with the back of a spoon to form pancakes.
- Cook until bubbles form on the surface of the pancakes, then flip and cook until the other side is golden brown.
- Continue until all of the batter has been utilized.
- Serve the sweet potato pancakes warm, drizzled with maple syrup.

Nutritional Values: Calories: 220, Protein: 6g, Fat: 7g, Carbohydrates: 34g, Fiber: 3g, Sugar: 7g, Sodium: 380mg

23. Kamut Porridge with Pears and Walnuts

Ingredients: 1 cup kamut grains, 2 cups water, 2 cups milk (dairy or plant-based), 2 ripe pears, peeled, cored, and diced, 1/4 cup chopped walnuts, 2 tbsp honey or maple syrup, 1/2 tsp cinnamon powder, pinch salt.

Preparation:

- Rinse the kamut grains under cold water.
- In a medium saucepan, combine kamut grains, water, and a pinch of salt. Bring to a boil, then reduce heat to low, cover, and simmer for 30-40 minutes or until kamut is tender.
- Boil the milk in another saucepan until it is warm.
- Once the kamut is cooked, stir in the warm milk, diced pears, chopped walnuts, honey (or maple syrup), and ground cinnamon. Cook over low heat, stirring occasionally, until the mixture thickens to your desired consistency.
- Remove from heat and let it sit for a few minutes to allow flavors to meld.
- Serve the kamut porridge warm, garnished with additional diced pears and a sprinkle of chopped walnuts.

Nutritional Values: Calories: 320, Protein: 10g, Fat: 8g, Carbohydrates: 55g, Fiber: 8g, Sugar: 18g, Sodium: 150mg

24. Baked Eggs with Tomatoes and Basil

Ingredients: 4 large eggs, 2 cups cherry tomatoes, halved, 2 tablespoons fresh basil, thinly sliced, 2 tablespoons olive oil, Salt and pepper, to taste, Grated Parmesan cheese (optional, for serving)

Preparation:

- Preheat the oven to 375°F (190°C).
- In a baking dish, drizzle 1 tablespoon of olive oil to coat the bottom.
- Arrange the halved cherry tomatoes in the dish.
- Create small wells in the tomatoes and carefully crack one egg into each well.

- Sprinkle the sliced basil over the eggs and tomatoes.
- Drizzle the remaining olive oil over the top and season with salt and pepper to taste.
- Cook for 12-15 minutes, so that the egg whites are set and the yolks are still somewhat runny, in an oven that has been preheated.
- Take it out from the oven and set aside for just a few minutes to cool.
- Serve the baked eggs with a sprinkle of grated Parmesan cheese if desired.

Nutritional Values: Calories: 220, Protein: 12g, Fat: 16g, Carbohydrates: 8g, Fiber: 2g, Sugar: 4g, Sodium: 160mg

25. Whole Wheat Crepes with Ricotta and Sugar-Free Jam

Ingredients:
For the Crepes: 1 cup whole wheat flour, 2 eggs, 1 1/2 cups milk (dairy or plant-based), 1/4 teaspoon salt, 2 tablespoons melted butter, Cooking spray or additional butter for greasing the pan
For the Filling: 1 cup ricotta cheese, Sugar-free jam or fruit compote of your choice, Fresh berries for garnish (optional), Mint leaves for garnish (optional)

Preparation:
For the Crepes:
- In a bowl, whisk together the whole-wheat flour, eggs, milk, and salt until well combined.
- Stir in the melted butter until the batter is smooth. Let it rest for at least 30 minutes in the refrigerator.
- Melt butter in a nonstick skillet or crepe pan over a medium-high flame. Grease lightly using a cooking spray or butter.
- Pour a small amount of batter into the center of the skillet, swirling to spread it thinly.
- Cook for one to two minutes per side, or until browned. Repeat with the remaining batter.

For the Filling:
- Spread a generous spoonful of ricotta cheese onto each crepe.
- Add a dollop of sugar-free jam or fruit compote in the center of the ricotta.
- Fold or roll the crepes and place them on a serving plate.

Serving:
1. Garnish the crepes with fresh berries and mint leaves if desired.
2. Serve immediately and enjoy your delicious and wholesome crepes!

Nutritional Values: Calories: 220, Protein: 12g, Fat: 10g, Carbohydrates: 22g, Fiber: 3g, Sugar: 5g, Sodium: 180mg

26. Pineapple Mint Smoothie

Ingredients: 1 cup fresh pineapple chunks, 1/2 banana, frozen, 1/2 cup Greek yogurt, 1/2 cup coconut water or pineapple juice, A handful of fresh mint leaves, Ice cubes (optional)

Preparation:
- In a blender, combine the fresh pineapple chunks, frozen banana, Greek yogurt, coconut water (or pineapple juice), and fresh mint leaves.
- To make a cooler smoothie, add a few ice cubes to the blender.
- Process the mixture at a high speed until it's creamy and smooth.
- Taste the smoothie and adjust the sweetness or thickness as needed by adding more banana or liquid.
- Pour the pineapple mint smoothie into glasses and garnish with a sprig of mint.

Nutritional Values: Calories: 180, Protein: 8g, Fat: 2g, Carbohydrates: 35g, Fiber: 5g, Sugar: 20g, Sodium: 45mg

27. Kefir Parfait with Fresh Fruit and Nuts

Ingredients: - 1 cup plain kefir, 1/2 cup granola, 1 cup mixed fresh fruit (berries, sliced banana, etc.), 2 tablespoons chopped nuts (almonds, walnuts, or your choice), 1 tablespoon of honey or maple syrup (optional), along with some fresh mint leaves for decoration.

Preparation:
- In a glass or a bowl, start by layering 1/4 cup of plain kefir at the bottom.
- Add 2 tablespoons of granola on top of the kefir layer.
- Place a portion of mixed fresh fruit (berries, sliced banana, etc.) over the granola.
- Sprinkle 1/2 tablespoon of chopped nuts over the fruit layer.
- Repeat the layers until the glass or bowl is filled, ending with a dollop of kefir on top.
- Drizzle honey or maple syrup over the parfait if you desire extra sweetness.
- For a blast of freshness, sprinkle with fresh mint leaves.
- Serve immediately and enjoy your delicious and nutritious kefir parfait!

Nutritional Values: Calories: 350, Protein: 12g, Fat: 15g, Carbohydrates: 45g, Fiber: 6g, Sugar: 20g, Sodium: 90mg

28. Rye Bread Sandwiches with Cheese and Avocado

Ingredients: 8 slices of rye bread, 1 large ripe avocado, sliced, 8 slices of your favorite cheese (cheddar, Swiss, or your preference), 1 tablespoon lemon juice, Salt and pepper, to taste, Fresh sprouts or lettuce leaves (optional, for garnish), Mustard or mayonnaise (optional, for spreading)

Preparation:
- Place the rye bread slices on a clean surface or a cutting board.
- In a bowl, toss the avocado slices with lemon juice to prevent browning. Season with salt and pepper.
- If desired, spread a thin layer of mustard or mayonnaise on one side of each slice of rye bread.
- On half of the bread slices, layer a slice of cheese, followed by avocado slices. Top with fresh sprouts or lettuce leaves if using.
- To make sandwiches, put the rest of the slices of bread on top.
- If desired, cut the sandwiches in half for easier handling.
- Serve the rye bread sandwiches immediately, or wrap them for later.

Nutritional Values: Calories: 350, Protein: 15g, Fat: 20g, Carbohydrates: 30g, Fiber: 8g, Sugar: 2g, Sodium: 480mg

29. Oatmeal with Strawberries and Chia Seeds

Ingredients: 1 cup old-fashioned oats, 2 cups milk (dairy or plant-based), 1/2 teaspoon vanilla extract, 1 cup fresh strawberries, sliced, 2 tablespoons chia seeds, 1-2 tablespoons honey or maple syrup (optional), Chopped nuts or coconut flakes for garnish (optional)

Preparation:

- In a saucepan, combine the oats and milk. Bring to a low boil over a medium-high flame.
- Mix in the vanilla essence while lowering the heat to low. Cook, stirring occasionally, until the oats are soft and the mixture has thickened.
- Remove the saucepan from heat and let it sit for a minute to cool slightly.
- In serving bowls, ladle the oatmeal.
- Top with sliced strawberries and sprinkle chia seeds over the strawberries.
- Sprinkle honey or maple syrup on the top if preferred for extra sweetness.
- Garnish with chopped nuts or coconut flakes if you prefer.
- Serve the oatmeal with strawberries and chia seeds immediately.

Nutritional Values: Calories: 300, Protein: 12g, Fat: 8g, Carbohydrates: 48g, Fiber: 9g, Sugar: 12g, Sodium: 80mg

30. Coconut Crepes with Strawberries

Ingredients:
For the Crepes: 1 cup all-purpose flour, 1 cup coconut milk, 1/2 cup water, 2 large eggs, 2 tablespoons melted coconut oil, 1 tablespoon sugar, 1/4 teaspoon salt
For the Filling: 2 cups fresh strawberries, sliced, Coconut flakes for garnish, Maple syrup or honey for drizzling

Preparation:
For the Crepes:

- In a blender, combine the all-purpose flour, coconut milk, water, eggs, melted coconut oil, sugar, and salt. Blend until smooth.
- Allow the mixture to cool down in the refrigerator for at least 30 minutes.
- Heat a non-stick skillet over medium heat and lightly grease it with coconut oil or cooking spray.
- Pour a small amount of batter into the skillet, swirling to spread it thinly. Sauté for two to three minutes per side, or until lightly golden. Repeat with the remaining batter.

For the Filling:

- Fill each coconut crepe with a generous portion of sliced strawberries.
- Fold or roll the crepes and place them on a serving plate.
- Garnish with additional strawberries, coconut flakes, and a drizzle of maple syrup or honey.

Nutritional Values: Calories: 250, Protein: 5g, Fat: 12g, Carbohydrates: 30g, Fiber: 3g, Sugar: 8g, Sodium: 180mg

31. Tapioca Pudding with Coconut Milk

Ingredients: 1/2 cup small pearl tapioca, 2 cups coconut milk, 1/2 cup sugar, 1/4 teaspoon salt, 1 teaspoon vanilla extract, Fresh fruit or toasted coconut for garnish (optional)

Preparation:

- Rinse the tapioca pearls under cold water.
- In a medium saucepan, combine the rinsed tapioca, coconut milk, sugar, and salt.
- Let the mixture sit for 15 minutes to allow the tapioca to soften.
- Place the saucepan over medium heat and bring the mixture to a simmer, stirring constantly to prevent sticking.
- Once it reaches a simmer, reduce the heat to low and continue to cook, stirring frequently, for 15-20 minutes or until the tapioca pearls are fully translucent.
- Once the heat is off, stir in the vanilla extract.
- Allow the pudding to cool for a few minutes before transferring it to serving bowls or glasses.
- Refrigerate the pudding for a minimum of 2 hours, or until it is cooled and set.
- Garnish with fresh fruit or toasted coconut before serving if desired.

Nutritional Values: Calories: 220, Protein: 2g, Fat: 10g, Carbohydrates: 30g, Fiber: 1g, Sugar: 18g, Sodium: 90mg

32. Yogurt Parfait with Blueberries and Granola

Ingredients: 2 cups Greek yogurt (plain or vanilla), 1 cup fresh blueberries, 1 cup granola, 2 tablespoons honey or maple syrup (optional), Fresh mint leaves for garnish (optional)

Preparation:

- In serving glasses or bowls, start by layering 1/4 cup of Greek yogurt at the bottom.
- Add a layer of fresh blueberries over the yogurt.
- Sprinkle 1/4 cup of granola on top of the blueberries.
- Repeat the layers until the glass or bowl is filled, ending with a dollop of Greek yogurt on top.
- Pour honey or maple syrup onto the parfait for extra sweetness if preferred.
- For a blast of freshness, sprinkle using fresh mint leaves.
- Serve the yogurt parfait with blueberries and granola immediately.

Nutritional Values: Calories: 300, Protein: 15g, Fat: 8g, Carbohydrates: 45g, Fiber: 5g, Sugar: 20g, Sodium: 80mg

33. Rye Toast with Avocado and Cherry Tomatoes

Ingredients: 4 slices rye bread, 2 ripe avocados, 1 cup cherry tomatoes, halved, 1 tablespoon lemon juice, Salt and pepper, to taste, Red pepper flakes (optional, for a spicy kick), Fresh basil or cilantro for garnish (optional)

Preparation:

- Toast the rye bread slices to your desired level of crispiness.
- While the bread is toasting, pit and scoop out the flesh of the avocados into a bowl.
- Mash the avocado with a fork, and mix in the lemon juice, salt, and pepper. Adjust seasoning to taste.
- Once the rye bread is toasted, spread the mashed avocado evenly over each slice.
- Top the avocado with halved cherry tomatoes, distributing them evenly.
- If you like a bit of heat, sprinkle red pepper flakes over the tomatoes.
- Garnish with fresh basil or cilantro for added flavor and freshness.
- Serve the rye toast with avocado and cherry tomatoes immediately.

Nutritional Values: Calories: 250, Protein: 6g, Fat: 15g, Carbohydrates: 28g, Fiber: 8g, Sugar: 3g, Sodium: 300mg

34. Spelt Porridge with Dried Apricots

Ingredients: 1 cup spelt grains, 2 cups water, 2 cups milk (dairy or plant-based), 1/2 cup dried apricots, chopped, 2 tablespoons honey or maple syrup, 1/2 teaspoon ground cinnamon, 1/4 teaspoon salt, Chopped nuts or seeds for garnish (optional)

Preparation:

- Rinse the spelt grains under cold water.
- In a medium saucepan, combine spelt grains, water, and a pinch of salt. Bring to a boil, then reduce heat to low, cover, and simmer for 30-40 minutes or until spelt is tender.
- Boil the milk in an independent saucepan until it is warm.
- Once the spelt is cooked, stir in the warm milk, chopped dried apricots, honey (or maple syrup), cinnamon, and salt. Cook over low heat, stirring occasionally, until the mixture thickens to your desired consistency.
- Remove from heat and let it sit for a few minutes to allow flavors to meld.
- Serve the spelt porridge warm, garnished with chopped nuts or seeds if desired.

Nutritional Values: Calories: 320, Protein: 10g, Fat: 8g, Carbohydrates: 55g, Fiber: 8g, Sugar: 18g, Sodium: 150mg

35. Zucchini Omelet with Fresh Mint

Ingredients: 3 large eggs, 1 small zucchini, grated, 2 tablespoons fresh mint, finely chopped, 1 tablespoon olive oil, Salt and pepper, to taste, 1/4 cup feta cheese, crumbled (optional), Cherry tomatoes, sliced, for garnish (optional)

Preparation:

- In a mixing basin, blend the eggs until well incorporated. Stir in the grated zucchini and chopped fresh mint. Season with salt and pepper.
- In a skillet with a nonstick coating over a medium-high flame, heat the olive oil.
- Put the egg mix into the hot skillet and distribute it evenly.
- Simmer for two to three minutes, or until the edges start to firm.
- If using, sprinkle crumbled feta cheese over one half of the omelet.
- Gently lift the other half of the omelet with a spatula and fold it over the cheese, creating a half-moon shape.
- Continue cooking for an additional 2-3 minutes or until the omelet is cooked through and slightly golden.
- Slide the zucchini omelet onto a plate and garnish with sliced cherry tomatoes if desired.
- Serve the omelet hot, either folded or rolled.

Nutritional Values: Calories: 250, Protein: 15g, Fat: 18g, Carbohydrates: 5g, Fiber: 2g, Sugar: 3g, Sodium: 250mg

36. Corn Pancakes with Maple Syrup

Ingredients: 1 cup cornmeal, 1 cup all-purpose flour, 1 tablespoon sugar, 1 tablespoon baking powder, 1/2 teaspoon salt, 1 cup milk (dairy or plant-based), 2 large eggs, 1/4 cup unsalted butter, melted, 1 cup corn kernels (fresh or frozen), Maple syrup, for serving

Preparation:

- Mix combined the cornmeal, all-purpose flour, sugar, baking powder, and salt in a big mixing basin.
- Stir combined the milk, eggs, and melted butter in a separate basin.
- Mix the wet and dry ingredients together until they are scarcely combined. Do not mix too much; a few lumps are acceptable.
- The corn kernels should be gently folded into the batter.

- Lightly butter a griddle or nonstick skillet over a medium-high flame.
- Pour 1/4 cup portions of batter onto the griddle, spreading them slightly with the back of a spoon to form pancakes.
- Cook until bubbles form on the surface of the pancakes, then flip and cook until the other side is golden brown.
- Till all of the batter has been utilized, keep going.
- Serve the corn pancakes warm, drizzled with maple syrup.

Nutritional Values: Calories: 220, Protein: 6g, Fat: 8g, Carbohydrates: 32g, Fiber: 3g, Sugar: 6g, Sodium: 380mg

37. Chia Seed Pudding with Mixed Berries

Ingredients: 1/4 cup chia seeds, 1 cup milk (dairy or plant-based), 1 tablespoon honey or maple syrup, 1/2 teaspoon vanilla extract, 1 cup mixed berries (strawberries, blueberries, raspberries), Granola for topping (optional)

Preparation:

- In a bowl, whisk together chia seeds, milk, honey (or maple syrup), and vanilla extract.
- Cover the bowl and refrigerate for at least 2 hours or overnight, allowing the chia seeds to absorb the liquid and create a pudding-like consistency.
- Before serving, stir the chia pudding well to ensure an even texture.
- In serving bowls or glasses, layer the chia pudding with a mixture of fruit.
- Optionally, top with granola for added crunch and texture.
- Serve the chia seed pudding with mixed berries chilled.

Nutritional Values: Calories: 220, Protein: 7g, Fat: 9g, Carbohydrates: 30g, Fiber: 10g, Sugar: 15g, Sodium: 80mg

38. Avocado Stuffed with Tomato and Egg

Ingredients: 2 ripe avocados, 2 large eggs, 1 large tomato, diced, 1 tablespoon fresh cilantro, chopped, 1 tablespoon lime juice, Salt and pepper, to taste, Red pepper flakes (optional, for a spicy kick)

Preparation:

- Preheat the oven to 375°F (190°C).
- Halve the avocados and scoop out the pits.
- To make a bigger well for the egg, take a small piece of flesh out of each avocado half.
- To keep the avocado halves steady, put them in a baking dish.
- In a bowl, mix together the diced tomato, fresh cilantro, lime juice, salt, and pepper.
- Spoon the tomato mixture into the wells of the avocados, creating a hollow space in the center.
- Crack one egg into each avocado half, letting it rest in the center of the tomato mixture.
- Add additional salt and pepper according to your liking.
- Optionally, add red pepper flakes for a touch of spiciness.
- Bake for 15 to 20 minutes, until all of the eggs are cooked to your preference, in an oven that has been preheated.
- Just before serving, take it out of the oven and allow it to chill for a few minutes.

Nutritional Values: Calories: 300, Protein: 8g, Fat: 25g, Carbohydrates: 15g, Fiber: 10g, Sugar: 2g, Sodium: 60mg

39. Whole Rye Toast with Avocado and Cherry Tomatoes

Ingredients: 4 slices whole rye bread, 2 ripe avocados, 1 cup cherry tomatoes, halved, 1 tablespoon lemon juice, Salt and pepper, to taste, Red pepper flakes (optional, for a spicy kick), Fresh basil or cilantro for garnish (optional)

Preparation:

- Toast the slices of whole rye bread to your desired level of crispiness.
- While the bread is toasting, pit and scoop out the flesh of the avocados into a bowl.
- Mash the avocado with a fork and mix in the lemon juice, salt, and pepper. Adjust seasoning to taste.
- Once the rye bread is toasted, spread the mashed avocado evenly over each slice.
- Top the avocado with halved cherry tomatoes, distributing them evenly.
- If you like a bit of heat, sprinkle red pepper flakes over the tomatoes.
- Garnish with fresh basil or cilantro for added flavor and freshness.
- Serve the whole rye toast with avocado and cherry tomatoes immediately.

Nutritional Values: Calories: 250, Protein: 6g, Fat: 15g, Carbohydrates: 28g, Fiber: 8g, Sugar: 3g, Sodium: 300mg

40. Oatmeal with Raspberries and Chia Seeds

Ingredients: 1 cup old-fashioned oats, 2 cups milk (dairy or plant-based), 1/2 teaspoon vanilla extract, 1 cup fresh raspberries, 2 tablespoons chia seeds, 1-2 tablespoons honey or maple syrup (optional), Sliced almonds or shredded coconut for garnish (optional)

Preparation:

- In a saucepan, combine the oats and milk. Simmer over a medium-low flame for a bit.
- Turn down to a low temperature and mix in the vanilla extract.
- Cook, stirring occasionally, until the oats are soft and the mixture has thickened.
- Remove the saucepan from heat and let it sit for a minute to cool slightly.
- In serving bowls, ladle the oatmeal.
- Top with fresh raspberries and sprinkle chia seeds over the raspberries.
- For extra sweetness, you can choose to pour maple syrup or honey on top.
- Garnish with sliced almonds or shredded coconut if you prefer.
- Serve the oatmeal with raspberries and chia seeds immediately.

Nutritional Values: Calories: 300, Protein: 10g, Fat: 8g, Carbohydrates: 48g, Fiber: 9g, Sugar: 12g, Sodium: 80mg

41. Buckwheat Pancakes with Maple Syrup

Ingredients: 1 cup buckwheat flour, 1/2 cup all-purpose flour, 1 tablespoon sugar, 1 teaspoon baking powder, 1/2 teaspoon baking soda, 1/4 teaspoon salt, 1 cup buttermilk, 1/2 cup milk (dairy or plant-based), 2 large eggs, 2 tablespoons unsalted butter, melted, Maple syrup, for serving

Preparation:

- In a large mixing bowl, whisk together the buckwheat flour, all-purpose flour, sugar, baking powder, baking soda, and salt.
- In a separate bowl, whisk together the buttermilk, milk, eggs, and melted butter.
- Add the wet mixture to the dry mixture and whisk just until incorporated. A few lumps are okay; don't overmix.
- Let the batter rest for about 10 minutes to allow the flours to absorb the liquid.
- Lightly grease and heat a nonstick skillet or griddle over a medium-high flame.
- Pour 1/4 cup portions of batter onto the griddle, spreading them slightly with the back of a spoon to form pancakes.
- Cook until bubbles form on the surface of the pancakes, then flip and cook until the other side is golden brown.
- Keep going until the batter is all used.
- Serve the buckwheat pancakes warm, drizzled with maple syrup.

Nutritional Values: Calories: 250, Protein: 8g, Fat: 8g, Carbohydrates: 35g, Fiber: 4g, Sugar: 5g, Sodium: 400mg

42. Tofu Scramble with Spinach and Sun-Dried Tomatoes

Ingredients: 1 block firm tofu, drained and crumbled, 2 tablespoons olive oil, 1 small onion, finely chopped, 2 cloves garlic, minced, 2 cups fresh spinach, chopped, 1/4 cup sun-dried tomatoes, chopped, 1 teaspoon turmeric powder, 1/2 teaspoon cumin, Salt and pepper, to taste, Fresh parsley for garnish (optional), Avocado slices for serving (optional), Toast or tortillas for serving

Preparation:

- Heat the olive oil in a big skillet over a medium-high flame.
- Sauté the chopped onions until they start to show through.
- Cook for a further one to two minutes after adding the garlic that has been minced and stirring.
- Add crumbled tofu to the skillet, spreading it evenly.
- Sprinkle turmeric and cumin over the tofu, stirring to incorporate and evenly distribute the spices.
- Cook for 5-7 minutes, allowing the tofu to absorb the flavors and develop a golden color.
- Sun-dried tomatoes and chopped spinach should be added to the skillet.
- Simmer until the tomatoes are tender and the spinach has wilted.
- Season with salt and pepper to taste. Adjust the seasoning as needed.
- Garnish with fresh parsley if desired.
- Serve the tofu scramble hot, with avocado slices on the side and your choice of toast or tortillas.

Nutritional Values: Calories: 250, Protein: 15g, Fat: 18g, Carbohydrates: 10g, Fiber: 4g, Sugar: 2g, Sodium: 350mg

43. Sweet Potato Pancakes with Maple Syrup

Ingredients: 1 cup cooked and mashed sweet potatoes, 1 cup all-purpose flour, 1 tablespoon brown sugar, 2 teaspoons baking powder, 1/2 teaspoon cinnamon, 1/4 teaspoon nutmeg, 1 cup milk (dairy or plant-based), 1 large egg, 2 tablespoons melted butter or oil, Maple syrup, for serving, Chopped pecans or walnuts for garnish (optional)

Preparation:

- In a large mixing bowl, combine mashed sweet potatoes, flour, brown sugar, baking powder, cinnamon, and nutmeg.
- Beat the egg, milk, and melted butter or oil in another bowl.
- Mixing until just mixed, pour the wet components into the dry ingredients. Avoid over-mixing; a few lumps are acceptable.
- Apply a thin layer of oil to a nonstick skillet or griddle before heating it to medium heat.
- Pour 1/4 cup portions of batter onto the griddle, spreading them slightly with the back of a spoon to form pancakes.
- Cook until bubbles form on the surface of the pancakes, then flip and cook until the other side is golden brown.
- Continue working until the batter is all used.
- Serve the sweet potato pancakes warm, drizzled with maple syrup and garnished with chopped nuts if desired.

Nutritional Values: Calories: 220, Protein: 6g, Fat: 8g, Carbohydrates: 32g, Fiber: 3g, Sugar: 8g, Sodium: 380mg

44. Fruit Salad with Fresh Mint

Ingredients: 2 cups strawberries, hulled and halved, 1 cup blueberries, 1 cup pineapple, diced, 1 cup grapes, halved, 2 kiwi peeled and sliced, 1 banana, sliced, 2 tablespoons fresh mint, chopped, 1 tablespoon honey (optional), 1 tablespoon lime juice

Preparation:

- In a large mixing bowl, combine strawberries, blueberries, diced pineapple, halved grapes, sliced kiwi, and sliced banana.
- Add chopped fresh mint to the bowl and gently toss the fruits and mint together.
- In a small bowl, whisk together honey (if using) and lime juice.
- Drizzle the honey-lime dressing over the fruit salad and toss again to coat the fruits evenly.
- Let the fruit salad marinate in the dressing for at least 10 minutes to enhance the flavors.
- Serve the fruit salad with a garnish of additional fresh mint if desired.

Nutritional Values: Calories: 150, Protein: 2g, Fat: 1g, Carbohydrates: 38g, Fiber: 6g, Sugar: 25g, Sodium: 5mg

45. Whole Wheat French Toast with Raspberries

Ingredients: 4 slices whole wheat bread, 2 large eggs, 1/2 cup milk (dairy or plant-based), 1 teaspoon vanilla extract, 1/2 teaspoon cinnamon, Pinch of salt, Butter or cooking oil for greasing the pan, Fresh raspberries for topping, Maple syrup for serving

Preparation:

- In a shallow dish, whisk together eggs, milk, vanilla extract, cinnamon, and a pinch of salt.
- Apply cooking oil or butter to a nonstick skillet or griddle before heating it to medium heat.
- Dip each slice of whole wheat bread into the egg mixture, ensuring both sides are coated.
- Place the coated bread slices on the hot griddle and cook until each side is golden brown and slightly crispy.
- Take the French toast from the griddle and put it onto a platter for dishing.
- Top the French toast with fresh raspberries.
- Apply a maple syrup drizzle right before serving.
- Optionally, sprinkle a bit of powdered sugar or add a dollop of whipped cream for extra sweetness.

Nutritional Values: Calories: 250, Protein: 10g, Fat: 8g, Carbohydrates: 35g, Fiber: 5g, Sugar: 10g, Sodium: 300mg

46. Pumpkin Pancakes with Cinnamon

Ingredients: 1 cup all-purpose flour, 1 tablespoon sugar, 1 teaspoon baking powder, 1/2 teaspoon baking soda, 1/2 teaspoon ground cinnamon, 1/4 teaspoon salt, 1/2 cup pumpkin puree, 1 cup buttermilk, 2 tablespoons of melted butter, 1 large egg, and serving maple syrup

Preparation:

- In a large mixing bowl, whisk together the flour, sugar, baking powder, baking soda, ground cinnamon, and salt.
- Melted butter, egg, buttermilk, and pumpkin puree should all be combined in a different bowl. Mix well.
- Add the wet mixture to the dry mixture and whisk just until incorporated. A few lumps are okay; don't overmix.
- Apply a thin layer of oil to a nonstick skillet or griddle before heating it to medium heat.
- Pour 1/4 cup portions of batter onto the griddle, spreading them slightly with the back of a spoon to form pancakes.
- Cook until bubbles form on the surface of the pancakes, then flip and cook until the other side is golden brown.
- Continue working until the batter is all used.
- Serve the pumpkin pancakes warm, drizzled with maple syrup.

Nutritional Values: Calories: 220, Protein: 6g, Fat: 8g, Carbohydrates: 32g, Fiber: 2g, Sugar: 8g, Sodium: 400mg

47. Egg Salad with Avocado and Spinach

Ingredients: 6 hard-boiled eggs, peeled and chopped, 1 ripe avocado, diced, 2 cups fresh spinach, chopped, 1/4 cup mayonnaise, 1 tablespoon Dijon mustard, 1 tablespoon fresh lemon juice, Salt and pepper, to taste, Whole grain bread or wraps, for serving

Preparation:

- In a large mixing bowl, combine the chopped hard-boiled eggs, diced avocado, and chopped fresh spinach.
- In a separate bowl, whisk together the mayonnaise, Dijon mustard, and fresh lemon juice until well combined.
- Pour the dressing over the egg mixture and toss gently to coat all the ingredients evenly.
- Season with salt and pepper, according to your liking. Adjust the seasoning as needed.
- To let the flavors in the egg salad, combine, refrigerate it for at least half an hour.

Nutritional Values: Calories: 300, Protein: 15g, Fat: 20g, Carbohydrates: 15g, Fiber: 6g, Sugar: 2g, Sodium: 400mg

48. Beet Smoothie with Ginger

Ingredients: 1 medium-sized beet, peeled and chopped, 1 cup frozen mixed berries (strawberries, blueberries, raspberries), 1 banana, peeled, 1 cup plain Greek yogurt, 1 tablespoon fresh ginger, grated, 1 tablespoon honey or maple syrup (optional), 1 cup water or coconut water, Ice cubes (optional)

Preparation:

- In a blender, combine the chopped beet, frozen mixed berries, peeled banana, Greek yogurt, grated fresh ginger, and honey or maple syrup if desired.
- Add water or coconut water to the blender to facilitate blending.
- Process the ingredients at a high speed until it becomes creamy and smooth.
- If the smoothie is too thick, you can add more liquid as needed.
- If desired, add ice cubes to the blender and blend again until the smoothie reaches your preferred consistency.
- Pour the beet smoothie into glasses and serve immediately.

Nutritional Values: Calories: 200, Protein: 10g, Fat: 2g, Carbohydrates: 40g, Fiber: 8g, Sugar: 25g, Sodium: 50mg

49. Oatmeal with Pears and Cinnamon

Ecco la ricetta formattata nel formato cookbook per l'"Oatmeal with Pears and Cinnamon":

Ingredients: 1 cup old-fashioned oats, 2 cups milk (dairy or plant-based), 2 ripe pears, peeled, cored, and diced, 1 teaspoon ground cinnamon, 1 tablespoon honey or maple syrup, Chopped nuts or seeds for garnish (optional)

Preparation:

- In a saucepan, combine the old-fashioned oats and milk. Heat to a simmer on a medium setting.
- Reduce the heat to low and add the diced pears and ground cinnamon to the saucepan.
- Stir well and let it simmer until the oats are cooked to your desired consistency and the pears are soft.
- Remove the saucepan from heat and stir in honey or maple syrup for sweetness.
- Let the oatmeal sit for a minute to cool slightly and allow the flavors to meld.
- Spoon the oatmeal into serving bowls.
- Optionally, garnish with chopped nuts or seeds for added texture and crunch.
- Serve the oatmeal with pears and cinnamon warm.

Nutritional Values: Calories: 250, Protein: 8g, Fat: 6g, Carbohydrates: 42g, Fiber: 7g, Sugar: 18g, Sodium: 80mg

50. Pepper Omelet with Onions and Basil

Ingredients: 3 large eggs, 1/2 cup bell peppers, thinly sliced, 1/4 cup onions, finely chopped, 2 tablespoons fresh basil, chopped, Salt and pepper, to taste, 1 tablespoon olive oil, Grated cheese for topping (optional)

Preparation:

- Break the eggs open and whisk them thoroughly in a bowl.
- In a nonstick skillet, warm the olive oil over a medium-high flame.
- Add sliced bell peppers and chopped onions to the skillet. Sauté until softened.
- Cover the skillet's sautéed vegetables with the beaten eggs.
- Allow the eggs to set slightly around the edges, then use a spatula to lift the edges and let the uncooked eggs flow underneath.
- Sprinkle chopped fresh basil over one half of the omelet.
- Season according to your liking with salt and pepper.
- Once the eggs are mostly set but still slightly runny on top, fold the omelet in half using the spatula.
- If desired, sprinkle grated cheese over the top of the folded omelet.
- Keep heating until the cheese melts and the eggs are set.
- Slide the pepper omelet onto a plate and serve hot.

Nutritional Values: Calories: 250, Protein: 15g, Fat: 18g, Carbohydrates: 8g, Fiber: 2g, Sugar: 4g, Sodium: 350mg

Chapter 7: Starters and snacks

50 Anti-inflammatory Appetizers and Snacks Recipes

Varied Selection of Recipes

There is a varied selection of recipes, from vegetable-based options such as hummus to light soups based on vegetable broth, up to snacks based on fruit and dried fruit. Also included are recipes for fish-based appetizers, such as smoked salmon rolls with cream cheese and lean protein delicacies such as chicken or tofu.

Easy to Prepare and Tasty

Each recipe is designed to be easy to prepare, making creating anti-inflammatory appetizers and snacks accessible even for those with no culinary experience. Furthermore, attention is placed on the goodness and satisfaction of taste, demonstrating that eating healthily does not mean giving up the pleasure of food.

Recipes Adaptable to Individual Needs

The recipes presented can be tailored to individual needs, allowing readers to customize entrees and snacks based on their food preferences, dietary restrictions and nutritional needs. This promotes flexibility in preparing anti-inflammatory meals and snacks.

Detailed Instructions and Common Ingredients

Each recipe comes with detailed preparation instructions and a list of common ingredients, making it easy to find the ingredients you need. This makes the cooking process easier and encourages readers to experiment with new anti-inflammatory dishes.

Anti-inflammatory appetizers and snacks and their preparation

1.Chickpea Hummus with Raw Vegetable Sticks

Ingredients:

For the Chickpea Hummus: 2 cups canned chickpeas (drained and rinsed), 1/3 cup tahini, 2 cloves garlic (minced), 1/4 cup fresh lemon juice (from about 1 large lemon), 2 tablespoons olive oil, 1/2 teaspoon ground cumin, Salt to taste, Water (as needed to adjust consistency).

For the Raw Vegetable Sticks: Carrot sticks, Cucumber sticks, Celery sticks, Bell pepper strips, Cherry tomatoes, Broccoli and cauliflower florets.

Preparation:

- Rinse and drain one can chickpeas.
- In a blender, combine the chickpeas, 2 tablespoons of tahini, the juice of one lemon, 2 tablespoons of olive oil, 1 clove of garlic, half a teaspoon of cumin powder, half a teaspoon of salt and a pinch of pepper.
- Blend the ingredients until smooth, adding water little by little if necessary.
- Cut raw vegetables into sticks, such as carrots, celery and peppers.
- Serve the hummus in a bowl with raw vegetables to use as dippers.

Nutritional Values: Calories, 150-200 kcal. Protein, 4-6 g. Fat, 8-10 g. Carbohydrates, 15-20 g. Fiber, 4-5 g.

2. Guacamole with Carrot Chips

Ingredients:

For the Guacamole: 2 ripe avocados (peeled, pitted, and mashed), 1 small onion (finely chopped), 2 cloves garlic (minced), 1 small tomato (diced), 1/4 cup fresh cilantro (chopped), Juice of 1 lime, Salt and black pepper (to taste).

For the Carrot Chips: 2 large carrots (peeled and cut into thin chips), 1 tablespoon olive oil, Salt and black pepper (to taste).

Preparation:

- In a mixing bowl, mash two ripe avocados.
- Add a small tomato, finely chopped, a quarter of a chopped red onion, the juice of one lime, and a handful of chopped fresh cilantro.
- Mix the ingredients until you get a creamy, well-combined guacamole.
- Cut the carrots into thin slices or sticks to make chips.
- Serve the guacamole beside the carrot chips

Nutritional Values: Calories, 150-200 kcal. Protein, 2-3 g. Fat, 12-14 g. Carbohydrates, 10-12 g. Fiber, 4-5 g.

3. Tomato and Basil Soup

Ingredients: 2 tablespoons olive oil, 1 onion (chopped), 2 cloves garlic (minced), 28 oz (800g) canned tomatoes, 1 cup vegetable broth, 1 teaspoon sugar, 1/2 cup fresh basil leaves, Optional: 1/2 cup heavy cream, salt and black pepper according to preference.

Preparation:

- In a saucepan, heat a little olive oil and fry a chopped onion and two crushed garlic cloves until golden.
- Add 6-8 ripe tomatoes cut into pieces and cook for a few minutes until they soften.
- Pour 4 cups of vegetable broth into the pot and bring to a boil.
- Add a bunch of fresh basil and cook for 10-15 minutes.
- Using an immersion blender to smooth out the soup.
- Dish this tomato and basil soup hot with fresh basil on top.

Nutritional Values: Calories, 150-200 kcal. Protein, 2-3 g. Fat, 8-10 g. Carbohydrates, 15-20 g. Fiber, 4-5 g.

4. Curry Turkey Meatballs

Ingredients:

For the Turkey Meatballs: 1 pound (450g) ground turkey, 1/4 cup breadcrumbs, 1/4 cup finely chopped onion, 2 cloves garlic (minced), 1 egg, 2 tablespoons curry powder, Salt and black pepper (to taste).

For the Curry Sauce: 1 can (14 oz) diced tomatoes, 1/2 cup coconut milk, 1 tablespoon curry powder, Salt and black pepper (to taste), Fresh cilantro for garnish (optional).

Preparation:

- In a bowl, mix 500g of ground turkey meat, half a chopped onion, two tablespoons of curry powder, half a cup of breadcrumbs, two eggs and a pinch of salt.
- Form evenly sized meatballs and place them on a baking tray lined with baking paper.
- Cook the meatballs in a preheated oven at 180°C for about 20-25 minutes or until golden brown and cooked through.
- Serve the curry turkey meatballs with a yogurt and garlic sauce if desired.

Nutritional Values: Calories, 250-300 kcal. Protein, 15-20 g. Fat, 10-12 g. Carbohydrates, 20-25 g. Fiber, 4-5 g.

5. Quinoa Salad with Cucumbers and Avocado

Ingredients:

For the Quinoa Salad: 1 cup quinoa (rinsed and cooked), 1 cucumber (diced), 2 ripe avocados (diced), 1/4 cup red onion (finely chopped), 1/4 cup fresh cilantro (chopped), 1/4 cup fresh parsley (chopped), Juice of 2 limes, 2 tablespoons olive oil, Salt and black pepper (to taste).

Preparation:

- Cook a cup of quinoa according to package instructions and let cool.
- Dice a cucumber and a ripe avocado and cut the cherry tomatoes in half.

- In a large bowl, combine the cooked quinoa, cucumber, avocado and cherry tomatoes.
- Make a light vinaigrette by mixing olive oil, lemon juice, salt, pepper and a pinch of garlic powder.
- Season the salad with the vinaigrette and mix well.
- Serve quinoa salad with cucumber and avocado as a fresh side dish or snack.

Nutritional Values: Calories, 300-350 kcal. Protein, 7-9 g. Fat, 18-20 g. Carbohydrates, 30-35 g. Fiber, 6-7 g.

6. Grilled Chicken Skewers with Yogurt Sauce

Ingredients:

For the Grilled Chicken Skewers: 1.5 pounds (680g) boneless, skinless chicken breasts (cut into cubes), 1/4 cup olive oil, 2 cloves garlic (minced), 1 teaspoon ground cumin, 1 teaspoon paprika, 1/2 teaspoon ground coriander, Salt and black pepper (to taste), Wooden skewers (soaked in water).

For the Yogurt Sauce: 1 cup Greek yogurt, 2 tablespoons fresh lemon juice, 1 clove garlic (minced), 1 tablespoon fresh mint (chopped), Salt and black pepper (to taste).

Preparation:

- Cut the chicken breast into cubes.
- In a bowl, mix 1 cup Greek yogurt, lemon juice, minced garlic, cumin, paprika, salt and pepper.
- Add the chicken to the marinade and let it rest in the refrigerator for at least 30 minutes.
- Grill the marinated chicken on skewers until cooked through.
- Prepare a yogurt sauce by mixing Greek yogurt, chopped fresh mint, garlic, salt and pepper.
- Serve the chicken skewers hot with the yogurt sauce.

Nutritional Values: Calories, 250-300 kcal. Protein, 20-25 g. Fat, 8-10 g. Carbohydrates, 20-25 g. Fiber, 3-4 g.

7. Hard Boiled Eggs with Smoked Paprika

Ingredients: 6 large eggs, 1/2 teaspoon smoked paprika, Salt and black pepper (to taste), Fresh chives for garnish (optional).

Preparation:

- Bring a pot of water to a boil.
- Add the eggs and cook them for approximately 9-12 minutes, depending on the desired degree of doneness.
- Drain the eggs and immediately immerse them in cold water to stop cooking.
- Gently peel and cut the eggs in half.
- Sprinkle the eggs with smoked paprika and a pinch of salt.
- Serve hard-boiled eggs with smoked paprika as a snack or appetizer.

Nutritional Values: Calories, 150-200 kcal. Protein, 12-14 g. Fat, 10-12 g. Carbohydrates, 2-3 g. Fiber, 0-1 g.

8. Melon Wrapped in Parma Ham

Ingredients: 1 ripe cantaloupe or honeydew melon, 6-8 slices of Parma ham or prosciutto

Preparation:

- Remove the seeds from the melon and cut it into slices or cubes.
- Wrap each piece of melon with a slice of Parma ham.
- Serve the melon wrapped in ham as a cool and refreshing appetizer.

Nutritional Values: Calories, 150-200 kcal. Protein, 6-8 g. Fat, 8-10 g. Carbohydrates, 12-15 g. Fiber, 1-2 g.

9. Smoked Salmon with Cucumber and Sour Cream

Ingredients: 8 slices of smoked salmon, 1 thinly sliced cucumber, 1/2 cup of sour cream, 1 tablespoon of chopped fresh dill, 1 lemon cut into wedges, freshly ground black pepper to taste.

Preparation:

- Cut the cucumber into thin slices.
- Spread a small amount of sour cream on each cucumber slice.
- Overlay a slice of smoked salmon on each slice of cucumber.
- Gently roll up the slices and hold them together with a toothpick.
- Serve smoked salmon with cucumber and sour cream as an elegant appetizer.

Nutritional Values: Calories, 250-300 kcal. Protein, 20-25 g. Fat, 15-20 g. Carbohydrates, 5-10 g. Fiber, 1-2 g.

10. Fresh Tomato Sauce with Basil

Ingredients: 6 ripe tomatoes (peeled, seeded, and diced), 2 cloves garlic (minced), 1/4 cup fresh basil (chopped), 2 tablespoons olive oil, Salt and black pepper (to taste).

Preparation:

- Cut the tomatoes into cubes and finely chop the basil and garlic.
- In a bowl, combine the tomatoes, basil, garlic, extra virgin olive oil, salt and pepper.
- Mix well and let rest for at least 15-30 minutes to allow the flavors to blend.
- Serve the fresh tomato sauce with basil as a condiment for bruschetta or as an accompaniment to crostini.

Nutritional Values: Calories, 50-75 kcal. Protein, 2-3 g. Fat, 2-3 g. Carbohydrates, 10-15 g. Fiber, 3-4 g.

11. Quinoa Salad with Cucumber and Avocado

Ingredients: 1 cup quinoa (rinsed and cooked), 1 cucumber (diced), 2 ripe avocados (diced), 1/4 cup red onion (finely chopped), 1/4 cup fresh cilantro (chopped), 1/4 cup fresh parsley (chopped), 2 lime juice, two tablespoons of olive oil, salt and black pepper (to taste).

Preparation:

- Cook a cup of quinoa according to package instructions and let cool.
- Dice a cucumber and a ripe avocado and cut the cherry tomatoes in half.
- In a large bowl, combine the cooked quinoa, cucumber, avocado and cherry tomatoes.
- Make a light vinaigrette by mixing olive oil, lemon juice, salt, pepper and a pinch of garlic powder.
- Season the salad with the vinaigrette and mix well.
- Serve quinoa salad with cucumber and avocado as a fresh side dish or snack.

Nutritional Values: Calories, 300-350 kcal. Protein, 7-9 g. Fat, 18-20 g. Carbohydrates, 30-35 g. Fiber, 6-7 g.

12. Guacamole with Wholemeal Nachos

Ingredients:

For the Guacamole: 3 ripe avocados, 1 small red onion (finely chopped), 2-3 cloves of garlic (minced), 2 ripe tomatoes (diced), 1/4 cup fresh cilantro (chopped), Juice of 2 limes, Salt and black pepper (to taste).

For the Wholemeal Nachos: Wholemeal tortilla chips (store-bought or homemade).

Preparation:

- In a mixing bowl, mash two ripe avocados.
- Add a small tomato, finely chopped, a quarter of a chopped red onion, the juice of one lime and a handful of chopped fresh cilantro.
- Mix the ingredients until you get a creamy, well-combined guacamole.

Serve guacamole with whole-grain nachos for a delicious appetizer.

Nutritional Values: Calories, 200-250 kcal. Protein, 4-5 g. Fat, 12-15 g. Carbohydrates, 20-25 g. Fiber, 4-5 g.

13. Black Bean and Corn Salad

Ingredients: 2 cups canned black beans (drained and rinsed), 2 cups corn kernels (fresh, frozen, or canned), 1 red bell pepper (diced), 1/2 red onion (finely chopped), 1/4 cup fresh cilantro (chopped), Juice of 2 limes, 2 tablespoons olive oil, 1 teaspoon ground cumin, Salt and black pepper (to taste).

Preparation:
- Drain and rinse one can of black beans and one can of sweet corn.
- Dice ripe tomatoes and red onion.
- In a large bowl, combine the black beans, corn, tomatoes and onion.
- Make a vinaigrette by mixing olive oil, red wine vinegar, minced garlic, cumin powder, salt and pepper.
- Season the salad with the vinaigrette and mix well.
- Serve the black bean and corn salad as a side or main course.

Nutritional Values: Calories, 200-250 kcal. Protein, 8-10 g. Fat, 2-3 g. Carbohydrates, 40-45 g. Fiber, 10-12 g.

14. Courgette flan

Ingredients: 2 large zucchinis (courgettes), grated, 2 shallots, finely chopped, 3 eggs, 1/2 cup heavy cream, 1/2 cup grated Parmesan cheese, 1/4 cup all-purpose flour, 2 tablespoons olive oil, 1 teaspoon dried thyme, Salt and black pepper to taste.

Preparation:
- Grate two courgettes and squeeze out the excess water.
- In a bowl, combine the grated zucchini, two eggs, grated cheese (such as Parmesan), salt, pepper and a sprinkle of nutmeg.
- Mix the ingredients well.
- Transfer the mixture to a baking tray and level the surface.
- Bake in a preheated oven at 180°C for about 25-30 minutes or until golden and cooked through.
- Serve the courgette flan as a side dish or appetizer.

Nutritional Values: Calories, 150-200 kcal. Protein, 5-6 g. Fat, 10-12 g. Carbohydrates, 10-12 g. Fiber, 2-3 g.

15. Eggplant rolls with Parmigiana

Ingredients: 2 large eggplants (thinly sliced lengthwise), 2 cups marinara sauce, 1 cup ricotta cheese, 1/2 cup grated Parmesan cheese, 1/4 cup fresh basil (chopped), 2 cups shredded mozzarella cheese, 2 tbsp of olive oil, salt, and black pepper (to taste).

Preparation:
- Cut the aubergines into thin slices and grill them lightly on both sides.
- In each slice of eggplant, place a portion of cheese (such as mozzarella) and a spoonful of tomato sauce.
- Roll up the stuffed aubergine slices and place them on a baking tray.
- Cover the rolls with more tomato sauce and cheese.
- Bake in a preheated oven at 180°C for approximately 15-20 minutes or until the cheese is melted and golden.
- Serve the aubergine parmigiana rolls as a main course or appetizer.

Nutritional Values: Calories, 250-300 kcal. Protein, 12-15 g. Fat, 18-20 g. Carbohydrates, 10-12 g. Fiber, 3-4 g.

16. Baked Sweet Chips with Spices

Ingredients: 4 sweet potatoes (peeled and thinly sliced into chips), 2 tablespoons olive oil, 1 teaspoon ground cumin, 1 teaspoon paprika, 1/2 teaspoon ground cinnamon, Salt and black pepper (to taste).

Preparation:
- Peel and cut the sweet potatoes into thin slices or sticks.
- In a bowl, combine the sweet potatoes with olive oil, cinnamon, smoked paprika, salt and pepper.
- Mix well to ensure the chips are well seasoned.
- Arrange the chips in a single layer on a baking tray lined with baking paper.
- Cook in a preheated oven at 200°C for approximately 20-25 minutes or until the chips are golden and crispy.
- Serve baked sweet potato chips with spices as a snack or side dish.

Nutritional Values: Calories, 150-200 kcal. Protein, 1-2 g. Fat, 5-6 g. Carbohydrates, 30-35 g. Fiber, 3-4 g.

17. Lean Meatballs with Tzatziki Sauce

Ingredients:

For the Lean Meatballs: 1 pound lean ground beef (or any lean meat of your choice), 1/4 cup breadcrumbs, 1/4 cup onion (finely chopped), 2 cloves garlic (minced), 1 teaspoon ground cumin, 1/2 teaspoon ground coriander, 1/4 cup fresh parsley (chopped), Salt and black pepper (to taste), Olive oil for cooking (if pan-frying).

For the Tzatziki Sauce: 1 cup Greek yogurt, 1 cucumber (finely grated and squeezed to remove excess liquid), 2 cloves garlic (minced), 1 tablespoon fresh dill (chopped), 1 tablespoon fresh mint (chopped), 1 tablespoon lemon juice, Salt and black pepper (to taste).

Preparation:
- In a bowl, mix lean ground beef, chopped onion, garlic, chopped fresh parsley, cumin, dried oregano, salt and pepper.
- Form small meatballs with the mixture.
- Cook the meatballs in a non-stick pan until golden and fully cooked.
- Meanwhile, prepare the tzatziki sauce by mixing Greek yogurt, grated cucumber, minced garlic, lemon juice, chopped fresh mint, salt and pepper.
- Serve the meatballs with tzatziki sauce as an appetizer or main course.

Nutritional Values: Calories, 250-300 kcal. Protein, 15-18 g. Fat, 12-15 g. Carbohydrates, 15-18 g. Fiber, 2-3 g.

18. Grilled Prawn Skewers

Ingredients: 1 pound large prawns (peeled and deveined), 2 cloves garlic (minced), 2 tablespoons olive oil, 1 lemon (juiced and zested), 1 tablespoon fresh parsley (chopped), Salt and black pepper (to taste), skewers made of wood (submerged in water for 30 minutes).

Preparation:
- In a bowl, combine peeled and peeled prawns with minced garlic, lemon juice, extra virgin olive oil, salt and pepper.
- Let the prawns marinate for about 15-30 minutes.
- Thread the marinated prawns onto skewers.
- Grill the shrimp on the hot grill until cooked through.
- Serve the grilled shrimp skewers as an appetizer or main course.

Nutritional Values: Calories, 150-200 kcal. Protein, 20-25 g. Fat, 2-3 g. Carbohydrates, 2-3 g. Fiber, 0-1 g.

19. Stuffed Tomatoes with Tuna and Olives

Ingredients: 4 large tomatoes, 1 can (6 ounces) tuna (drained and flaked), 1/4 cup black olives (pitted and chopped), 1/4 cup green olives (pitted and chopped), 2 cloves garlic (minced), 2 tablespoons fresh parsley (chopped), 2 tablespoons olive oil, Salt and black pepper (to taste).
Preparation:
- Cut off the tops of the tomatoes and carefully empty them.
- In a bowl, mix drained tuna, sliced black olives, capers, chopped fresh parsley, olive oil, lemon juice, salt and pepper.
- Fill the tomatoes with the tuna filling.
- Serve the stuffed tomatoes with tuna and olives as an appetizer or side dish.

Nutritional Values: Calories, 200-250 kcal. Protein, 10-12 g. Fat, 10-12 g. Carbohydrates, 15-18 g. Fiber, 3-4 g.

20. Chickpea Salad with Parsley and Lemon

Ingredients: 2 cans (15 ounces each) chickpeas (drained and rinsed), 1/2 cup fresh parsley (chopped), 1 lemon (juiced and zested), 2 tablespoons olive oil, 2 cloves garlic (minced), Salt and black pepper (to taste).
Preparation:
- Drain and rinse the cooked chickpeas.
- In a bowl, combine the chickpeas, chopped fresh parsley, grated lemon zest, lemon juice, extra virgin olive oil, salt and pepper.
- Mix the ingredients well.
- Serve the chickpea salad with parsley and lemon as a side dish or main course.

Nutritional Values: Calories, 150-200 kcal. Protein, 5-7 g. Fat, 5-6 g. Carbohydrates, 20-25 g. Fiber, 6-7 g.

21. Chicken and Lettuce Roll with Peanut Sauce

Ingredients:
For the Chicken and Lettuce Roll: 2 boneless, skinless chicken breasts, 8 large lettuce leaves (such as iceberg or butter lettuce), 1 cucumber (julienned), 1 carrot (julienned), 1 red bell pepper (julienned), 1/2 cup fresh cilantro leaves.
For the Peanut Sauce: 1/2 cup peanut butter, 2 tablespoons soy sauce, 2 tablespoons honey, 1 tablespoon rice vinegar, 1 clove garlic (minced), 1/2 teaspoon fresh ginger (grated), 1/4 cup warm water (adjust for desired consistency).
Preparation:
- Cook the thinly sliced chicken in a pan until cooked through.
- Prepare the peanut sauce by mixing peanut butter, soy sauce, lime juice, minced garlic and a pinch of crushed red chili pepper.
- Arrange lettuce leaves on a work surface and place a slice of cooked chicken in the center of each leaf.
- Add striped peppers and pour peanut sauce over the top.
- Roll the lettuce leaves around the filling to form the chicken and lettuce rolls.
- Serve chicken rolls with peanut sauce as an appetizer or main course.

Nutritional Values: Calories, 250-300 kcal. Protein, 15-18 g. Fat, 12-15 g. Carbohydrates, 20-25 g. Fiber, 3-4 g.

22. Tzatziki Sauce with Cucumber Sticks

Ingredients:
For the Tzatziki Sauce: 1 cup Greek yogurt, 1 cucumber (finely grated), 2 cloves garlic (minced), 2 tablespoons fresh dill (chopped), 1 tablespoon fresh mint (chopped), 1 tablespoon olive oil, 1 tablespoon lemon juice, Salt and black pepper (to taste).

For the Cucumber Sticks: 2 cucumbers (cut into sticks).
Preparation:
- Squeeze the extra water from a cucumber.
- In a bowl, combine the grated cucumber, Greek yogurt, minced garlic, lemon juice, chopped fresh mint, salt and pepper.
- Mix well to obtain the tzatziki sauce.
- Cut the cucumber into sticks and serve with tzatziki sauce as a snack or appetizer.

Nutritional Values: Calories, 50-75 kcal. Protein, 2-3 g. Fat, 4-5 g. Carbohydrates, 3-4 g. Fiber, 1-2 g.

23. Baked Kale Chips

Ingredients: 1 bunch of kale (stems removed and leaves torn into bite-sized pieces), 1-2 tablespoons olive oil, Salt (to taste), Black pepper (to taste).
Preparation:
- Wash and dry the kale leaves and cut them into pieces.
- In a bowl, combine the cabbage leaves with olive oil, sweet paprika, salt and pepper.
- Arrange the leaves on a baking sheet in a single layer.
- Cook in a preheated oven at 180°C for approximately 15-20 minutes or until the chips are crispy.
- Serve baked kale chips as a healthy snack.

Nutritional Values: Calories, 50-75 kcal. Protein, 2-3 g. Fat, 3-4 g. Carbohydrates, 7-8 g. Fiber, 2-3 g.

24. Bruschetta with Tomato and Fresh Basil

Ingredients: 4 slices of rustic bread, 2 ripe tomatoes (diced), 1/4 cup fresh basil leaves (chopped), 2 cloves garlic (peeled and halved), 2 tablespoons extra-virgin olive oil, Salt and black pepper (to taste), Balsamic vinegar (optional, for drizzling).
Preparation:
- Cut slices of crusty bread (such as baguette) and toast them lightly.
- Cut ripe tomatoes into cubes and chop some fresh basil.
- Peel a clove of garlic and rub it on the toasted slices of bread.
- Distribute the tomato cubes and basil leaves over the toasted bread slices.
- Season with extra virgin olive oil, salt and pepper.
- Serve the bruschetta as an appetizer.

Nutritional Values: Calories, 150-200 kcal. Protein, 4-5 g. Fat, 5-6 g. Carbohydrates, 20-25 g. Fiber, 3-4 g.

25. Steamed Broccoli Salad

Ingredients: 2 heads of broccoli (cut into florets), 1/4 cup red onion (finely chopped), 1/4 cup raisins, 1/4 cup sunflower seeds, 2 tablespoons extra-virgin olive oil, 2 tablespoons red wine vinegar, 1 teaspoon honey, Salt and black pepper (to taste).
Preparation:
- Blanch the broccoli in boiling salted water for a few minutes, then drain and leave to cool.
- Prepare a vinaigrette by mixing extra virgin olive oil, red wine vinegar, mustard, minced garlic, salt and pepper.
- Season the broccoli with the vinaigrette and serve as a side dish.

Nutritional Values: Calories, 50-75 kcal. Protein, 2-3 g. Fat, 1-2 g. Carbohydrates, 10-12 g. Fiber, 4-5 g.

26. Baby Carrots with Beetroot Hummus

Ingredients: 1 cup baby carrots,1 cup beetroot hummus, Fresh parsley leaves for garnish (optional)
Preparation:

- Blanch the baby carrots in salted water until tender, then drain and leave to cool.
- Make beetroot hummus by blending cooked beets, cooked chickpeas, garlic, lemon juice, tahini, salt and pepper.
- Serve baby carrots with beetroot hummus as an appetizer or snack.

Nutritional Values: Calories, 100-125 kcal. Protein, 2-3 g. Fat, 3-4 g. Carbohydrates, 15-18 g. Fiber, 4-5 g.

27. Smoked Fish with Cucumber Slices

Ingredients: 8 ounces smoked fish (such as salmon or mackerel), 1 cucumber (thinly sliced), 2 tablespoons fresh dill (chopped), 2 tablespoons lemon juice, 2 tablespoons extra-virgin olive oil, Salt and black pepper (to taste).

Preparation:

- Cut smoked fish (such as salmon) into thin slices.
- Cut the cucumber into tiny slices as well.
- Overlay the smoked fish slices on the cucumber slices.
- Serve the smoked fish with cucumber slices as an appetizer.

Nutritional Values: Calories, 150-200 kcal. Protein, 15-18 g. Fat, 8-10 g. Carbohydrates, 5-7 g. Fiber, 2-3 g.

28. Avocado and Tomato Salad

Ingredients: 2 ripe avocados (diced), 2 ripe tomatoes (diced), 1/4 cup red onion (finely chopped), 2 tablespoons fresh cilantro (chopped), 2 tablespoons extra-virgin olive oil, 1 tablespoon lime juice, Salt and black pepper (to taste).

Preparation:

- Cut avocado into cubes and ripe tomatoes into cubes.
- Add chopped red onion.
- Season with extra virgin olive oil, lemon juice, salt and pepper.
- Serve the avocado and tomato salad as a side dish or appetizer.

Nutritional Values: Calories, 150-200 kcal. Protein, 2-3 g. Fat, 12-15 g. Carbohydrates, 10-12 g. Fiber, 5-6 g.

29. Garnish of Peppers Stuffed with Brown Rice

Ingredients: 4 bell peppers (any color), 1 cup cooked brown rice, 1/2 cup black beans (cooked and drained), 1/2 cup corn kernels (fresh or frozen), 1/4 cup red onion (finely chopped), 1/4 cup diced tomatoes, 1/4 cup shredded cheddar cheese (optional), 2 tablespoons fresh cilantro (chopped), 2 tablespoons olive oil, 1 teaspoon chili powder, Salt and black pepper (to taste).

Preparation:

- Brown rice should be cooked according to package recommendations.
- Remove the tops of the peppers and the seeds.
- Fill the peppers with cooked rice, chopped vegetables (such as courgettes, tomatoes) and spices to taste.
- Cook the stuffed peppers in the oven at 180°C for about 30-40 minutes or until the peppers are tender.
- Serve the stuffed peppers as a side dish or main course.

Nutritional Values: Calories, 200-250 kcal. Protein, 6-7 g. Fat, 3-4 g. Carbohydrates, 40-45 g. Fiber, 4-5 g.

30. Stuffed Eggs with Tuna and Capers

Ingredients: 6 hard-boiled eggs, 1 can (5 ounces) tuna (drained), 2 tablespoons mayonnaise, 1 tablespoon capers (finely chopped), 1 tablespoon fresh parsley (finely chopped), 1 teaspoon Dijon mustard, Paprika for garnish (optional), salt and black pepper according to preference.

Preparation:

- Peel and cut the hard-boiled eggs in half.
- Remove the egg yolks and mix them with drained tuna, capers, mayonnaise, salt and pepper.
- Fill the egg halves with the prepared filling.
- Decorate with chopped fresh parsley.
- Serve stuffed eggs as an appetizer or snack.

Nutritional Values: Calories, 150-200 kcal. Protein, 10-12 g. Fat, 10-12 g. Carbohydrates, 1-2 g. Fiber, 1-2 g.

31. Maple Bacon with Pecans

Ingredients: 6 slices of bacon, 1/4 cup pecan halves, 2 tablespoons maple syrup, 1/2 teaspoon ground cinnamon, Pinch of cayenne pepper (optional for a spicy kick).

Preparation:

- Arrange slices of bacon on a baking tray.
- Brush the slices with maple syrup and sprinkle with toasted pecans.
- Cook in a preheated oven at 180°C for approximately 10-15 minutes or until the bacon is crispy.
- Serve maple bacon with pecans as an appetizer or snack.

Nutritional Values: Calories, 200-250 kcal. Protein, 5-7 g. Fat, 15-18 g. Carbohydrates, 10-12 g. Fiber, 2-3 g.

32. Cucumber Tzatziki with Lemon Chicken

Ingredients: 2 boneless, skinless chicken breasts, 1 lemon (zested and juiced), 2 cloves garlic (minced), 1 cup plain Greek yogurt, 1/2 cucumber (grated and excess water squeezed out), 1 tablespoon fresh dill (chopped), 1 tablespoon fresh mint (chopped), Salt and black pepper (to taste), Olive oil for cooking.

Preparation:

- Prepare the chicken by marinating pieces of chicken breast in lemon juice, minced garlic, oregano, olive oil, salt and pepper.
- Cook the chicken on a hot grill until cooked through.
- For the tzatziki, grate a cucumber and squeeze out the excess water.
- Mix the grated cucumber with Greek yogurt, minced garlic, lemon juice, chopped fresh mint, salt and pepper.
- Serve the lemon chicken with tzatziki as a side or main course.

Nutritional Values: Calories, 250-300 kcal. Protein, 20-25 g. Fat, 10-12 g. Carbohydrates, 20-25 g. Fiber, 4-5 g.

33. Baked Sweet Potatoes with Rosemary

Ingredients: 4 medium-sized sweet potatoes, 2 tablespoons olive oil, 2 teaspoons fresh rosemary (chopped), Salt and black pepper (to taste).

Preparation:

- Make thin slices of the sweet potatoes.
- Season the potato slices with olive oil, chopped fresh rosemary, salt and pepper.
- Place the potato pieces on a baking pan in a single layer.
- Cook in a preheated oven at 180°C for approximately 20-30 minutes or until the potatoes are tender and slightly crispy.
- Serve the baked sweet potatoes as a side dish.

Nutritional Values: Calories, 150-200 kcal. Protein, 2-3 g. Fat, 1-2 g. Carbohydrates, 35-40 g. Fiber, 5-6 g.

34. Wholemeal Bread Crostini with Goat's Cheese

Ingredients: 4 slices wholemeal bread, 4 oz (about 113 grams) goat's cheese, 1 clove garlic (peeled and cut in half), 2 tablespoons extra-virgin olive oil, Fresh basil leaves for garnish (optional), Salt and black pepper to taste.

Preparation:

- Toast slices of wholemeal bread until golden brown.
- Spread creamy goat cheese on toasted bread slices.
- Drizzle honey over the goat cheese.
- Serve the crostini as an appetizer or snack.

Nutritional Values: Calories, 150-200 kcal. Protein, 5-6 g. Fat, 8-10 g. Carbohydrates, 15-18 g. Fiber, 2-3 g.

35. Beetroot Salad with Toasted Almonds

Ingredients: 4 medium-sized beetroots, 1/2 cup almonds (toasted and chopped), 2 tablespoons olive oil, 2 tablespoons balsamic vinegar, Salt and black pepper to taste, Fresh parsley for garnish (optional).

Preparation:

- Peel and dice cooked beets.
- Dry toast almonds in a pan until golden brown.
- Mix the beets with the toasted almonds.
- Season with a vinaigrette made of extra virgin olive oil, balsamic vinegar, minced garlic, salt and pepper.
- Serve the beetroot salad as a side dish or appetizer.

Nutritional Values: Calories, 200-250 kcal. Protein, 4-5 g. Fat, 10-12 g. Carbohydrates, 20-25 g. Fiber, 4-5 g.

36. Baked aubergine meatballs

Ingredients: 2 large aubergines (eggplants), 1 pound (about 450 grams) ground beef or your preferred meat substitute, 1/2 cup breadcrumbs, 1/4 cup grated Parmesan cheese, 1/4 cup chopped fresh parsley, 1 egg, 1 small onion (finely chopped), 2 cloves garlic (minced), 1 can (14 ounces) crushed tomatoes, 1 teaspoon dried oregano, Salt and black pepper to taste, Olive oil for greasing.

Preparation:

- Cook sliced aubergines on the grill until golden brown.
- Chop the grilled aubergines and mix them with breadcrumbs, grated cheese, chopped garlic, chopped fresh parsley, salt and pepper.
- Form small meatballs with the mixture.
- Cook the aubergine meatballs in the oven at 180°C for about 15-20 minutes or until they are golden and cooked.
- Serve the aubergine meatballs as an appetizer or side dish.

Nutritional Values: Calories, 200-250 kcal. Protein, 8-10 g. Fat, 10-12 g. Carbohydrates, 20-25 g. Fiber, 5-6 g.

37. Lentil Soup with Turmeric

Ingredients: 1 cup red or brown lentils, rinsed and drained, 1 onion, chopped, 2 cloves garlic, minced, 1 carrot, diced, 1 celery stalk, diced, 1 teaspoon ground turmeric, 1 teaspoon ground cumin, 6 cups vegetable or chicken broth, 2 tablespoons olive oil, Salt and black pepper to taste, Fresh cilantro leaves for garnish, Lemon wedges for serving.

Preparation:

- Fry chopped onion in a pan with olive oil until golden brown.
- Add rinsed red lentils, turmeric, vegetable broth and other spices to taste.
- Cook the soup until the lentils are tender.
- Serve lentil soup as a main course or side dish.

Nutritional Values: Calories, 150-200 kcal. Protein, 6-8 g. Fat, 2-3 g. Carbohydrates, 25-30 g. Fiber, 8-10 g.

38. Chilli and Lime Sauce with Shrimp

Ingredients: 1 pound large shrimp, peeled and deveined, 2 tablespoons olive oil, 2 cloves garlic, minced, 1 red chili, thinly sliced, Zest and juice of 2 limes, 2 tablespoons fresh cilantro, chopped, Salt and pepper to taste.

Preparation:

- Sauté peeled shrimp in a pan with olive oil until cooked through.
- Make a sauce by mixing chopped red chillies, lime juice, minced garlic, sugar and soy sauce.
- Pour the sauce over the shrimp and mix well.
- Serve the chili lime sauce with shrimp as an appetizer or main course.

Nutritional Values: Calories, 150-200 kcal. Protein, 20-25 g. Fat, 5-6 g. Carbohydrates, 8-10 g. Fiber, 2-3 g.

39. Spinach Salad with Strawberries and Almonds

Ingredients: Fresh spinach leaves (2 cups), Strawberries (sliced, 1/2 cup), Sliced almonds (1/4 cup), Red onion (thinly sliced, 2 tablespoons), Feta cheese (crumbled, 2 tablespoons), Balsamic vinaigrette dressing (2 tablespoons).

Preparation:

- Wash and dry fresh spinach leaves.
- Add sliced strawberries and toasted almonds.
- Season with a vinaigrette made of olive oil, balsamic vinegar, mustard, honey, salt and pepper.
- Serve the spinach salad as a side dish or appetizer.

Nutritional Values: Calories, 200-250 kcal. Protein, 6-8 g. Fat, 12-15 g. Carbohydrates, 20-25 g. Fiber, 5-6 g.

40. Stuffed Eggs with Avocado and Paprika

Ingredients: Eggs (hard-boiled, 6), Avocado (ripe, 2), Lemon juice (1 tablespoon), Paprika (1/2 teaspoon), Salt (to taste), Black pepper (to taste).

Preparation:

- Peel and cut the hard-boiled eggs in half.
- Remove the egg yolks and mix them with mashed avocado, smoked paprika, chopped fresh parsley, salt and pepper.
- Fill the egg halves with the prepared filling.
- Serve stuffed eggs as an appetizer or snack.

Nutritional Values: Calories, 150-200 kcal. Protein, 6-8 g. Fat, 10-12 g. Carbohydrates, 4-6 g. Fiber, 3-4 g.

41. Bruschetta with Pesto and Dried Tomato

Ingredients: Baguette (1), Pesto sauce (1/2 cup), Dried tomatoes (chopped, 1/4 cup), Olive oil (1 tablespoon), Fresh basil leaves (for garnish).

Preparation:

- Toast thick bread slices till golden brown.
- Spread pesto over the toasted bread slices.
- Add chopped dried tomatoes on top of the pesto.
- Serve as an appetizer or snack.

Nutritional Values: Calories, 150-200 kcal. Protein, 4-5 g. Fat, 8-10 g. Carbohydrates, 15-18 g. Fiber, 2-3 g.

42. Chinese Cabbage Salad with Peanuts

Ingredients: Chinese cabbage (1 head), Carrots (2, grated), Peanuts (1/2 cup, crushed), Green onions (3, chopped), Cilantro leaves (1/4 cup, chopped), Soy sauce (2 tablespoons), Rice vinegar (2 tablespoons), Sesame oil (1 tablespoon), Sugar (1 tablespoon), Salt (1/2 teaspoon), Red pepper flakes (1/4 teaspoon, optional).

Preparation:

- Bok choy should be cut into thin pieces.
- Roast peanuts in a pan without oil until golden brown.
- Mix the bok choy with the roasted peanuts.
- Prepare a vinaigrette by mixing sesame oil, rice vinegar, minced garlic, sugar, salt and pepper.
- Before serving, drizzle the vinaigrette over the salad.

Nutritional Values: Calories, 200-250 kcal. Protein, 6-8 g. Fat, 15-18 g. Carbohydrates, 12-15 g. Fiber, 3-4 g.

43. Grilled Chicken with Pepper Sauce

Ingredients: Chicken breasts (4, boneless and skinless), Red bell pepper (1, finely chopped), Yellow bell pepper (1, finely chopped), Green bell pepper (1, finely chopped), Onion (1, finely chopped), Garlic (2 cloves, minced), Olive oil (2 tablespoons), Paprika (1 teaspoon), Red pepper flakes (1/4 teaspoon, optional for extra heat), Salt (1/2 teaspoon), Black pepper (1/4 teaspoon), Chicken broth (1 cup), Heavy cream (1/2 cup), Fresh parsley (2 tablespoons, chopped, for garnish).

Preparation:
- Marinate the chicken breast in olive oil, minced garlic, chopped parsley, salt and pepper.
- Cook the chicken breast on the grill until cooked through.
- Make the sauce by blending roasted peppers, garlic, parsley, olive oil, salt and pepper.
- Serve the grilled chicken with the pepper sauce.

Nutritional Values: Calories, 250-300 kcal. Protein, 30-35 g. Fat, 10-12 g. Carbohydrates, 5-8 g. Fiber, 2-3 g.

44. Green Bean and Almond Salad

Ingredients: Green beans (250g, trimmed and blanched), Almonds (1/2 cup, toasted), Red onion (1/4 cup, finely chopped), Olive oil (2 tablespoons), Red wine vinegar (2 tablespoons), Dijon mustard (1 teaspoon), Honey (1 teaspoon), Salt (1/2 teaspoon), Black pepper (1/4 teaspoon), Fresh parsley (2 tablespoons, chopped, for garnish).

Preparation:
- Steam the mung beans until tender, then let them cool.
- Dry toast almonds in a pan until golden brown.
- Mix the green beans with the toasted almonds.
- Season with a vinaigrette made of olive oil, red wine vinegar, mustard, minced garlic, salt and pepper.
- Serve the green bean salad as a side dish or appetizer.

Nutritional Values: Calories, 150-200 kcal. Protein, 4-6 g. Fat, 10-12 g. Carbohydrates, 10-12 g. Fiber, 4-5 g.

45. Sun-Dried Tomatoes Stuffed with Olives and Capers

Ingredients: Sun-Dried Tomatoes (10 pieces), Green Olives (1/2 cup, pitted), Feta Cheese (1/2 cup, crumbled), Extra Virgin Olive Oil (2 tablespoons), Fresh Basil Leaves (10 leaves, for garnish), Balsamic Vinegar (1 tablespoon), Ground Black Pepper (1/4 teaspoon).

Preparation:
- Cut the sun-dried tomatoes in half and remove the seeds.
- Prepare a mixture by chopping olives, capers, garlic, parsley, olive oil, salt, and pepper.
- Fill the halves of the sun-dried tomatoes with the prepared mixture.
- Serve the stuffed sun-dried tomatoes as an appetizer or snack.

Nutritional Values: Calories, 50-70 kcal. Protein, 1-2 g. Fat, 4-6 g. Carbohydrates, 3-4 g. Fiber, 1-2 g.

46. Ham and Asparagus Rolls

Ingredients: Ham Slices (8 slices), Asparagus Spears (16 spears), Cream Cheese (1/2 cup, softened), Lemon Juice (1 tablespoon), Salt (1/4 teaspoon), Black Pepper (1/4 teaspoon), Fresh Chives (2 tablespoons, chopped), Toothpicks (for securing the rolls).

Preparation:
- Steam the asparagus until tender, then leave to cool.
- Wrap each asparagus with a slice of raw ham.
- Serve the ham and asparagus rolls as an appetizer or snack.

Nutritional Values: Calories, 150-200 kcal. Protein, 10-12 g. Fat, 8-10 g. Carbohydrates, 8-10 g. Fiber, 2-3 g.

47. Celery and Apple Salad

Ingredients: Celery Stalks (4 stalks, thinly sliced), Apples (2, cored and diced), Walnuts (1/2 cup, chopped), Raisins (1/4 cup), Lemon Juice (2 tablespoons), Mayonnaise (1/4 cup), Greek Yogurt (1/4 cup), Honey (1 tablespoon, optional for sweetness), Salt (1/4 teaspoon), Black Pepper (1/4 teaspoon).

Preparation:
- Cut the celery into thin slices and the apples into cubes.
- Dry toast walnuts in a pan until golden brown.
- Stir in the celery, apples and toasted walnuts.
- Season with a vinaigrette made of olive oil, lemon juice, mustard, honey, salt and pepper.
- Serve the celery and apple salad as a side dish or appetizer.

Nutritional Values: Calories, 80-100 kcal. Protein, 1-2 g. Fat, 0-1 g. Carbohydrates, 20-25 g. Fiber, 3-4 g.

48. Roasted Tomato Sauce with Chilli

Ingredients: Tomatoes (6 large, ripe), Red Chilli (1, dried or fresh, adjust to taste), Garlic Cloves (4), Olive Oil (2 tablespoons), Salt (1 teaspoon, or to taste), Black Pepper (1/2 teaspoon, or to taste), Sugar (1 teaspoon, optional), Fresh Basil Leaves (a handful, for garnish).

Preparation:
- Roast ripe tomatoes in the oven until golden, then let them cool.
- Blend the roasted tomatoes with fresh chili pepper, minced garlic, olive oil, salt and pepper.
- Heat the sauce in a pan and serve it as a sauce for pasta or main dishes.

Nutritional Values: Calories, 70-90 kcal. Protein, 2-3 g. Fat, 3-4 g. Carbohydrates, 10-12 g. Fiber, 2-3 g.

49. Turkey Meatballs with Parsley

Ingredients: Ground Turkey (1 pound), Bread Crumbs (1/2 cup), Fresh Parsley (1/4 cup, chopped), Egg (1), Onion (1/2, finely chopped), Salt (1 teaspoon), Black Pepper (1/2 teaspoon), Olive Oil (2 tablespoons).

Preparation:
- Mix ground turkey meat with chopped fresh parsley, chopped onion, chopped garlic, black pepper, salt and eggs.
- Form small meatballs with the mixture.
- Cook turkey meatballs in a pan with olive oil until cooked through.
- Serve the meatballs as an entree or an appetizer.

Nutritional Values: Calories, 150-200 kcal. Protein, 15-18 g. Fat, 6-8 g. Carbohydrates, 8-10 g. Fiber, 1-2 g.

50. Baked Zucchini Chips

Ingredients: Zucchini (2 medium), Olive Oil (2 tablespoons), Grated Parmesan Cheese (1/4 cup), Breadcrumbs (1/4 cup), Salt (1/2 teaspoon), Black Pepper (1/4 teaspoon), Garlic Powder (1/4 teaspoon), Paprika (1/4 teaspoon), Cayenne Pepper (1/4 teaspoon, optional).

Preparation:
- Cut courgettes into thin slices.
- Season the zucchini slices with olive oil, sweet paprika, garlic powder, salt and pepper.
- Arrange the slices of zucchini on a baking pan in a single layer.
- Cook in a preheated oven at 180°C for approximately 15-20 minutes or until the chips are golden and crispy.
- As a snack or side dish, serve the zucchini chips.

Nutritional Values: Calories, 60-80 kcal. Protein, 2-3 g. Fat, 3-4 g. Carbohydrates, 8-10 g. Fiber, 2-3 g.

Chapter 8: Main dishes

100 Anti-Inflammatory Main Dish Recipes

This chapter is a vital resource for those looking to follow an anti-inflammatory diet to improve their health and well-being. The 100 main dish recipes offer a variety of tasty and nutritious options that suit different tastes and dietary preferences. Each recipe has been carefully developed and curated by experts to ensure they comply with the principles of an anti-inflammatory diet. These recipes include ingredients that are known for their anti-inflammatory properties and their contribution to maintaining good health. Within this chapter, you will find main dishes that include lean proteins such as chicken, fish, turkey and legumes. Creative and tasty preparations will be presented, allowing you to enjoy a wide range of flavors and combinations of ingredients. Each recipe will be accompanied by detailed preparation and cooking instructions, to make the cooking process as simple as possible. The anti-inflammatory main dish recipes will be divided into categories based on protein types and dietary preferences, ensuring you can easily find dishes that fit your needs and nutritional goals. This chapter will give you balanced, delicious meal options that will help you successfully follow an anti-inflammatory diet while enjoying a variety of tasty foods. Whether you're looking for recipes for lunch or dinner, this chapter will be a valuable resource for incorporating anti-inflammatory eating habits into your daily routine and improving your overall health.

Main dishes

1. Lemon Chicken with Broccoli

Ingredients:4 chicken breasts, 2 lemons, juiced, 2 tablespoons olive oil, 3 cloves garlic, minced, 1 bunch broccoli, Salt and freshly ground black pepper to taste, chopped fresh parsley for garnish

Preparation:

- In a large bowl, mix the lemon juice, olive oil, minced garlic, salt and pepper. This marinade will be used to flavor the chicken.
- Make sure the chicken breasts are fully coated in the marinade.
- Cover the bowl and leave to marinate in the refrigerator for at least 30 minutes. Over a medium-high flame, prepare a grill or a nonstick skillet.
- Cook the marinated chicken breasts for about 6-8 minutes per side or until browned and cooked through. The cooking time will vary according on the size of the chicken.
- While the chicken is cooking, also cook the broccoli on the grill or in a separate pan with a drizzle of olive oil, salt and pepper.
- Cook for about 5-7 minutes or until tender and lightly browned.
- Serve the lemon chicken with broccoli as a side dish. Garnish with chopped fresh parsley and squeeze some additional lemon over the chicken for an extra touch of freshness.

Nutritional Values: Calories: 350-400 kcal, Protein: 25-30 g, Fat: 15-20 g, Carbohydrates: 20-25 g, Fiber: 4-5 g

2. Grilled Salmon with Avocado Sauce

Ingredients: 4 salmon fillets, 2 ripe avocados, 1 lemon, juiced, 2 tablespoons olive oil, 2 cloves garlic, minced, Salt and freshly ground black pepper to taste, chopped fresh parsley for garnish

Preparation:

- Mix the avocados with a fork in a mixing dish until homogeneous.
- Combine the lemon juice, olive oil, minced garlic, salt, and pepper in a mixing bowl. Mix until the sauce is homogeneous.
- Heat a grill to medium-high heat. Brush the salmon fillets lightly with olive oil and grill them for about 4-5 minutes per side or until marked and cooked through.
- Top the cooked salmon with the avocado sauce. Garnish with chopped fresh parsley and squeeze in some additional lemon, if desired.

Nutritional Values: Calories: 350-400 kcal, Protein: 25-30 g, Fat: 20-25 g, Carbohydrates: 10-15 g, Fiber: 3-4 g

3. Turkey Tacos with Fresh Tomato Salsa

Ingredients:500g ground turkey meat, 1 red onion, finely chopped, 2 ripe tomatoes, diced, 1 red pepper, diced, 2 garlic cloves, chopped, 1 teaspoon cumin powder, 1 teaspoon paprika smoked, Salt and freshly ground black pepper to taste, Lettuce leaves or tortillas to serve, Sliced avocado to garnish, Chopped fresh coriander to garnish

Preparation:

- In a non-stick pan, heat a drizzle of olive oil over medium heat.
- Sauté the sliced garlic and onion till golden.
- Add the ground turkey to the pan and cook until well cooked and crumbly.
- Add cumin, paprika, salt and black pepper. Mix well.
- Meanwhile, prepare the fresh tomato sauce by mixing the diced tomatoes and red pepper in a bowl.
- Add salt and pepper to taste. Reheat tortillas or prepare lettuce leaves to make tacos.
- Fill tortillas or lettuce leaves with ground turkey and fresh tomato salsa. Garnish with slices of avocado and freshly chopped cilantro if desired.
- Nutritional Values: Calories: 300-350 kcal, Protein: 20-25 g, Fat: 10-12 g, Carbohydrates: 25-30 g, Fiber: 4-5 g

4. Beef Steak with Chimichurri

Ingredients:

4 beef steaks (any cut you prefer), 1 bunch fresh parsley, chopped, 3 cloves garlic, minced, 1/2 cup olive oil, 1/4 cup red wine vinegar, 1 teaspoon dried oregano, 1/2 teaspoon dried red chili (optional), Salt and freshly ground black pepper to taste

Preparation:

- In a bowl, mix the chopped fresh parsley, minced garlic, olive oil, red wine vinegar, dried oregano, dried red chili pepper (if desired), salt and black pepper. This will be the chimichurri sauce.
- Grill beef steaks over medium-high heat for approximately 4-5 minutes per side or until desired doneness.
- When the steaks are done, let them rest for a few minutes before slicing.
- Serve sliced steaks with chimichurri sauce on top. This sauce will add a fresh and aromatic touch to the meat.

Nutritional Values: Calories: 350-400 kcal, Protein: 25-30 g, Fat: 20-25 g, Carbohydrates: 5-10 g, Fiber: 2-3 g

5. Chicken Curry with Coconut Milk

Ingredients: 4 chicken breasts, cut into cubes, 1 onion, finely chopped, 2 cloves of garlic, chopped, 1 red pepper, cut into strips, 2 tablespoons red curry paste, 400 ml coconut milk, 2 tablespoons olive oil, salt and freshly ground black pepper to taste, chopped fresh coriander to garnish, cooked basmati rice to serve

Preparation:
- Warm the olive oil in a big skillet over a medium-high flame. Sauté the sliced onion and garlic till golden.
- Add the chicken breast cubes to the pan and cook until golden brown on all sides.
- Add the red curry paste and mix well with the chicken for about 1 minute or until the flavors blend.
- Add the red pepper cut into strips and the coconut milk.
- Mix well and cook over medium heat for about 10-15 minutes or until the chicken is cooked and the sauce has thickened.
- Serve chicken curry with coconut milk over cooked basmati rice.
- Garnish with chopped fresh cilantro for a touch of freshness.

Nutritional Values: Calories: 350-400 kcal, Protein: 20-25 g, Fat: 20-25 g, Carbohydrates: 10-15 g, Fiber: 2-3 g

6. Tomato Lentil Soup

Ingredients: 1 cup dried lentils, 1 onion, chopped, 2 cloves garlic, chopped, 2 carrots, diced, 2 celery sticks, diced, 1 can (400g) chopped tomatoes, 1 teaspoon dried oregano, 1 teaspoon dried basil, 4 cups vegetable broth, Salt and freshly ground black pepper to taste, Olive oil for sautéing

Preparation:
- Warm some olive oil in a big saucepan over medium heat. Add the onion, garlic, carrots and celery. Sauté until the vegetables become tender.
- Add the dried lentils and mix well with the vegetables.
- Add the chopped tomatoes, oregano, basil, vegetable broth, salt and black pepper.
- Bring to a boil after thoroughly mixing.
- Reduce the heat and simmer for about 25-30 minutes or until the lentils are soft.
- Serve the soup hot, possibly garnished with fresh basil.

Nutritional Values: Calories: 250-300 kcal, Protein: 10-15 g, Fat: 5-7 g, Carbohydrates: 40-45 g, Fiber: 10-12 g

7. Baked Trout Fillet with Aromatic Herbs

Ingredients: 4 trout fillets, juice of 1 lemon, 2 tablespoons chopped fresh parsley, 2 tablespoons chopped fresh chives, 2 tablespoons chopped fresh tarragon (optional), Salt and freshly ground black pepper to taste, Lemon slices for garnish

Preparation:
- Heat the temperature of the oven to 180°C and butter a baking sheet lightly.
- Place the fillets of fish on a baking pan.
- Sprinkle the lemon juice evenly over the trout fillets. Mix the parsley, chives and tarragon (if using) in a bowl.
- Spread this herb mixture over the trout fillets. Garnish with salt and black pepper according to preference.
- Bake in the preheated oven for about 15-20 minutes or until the fish is cooked through and flakes easily with a fork. Serve the baked trout fillet with lemon slices as a garnish.

Nutritional Values: Calories: 250-300 kcal, Protein: 20-25 g, Fat: 15-20 g, Carbohydrates: 5-10 g, Fiber: 1-2 g

8. Quinoa Meatballs with Spinach

Ingredients: 1 cup cooked quinoa, 200 g fresh spinach, cooked and squeezed, 1 egg, 1/4 cup wholemeal breadcrumbs, 2 tablespoons grated cheese (optional), 1 clove of minced garlic, 1 teaspoon paprika sweet, Salt and freshly ground black pepper to taste, Olive oil for frying

Preparation:
- In a large bowl, mix cooked quinoa, cooked spinach, egg, breadcrumbs, grated cheese (if using), garlic, paprika, salt and pepper.
- Mix well until a homogeneous mixture is obtained. Form meatballs with the dough.
- If the dough is too wet, you can add a little more breadcrumbs.
- Temperature some olive oil in a nonstick skillet over a medium-high flame.
- Cook meatballs until golden brown on both sides, about 3-4 minutes per side.
- Serve the quinoa meatballs with hot spinach, perhaps accompanied by a sauce or cream of your choice.

Nutritional Values: Calories: 300-350 kcal, Protein: 15-20 g, Fat: 10-15 g, Carbohydrates: 30-35 g, Fiber: 5-6 g

9. Roasted Duck Breast with Cherry Sauce

Ingredients: 2 duck breasts, Salt and freshly ground black pepper to taste, 1 cup fresh cherries, pitted and halved, 1/4 cup brown sugar, 1/4 cup red wine vinegar, 1/2 teaspoon ground cinnamon

Preparation:
- Preheat the oven to 200°C. Score the skin of the duck breasts with a sharp knife, making diagonal incisions. This will aid in the release of fat when cooking.
- Salt and pepper the duck breasts on both sides. Warm up a skillet with nonstick coating over medium-high heat.
- Arrange the duck's breasts skin side up in the pan.
- Cook for 5-6 minutes or until the skin is golden and crispy.
- Turn the duck breasts and cook for another 3-4 minutes.
- Transfer the duck breasts to a baking tray and cook in the preheated oven for about 10-15 minutes for medium-rare or longer for well-done.
- Keep in mind that cooking times may vary depending on the size of the duck breasts and your cooking preferences.
- Meanwhile, prepare the cherry sauce.
- In a saucepan, combine the cherries, brown sugar, red wine vinegar and cinnamon.
- Cook over medium-low heat until the cherries fall apart and the sauce thickens slightly.
- Once cooked, cut the duck breasts into thin slices and serve with the cherry sauce on top.

Nutritional Values: Calories: 400-450 kcal, Protein: 20-25 g, Fat: 25-30 g, Carbohydrates: 15-20 g, Fiber: 1-2 g

10. Grilled Pork with Cranberry Sauce

Ingredients:4 pork chops, Salt and freshly ground black pepper to taste,1 cup fresh cranberries,1/4 cup sugar,1/4 cup orange juice,1 tablespoon balsamic vinegar,1 teaspoon of chopped fresh rosemary

Preparation:
- Preheat grill to medium-high heat. Salt and pepper the pork chops on both sides.
- In a saucepan, combine the cranberries, sugar, orange juice, balsamic vinegar and rosemary.

- Bring everything to the boil, then reduce the heat and leave to simmer for about 10-15 minutes or until the sauce thickens slightly.
- Grill the pork chops on the preheated grill for about 4-5 minutes per side or until cooked through and have nice streaks from the grill. Serve pork chops hot with cranberry sauce on top.

Nutritional Values: Calories: 300-350 kcal, Protein: 20-25 g, Fat: 10-15 g, Carbohydrates: 15-20 g, Fiber: 1-2 g

11. Quinoa Salad with Chickpeas and Olives

Ingredients: 1 cup quinoa, 2 cups water, 1 can chickpeas, rinsed and drained, 1/2 cup black olives, pitted and sliced, 1/2 cup green olives, pitted and sliced, Grated zest of 1 lemon, Juice of 2 lemons, 2 tablespoons of extra virgin olive oil, Salt and black pepper to taste. Fresh basil leaves for garnish (optional)

Preparation:
- Rinse the quinoa under cold running water. In a saucepan, bring 2 cups of water to a boil, then add the quinoa.
- Reduce the heat, cover and simmer for about 15 minutes or until the quinoa absorbs the water and is tender. Drain the quinoa and place it in a large bowl.
- Add the chickpeas, black olives, green olives, grated lemon zest and lemon juice.
- Pour in the olive oil and mix all the ingredients well. To taste, add salt and pepper according to preference.
- Allow it cool for at least 30 minutes in the fridge until serving.
- If desired, sprinkle with new basil leaves.

Nutritional Values: Calories: 300-350 kcal, Protein: 10-15 g, Fat: 10-12 g, Carbohydrates: 40-45 g, Fiber: 8-10 g

12. Baked Salmon with Walnut Crust

Ingredients:4 salmon fillets,1 cup chopped walnuts,1/4 cup chopped fresh parsley,2 tablespoons Dijon mustard,2 tablespoons honey, 2 tablespoons olive oil, Salt and black pepper to taste, Lemon slices for garnish

Preparation:
- Preheat the oven to 200°C and line. On a baking tray with baking paper. In a bowl, mix the chopped walnuts, parsley, Dijon mustard, honey and olive oil.
- Place the salmon fillets on the baking sheet and spread with the nut mixture.
- Cook for 12-15 minutes, so that the salmon flakes easily with a fork, in a preheated oven. Garnish the cooked fish with lemon wedges.

Nutritional Values: Calories: 350-400 kcal, Protein: 25-30 g, Fat: 20-25 g, Carbohydrates: 5-10 g, Fiber: 2-3 g

13. Paprika Chicken with Peppers

Ingredients: 4 chicken breasts, 2 tablespoons sweet paprika, 1 tablespoon olive oil, 1 red onion, thinly sliced, 2 red peppers, cut into strips, 1/2 cup chicken broth, Salt and black pepper to pleasure, chopped fresh parsley for garnish (optional)

Preparation:
- In a bowl, mix the sweet paprika, salt and black pepper. Then, sprinkle the chicken breasts with this mixture.
- Heat the olive oil in a nonstick skillet over medium-high heat.
- Add chicken breasts and cook for 5-6 minutes per side or until browned and cooked through.
- Take the chicken out of the pan and set it away. In the same pan, add the red onion and red peppers.

- Cook for 3-4 minutes or until soft. Put the chicken stock to a boil in the pan.
- Reduce heat and simmer for another 5 minutes or until sauce thickens. Add the chicken and sauce to the pan and heat for 2-3 minutes.
- If desired, sprinkle with minced fresh parsley.

Nutritional Values: Calories: 300-350 kcal, Protein: 20-25 g, Fat: 10-15 g, Carbohydrates: 10-15 g, Fiber: 2-3 g

14. Grilled Tofu with Chili Sauce

Ingredients: 1 block extra-firm tofu, drained and cut into thick slices, 2 tablespoons soy sauce, 2 tablespoons sesame oil, 2 teaspoons rice vinegar, 1 teaspoon sugar, 1 teaspoon chili sauce (or more depending on your taste), 1 teaspoon grated fresh ginger, 1 finely chopped clove of garlic, toasted sesame seeds for garnish (optional), chopped chives for garnish (optional)

Preparation:
- In a small bowl, mix the soy sauce, sesame oil, rice vinegar, sugar, chili sauce, grated ginger and minced garlic to make the marinade.
- Place the tofu slices on a shallow plate and pour the marinade over them. Leave to marinate for at least 15-30 minutes.
- Preheat a grill or nonstick skillet over medium-high heat.
- Cook the tofu marinades for about 2-3 minutes per side or until golden brown and crispy.
- Serve the grilled tofu hot and garnish with toasted sesame seeds and chopped chives, if desired.

Nutritional Values: Calories: 200-250 kcal, Protein: 15-20 g, Fat: 10-12 g, Carbohydrates: 15-20 g, Fiber: 2-3 g

15. Tuna Steak with Mango Salsa

Ingredients: 4 tuna steak fillets, 2 ripe mangoes, peeled and diced, 1 red onion, finely chopped, 1 red chili pepper, seeded and finely chopped, Juice of 2 limes, 2 tablespoons chopped fresh coriander, Salt and black pepper to taste

Preparation:
- Preheat grill to medium-high heat.
- Cook the tuna steak fillets on the grill for about 2-3 minutes per side or until cooked through but still pink inside. Take them off the grill and set them aside.
- In a bowl, mix the mango cubes, red onion, chili pepper, lime juice and coriander. Sprinkle according to preference with salt and pepper.
- Serve tuna steak fillets with mango salsa on top.

Nutritional Values: Calories: 350-400 kcal, Protein: 25-30 g, Fat: 10-15 g, Carbohydrates: 15-20 g, Fiber: 2-3 g

16. Curry Chicken Meatballs

Ingredients: 500g minced chicken, 1 egg, 1/4 cup breadcrumbs, 2 tablespoons curry powder, 1 tablespoon olive oil, Salt and black pepper to taste, Chopped fresh chives for garnish (optional)

Preparation:
- In a bowl, mix the ground chicken, egg, breadcrumbs, curry powder, salt and black pepper.
- Form evenly sized meatballs with the mixture.
- Heat the olive oil in a nonstick skillet over medium-high heat.
- Cook chicken meatballs until cooked through and golden brown, about 5-7 minutes per side.
- Serve the meatballs hot and garnish with chopped chives, if desired.

Nutritional Values: Calories: 300-350 kcal, Protein: 15-20 g, Fat: 10-15 g, Carbohydrates: 20-25 g, Fiber: 2-3 g

17. Zucchini Spaghetti with Basil Pesto

Ingredients:4 medium courgettes,2 cups fresh basil leaves,1/2 cup toasted walnuts,1/2 cup extra virgin olive oil,2 cloves garlic, minced,1/2 cup Parmesan cheese- Grated Reggiano cheese, Salt and black pepper to taste, Grated zest of 1 lemon (optional), Additional Parmigiano-Reggiano cheese for garnish (optional)

Preparation:

- Use a spiralizer or vegetable peeler to create zucchini spaghetti.
- In a food processor, blend basil leaves, toasted walnuts, olive oil, garlic, Parmigiano-Reggiano cheese, salt and black pepper until smooth pesto.
- Season the courgette spaghetti with the basil pesto and mix well.
- If desired, garnish with grated lemon zest and additional Parmigiano-Reggiano cheese.

Nutritional Values: Calories: 250-300 kcal, Protein: 5-10 g, Fat: 20-25 g, Carbohydrates: 15-20 g, Fiber: 3-4 g

18. Mustard Salmon with Asparagus

Ingredients:4 salmon fillets, 1/4 cup Dijon mustard, 2 tablespoons honey, 1 tablespoon lemon juice, 1 clove garlic, finely chopped, 1 bunch asparagus, Salt and black pepper to taste, Olive oil

Preparation:

- Preheat the oven to 200°C. Using parchment paper to prepare a baking sheet.
- In a bowl, mix the Dijon mustard, honey, lemon juice, minced garlic, salt and black pepper.
- Place the salmon fillets on the prepared baking sheet and brush with the mustard mixture.
- Arrange the asparagus around the salmon, sprinkle with olive oil, salt and black pepper.
- Bake in the preheated oven for about 12 to 15 minutes, or until the salmon flakes easily with a fork and the asparagus is tender.
- Serve the mustard salmon with asparagus.

Nutritional Values: Calories: 350-400 kcal, Protein: 25-30 g, Fat: 20-25 g, Carbohydrates: 10-15 g, Fiber: 4-5 g

19. Beef Steak with Rosemary

Ingredients: 4 beef steaks (about 200 g each), 2 tablespoons chopped fresh rosemary, 2 tablespoons extra virgin olive oil, Salt and black pepper to taste

Preparation:

- Preheat grill or nonstick skillet over medium-high heat. Brush both sides of the beef steaks with olive oil.
- Sprinkle fresh rosemary, salt and black pepper on both sides of the steaks.
- Cook the steaks on the grill or in the pan for about 3-4 minutes per side for medium-rare, or longer if you prefer a different doneness.
- Allow for a few minutes of resting time before presenting the steaks.

Nutritional Values: Calories: 350-400 kcal, Protein: 25-30 g, Fat: 20-25 g, Carbohydrates: 5-10 g, Fiber: 2-3 g

20. Grilled Chicken with Peppers and Onions

Ingredients:4 chicken breasts,2 peppers, cut into strips,2 onions, sliced,2 tablespoons extra virgin olive oil,2 teaspoons paprika
Salt and black pepper to taste, chopped fresh parsley for garnish (optional)

Preparation:

- Preheat grill to medium-high heat.
- In a bowl, mix the peppers, onions, olive oil, paprika, salt and black pepper.
- Grill chicken breasts until cooked through and browned, about 6 to 7 minutes per side.
- During the last few minutes of cooking, add the pepper and onion mixture to the grill and cook until tender and lightly charred.
- Serve the grilled chicken with the pepper and onion sauce, garnishing with chopped fresh parsley if desired.

Nutritional Values: Calories: 250-300 kcal, Protein: 25-30 g, Fat: 10-15 g, Carbohydrates: 10-15 g, Fiber: 2-3 g

21. Cotechino with Lentils and Spinach

Ingredients: 4 thick slices of cotechino, 2 cups of dried lentils, 200 g of fresh spinach, 2 cloves of garlic, finely chopped, 2 tablespoons of extra virgin olive oil, Salt and black pepper to taste.

Preparation:

- Cook the cotechino in boiling water following the instructions on the package (generally for 1-2 hours).
- Meanwhile, rinse the lentils under running water and cook in boiling salted water until tender but not mushy, usually 20-25 minutes.
- School them. Warm the olive oil in a pan over a medium-high flame.
- Fry the minced garlic until fragrant. Add fresh spinach to the pan and cook until wilted and reduced in volume.
- Add the cooked lentils to the spinach, mix well and cook for a few minutes until combined.
- Cut the cotechino into thick slices and serve it hot over a bed of lentils and spinach.

Nutritional Values: Calories: 350-400 kcal, Protein: 15-20 g, Fat: 10-15 g, Carbohydrates: 40-45 g, Fiber: 10-12 g

22. Fish Tacos with Mango Salsa

Ingredients:500g fish fillets (e.g. tilapia or cod),1 tablespoon olive oil,1 teaspoon paprika,1 teaspoon cumin,1/2 teaspoon cayenne pepper (optional), Salt and pepper black to taste, 8 corn or flour tortillas, 2 cups chopped green cabbage, 1 ripe mango, peeled and diced, 1/2 red onion, finely chopped, Juice of 1 lime, chopped fresh cilantro for garnish (optional)

Preparation:

- In a bowl, combine the olive oil, paprika, cumin, cayenne (if desired), salt, and black pepper.
- Brush the mixture over the fish fillets and let them marinate for at least 30 minutes.
- Heat a non-stick pan over medium-high heat and cook the fish fillets for 3-4 minutes per side or until cooked through.
- Cut the fish into smaller pieces and assemble the tacos with the fish, cabbage, mango, red onion and a little lime juice.
- Garnish with fresh cilantro if desired.

Nutritional Values: Calories: 300-350 kcal, Protein: 20-25 g, Fat: 10-15 g, Carbohydrates: 30-35 g, Fiber: 5-6 g

23.Turkey Meatballs with Tzatziki Sauce

Ingredients: 500g minced turkey meat, 1 egg, 1/4 cup breadcrumbs, 1/4 cup finely chopped red onion, 1/4 cup chopped fresh parsley, 1 chopped clove of garlic, 1 teaspoon dried oregano, Salt and ground black pepper (to taste), 1 cup Greek yogurt, 1 cucumber (peeled, seeded and grated), 1 teaspoon chopped fresh mint, 1 teaspoon fresh lemon juice, Salt and ground black pepper (to taste).

Preparation:

- In a large bowl, combine the ground turkey, egg, breadcrumbs, red onion, parsley, garlic, oregano, salt and ground black pepper.
- Thoroughly combine to get a homogenous mixture. Form similar sized meatballs, using wet hands to prevent the mixture from sticking to your fingers.
- A non-stick pan should be heated to medium-high heat before adding a drizzle of olive oil.
- Cook the meatballs in the pan, turning occasionally, until they are golden brown and evenly cooked. It will take about 10-12 minutes.
- Meanwhile, prepare the tzatziki sauce. In a bowl, mix the Greek yogurt, grated cucumber, chopped fresh mint and lemon juice.
- To taste, add salt and ground black pepper for seasoning.
- Serve the meatballs hot accompanied by fresh tzatziki sauce. You can use it as a sauce for meatballs or as a side dish.

Nutritional Values: Calories: 300-350 kcal, Protein: 20-25 g, Fat: 10-15 g, Carbohydrates: 10-15 g, Fiber: 1-2 g

24.Duck breast with pink pepper

Ingredients: 2 duck breasts, salt, freshly ground black pepper, 2 tablespoons pink peppercorns, 1 tablespoon olive oil, 1/2 cup chicken broth, 1/4 cup fresh cream, 1 tablespoon of cold butter.

Preparation:

- Dry the duck breasts well with absorbent paper and make checkerboard cuts on the skin without cutting the meat.
- Make sure to season the breasts of duck with freshly ground black salt and black pepper.
- Lightly crush the pink peppercorns with the flat side of a knife.
- In a skillet with nonstick over medium-high heat, heat the olive oil. Add the duck breasts, skin side down, and cook for 6-8 minutes until the skin is golden brown and crispy.
- Turn the duck breasts and cook for another 2-4 minutes on the opposite side to reach the desired doneness.
- Remove the duck breasts from the pan and let them rest on a warm plate covered with foil.
- In the same pan, pour the chicken broth and scrape the bottom with a wooden spoon to release the juices and cooking residues.
- Bring the stock to the boil and cook for a few minutes until it reduces slightly.
- Add the fresh cream and crushed pink pepper, then cook over medium-low heat until the sauce thickens slightly.
- Remove the pan from the heat and stir the cold butter into the sauce to make it creamy.
- Cut the duck breasts into thin slices and arrange them on individual plates.
- Pour the pink pepper sauce over the duck slices. Serve immediately with any side dishes you like, such as mashed potatoes, steamed asparagus or salad.

Nutritional Values: Calories: 400-450 kcal, Protein: 20-25 g, Fat: 25-30 g, Carbohydrates: 5-10 g, Fiber: 1-2 g

25.Trout fillet with lemon and parsley sauce

Ingredients: 4 trout fillets, salt, freshly ground black pepper, flour for breading, 2 tablespoons butter, 2 tablespoons olive oil, juice of 2 lemons, 1/4 cup chopped fresh parsley, thin slices of lemon to decorate.

Preparation:

- Start by preparing the trout fillets. Wash them carefully under running water and dry them with absorbent paper.
- Check for any thorns remaining and remove them with kitchen tongs.
- Season the trout fillets with salt and freshly ground black pepper on both sides.
- Dredge the fillets in the flour, shaking them slightly to remove the excess flour.
- In a large nonstick skillet, heat the butter and olive oil over medium heat.
- Add the trout fillets to the pan and cook for about 3-4 minutes per side, until golden and crispy.
- Remove the trout fillets from the pan and set aside. In the same pan, add the juice of the lemons and the chopped parsley.
- Cook for a couple of minutes until the parsley becomes aromatic and the liquid reduces slightly.
- Place the trout fillets in the pan with the lemon and parsley sauce, turning them gently to cover them with the sauce.
- Cook for a further 2-3 minutes until the trout fillets are heated through and completely coated in the sauce.
- Transfer the trout fillets to a serving plate and decorate with thin slices of lemon. While the fish is still hot, serve immediately.

Nutritional Values: Calories: 250-300 kcal, Protein: 20-25 g, Fat: 15-20 g, Carbohydrates: 5-10 g, Fiber: 1-2 g

26.Chicken Curry with Chickpeas and Spinach

Ingredients: Chicken Curry with Chickpeas and Spinach (Medium Servings): 1.5 pounds (680g) boneless, skinless chicken thighs (cut into bite-sized pieces), 2 tablespoons vegetable oil, 1 large onion (finely chopped), 3 cloves garlic (minced), 1 tablespoon fresh ginger (minced), 2 tablespoons curry powder, 1 teaspoon ground cumin, 1 teaspoon ground coriander, 1/2 teaspoon ground turmeric, 1/2 teaspoon paprika, 1/4 teaspoon cayenne pepper (adjust to taste), Salt and black pepper (to taste), 1 can (15 oz) chickpeas (drained and rinsed), 1 can (14 oz) diced tomatoes, 1 cup coconut milk, 2 cups fresh spinach leaves, Fresh cilantro leaves for garnish (optional).

Preparation:

- Heat in a large skillet over medium-high heat. Add the chopped onion and minced garlic and fry until golden and fragrant.
- Add the chicken breast cubes and cook until golden brown on all sides.
- Add curry powder and chilli powder and mix well to flavor the chicken.
- Pour the canned diced tomatoes and drained chickpeas into the pan. Mix everything together.
- Reduce the heat and simmer over medium-low heat for about 15-20 minutes, until the chicken is cooked and the flavors have blended.
- Add fresh spinach to the pan and stir until wilted and reduced in volume. Mix well after pouring the coconut milk into the pan.
- Cook for a further 5-7 minutes until the chicken is tender and the sauce has thickenedSprinkle pepper and salt according to your taste

- Serve the chicken curry with chickpeas and spinach hot, preferably over basmati rice or couscous.

Nutritional Values: Calories: 350-400 kcal, Protein: 20-25 g, Fat: 15-20 g, Carbohydrates: 20-25 g, Fiber: 5-6 g

27. Baked Salmon with Lemon and Dill Sauce

Ingredients: Baked Salmon with Lemon and Dill Sauce (Medium Servings): For the Baked Salmon: 4 salmon fillets, 2 tablespoons olive oil, 2 cloves garlic (minced), 1 teaspoon dried dill, Salt and black pepper to taste, Slices of lemon for garnish. For the Lemon and Dill Sauce: 1/2 cup Greek yogurt, 2 tablespoons fresh dill (chopped), Zest and juice of 1 lemon, 1 tablespoon Dijon mustard, Salt and black pepper to taste.

Preparation:

- Line the oven with baking paper after preheating it to 200°C. In a bowl, mix the olive oil, minced garlic, lemon juice, and chopped dill.
- Add salt and pepper to tastePrepare the pan and place the salmon fillets. Pour the lemon dill sauce evenly over the salmon fillets.
- Cut a few lemon slices and place them on top of the fish for additional presentation.
- Cover the baking dish with foil and cook the salmon in the preheated oven for about 15 to 20 minutes, or until the salmon flakes easily with a fork and has a light pink hue in the center.
- Serve baked salmon with hot lemon-dill sauce, garnished with additional lemon slices and dill sprigs.

Nutritional Values : Calories : 350-400 kcal, Protein: 25-30 g Fat: 20-25 g, Carbohydrates: 5-10 g, Fiber: 2-3 g

28.Quinoa Meatballs with Peppers

Ingredients: Quinoa Meatballs with Peppers (Medium Servings): For the Quinoa Meatballs: 1 cup cooked quinoa, 1 cup black beans (mashed), 1/2 cup breadcrumbs, 1/4 cup grated Parmesan cheese, 1/4 cup chopped fresh parsley, 1 egg, 2 cloves garlic (minced), 1 teaspoon cumin, 1/2 teaspoon chili powder, Salt and black pepper to taste. For the Peppers: 2 bell peppers (cut into strips), 2 tablespoons olive oil, 1 teaspoon paprika, Salt and black pepper to taste.

Preparation:

- In a large bowl, combine the cooked quinoa, chopped peppers, chopped onion, minced garlic, grated cheese (you can use your choice of cheese such as pecorino or parmesan), chopped parsley and breadcrumbs. TO
- add the eggs and mix well to combine all the ingredients.
- Season with salt and pepper to taste.
- With wet hands, shape the mixture into small round patties.
- Heat some olive oil in a nonstick skillet over medium-high heat.
- Cook the quinoa meatballs in the pan until golden and crispy on all sides, about 3-4 minutes per side.
- To eliminate excess oil, drain them using absorbent paper.
- Serve the quinoa meatballs with peppers hot as a main course or as a side dish, accompanying them with a sauce of your choice.

Nutritional Values: Calories: 300-350 kcal, Protein: 15-20 g, Fat: 10-15 g, Carbohydrates: 20-25 g, Fiber: 3-4 g

29. Mustard Pork with Cabbage

Ingredients: Mustard Pork with Cabbage (Medium Servings): For the Mustard Pork: 1 pound (450g) pork tenderloin, sliced into medallions, 2 tablespoons Dijon mustard, 1 tablespoon olive oil, 2 cloves garlic minced, Pepper and salt to taste along with 1 tablespoon of dried thyme. For the Cabbage: 1 small cabbage, thinly sliced, 2 tablespoons butter, 1 onion, chopped, 1/4 cup chicken broth, 1 teaspoon caraway seeds (optional), Salt and black pepper to taste.

Preparation:

- In a large pan, heat some olive oil over medium heat. Bring to golden brown on both sides after adding the pork slices.
- Transfer them to a plate and cover them to keep them warm. In the same pan put chopped garlic and onion.
- Sauté until golden and aromatic. Add the green cabbage cut into strips and the dried thyme.
- Stir well and cook the cabbage until softened, about 5-7 minutes.
- Pour the chicken stock into the pan and add the Dijon mustard. Stir to create a creamy sauce.
- Return the pork slices to the pan and cook for another couple of minutes to heat through.
- Add pepper and salt after tasting. Serve mustard pork with hot cabbage as a main course.

Nutritional Values: Calories: 300-350 kcal, Protein: 20-25 g, Fat: 10-15 g, Carbohydrates: 15-20 g, Fiber: 4-5 g

30.Turmeric Tofu with Broccoli

Ingredients: 14 oz (400g) firm tofu, cubed, 1 tablespoon olive oil, 1 teaspoon turmeric powder, Salt and black pepper to taste, 2 cups broccoli florets, 1 tablespoon olive oil, 1/2 teaspoon turmeric powder, Salt and black pepper to taste.

Preparation:

- In a bowl, mix the diced tofu with the turmeric powder, soy sauce, and grated ginger.
- Marinate for at least 15-20 minutes. Place sesame oil in a large pan and let heat. Add the minced garlic and chopped broccoli. Sauté for about 5 minutes until the broccoli is tender.
- Set the broccoli aside after removing it from the pan. In the same pan, add a little oil if necessary and cook the marinated tofu until golden brown on all sides.
- Add the previously cooked broccoli to the pan with the tofu and mix well to blend the flavors.
- According to your taste, add pepper and salt. Serve the turmeric tofu with broccoli as a main course, preferably with basmati rice or noodles.

Nutritional Values: Calories: 250-300 kcal, Protein: 15-20 g, Fat: 10-12 g, Carbohydrates: 20-25 g, Fiber: 4-5 g

31.Grilled Tuna Steak with Avocado Sauce

Ingredients: Tuna steaks (2 steaks), olive oil (2 tablespoons), lemon juice (1 teaspoon), dried oregano (1 teaspoon), salt (to taste), black pepper (to taste), ripe avocado (1), Greek yogurt (1/4 cup), garlic (1 clove, minced), fresh cilantro (1 tablespoon, chopped), lime juice (1 tablespoon), salt (to taste), black pepper (to taste).

Preparation:

- Preheat grill to medium-high heat. Brush the tuna steak with a little olive oil and season with salt and pepper to taste.
- Place the tuna steak on the hot grill and cook for 2-3 minutes per side, or until cooked through but still pink inside.
- While the tuna cooks, prepare the avocado salsa. In a bowl, mash the ripe avocado with a fork and mix with the lime juice, minced garlic and chopped fresh cilantro.

- Add salt and pepper to taste. Once cooked, remove the tuna from the grill and thinly slice it.
- Serve the grilled tuna steak with the avocado salsa on top as a condiment.

Nutritional Values: Calories: 350-400 kcal Protein: 25-30 g, Fat: 20-25 g, Carbohydrates: 10-15 g, Fiber: 4-5 g

32.Grilled Chicken with Quinoa Salad

Ingredients: Trout fillets (2 medium fillets), Olive oil (2 tablespoons), Salt (1/2 teaspoon), Black pepper (1/2 teaspoon), Paprika (1/2 teaspoon), Lemon zest (1 teaspoon), Fresh basil leaves (1/2 cup), Ripe tomatoes (2 medium), Garlic (2 cloves), Olive oil (2 tablespoons), Balsamic vinegar (1 tablespoon), Salt (1/2 teaspoon), Black pepper (1/2 teaspoon).

Preparation:
- Cook the quinoa according to the package instructions. Let it cool. Heat a grill or nonstick skillet over medium-high heat.
- Season the chicken breast with olive oil, salt and pepper.
- Grill the chicken breast until it is cooked through and has nice streaks from the grill. This usually takes about 6-7 minutes per side, depending on the thickness of the chicken breast.
- Make sure the chicken reaches an appropriate internal temperature of 165°F.
- While the chicken cooks, prepare the quinoa salad. In a bowl, combine the cooked quinoa, the cherry tomatoes cut in half, the diced cucumbers, the sliced black olives and the chopped fresh parsley.
- Add lemon, pepper, olive oil and salt to the salad and mix everything well.
- Once the chicken is cooked, cut it into thin slices. Serve the chicken breast slices over the quinoa, garnishing with additional fresh herbs if desired.

Nutritional Values: Calories: 300-350 kcal, Protein: 20-25 g, Fat: 10-15 g, Carbohydrates: 25-30 g, Fiber: 4-5 g

33.Duck Breast with Orange Sauce

Ingredients: For the Duck Breast: 2 duck breasts, Salt and black pepper to taste

For the Orange Sauce: 1 cup fresh orange juice, Zest of 1 orange, 2 tablespoons honey, 2 cloves garlic, minced, 1/4 cup chicken broth, 2 tablespoons butter, Salt and black pepper to taste

Preparation:
- Preheat the oven to 180°C. Score the skin of the duck breasts with a sharp knife to create a checkerboard pattern without cutting the meat.
- In a pan over medium heat, melt the brown sugar until golden caramel. Add the orange juice, red wine vinegar, grated ginger and caramel soy sauce.
- Cook until everything is reduced by half and thickens slightly. Place a skillet over medium-high heat.
- There is no need to add oil, as the duck will release its fat.
- Cook the duck breasts, skin side down, for about 4-5 minutes until the skin is crisp and golden.
- Turn the breasts and cook for another 2-3 minutes.
- Transfer the duck breasts to the oven rack and cook them for about 8-10 minutes for medium-rare or longer if you prefer more well done cooking. Sauce:
- Add the orange sauce over the freshly baked duck breasts. Let the duck breasts rest for a few minutes before cutting them into thin slices.

- Serve the duck breast with the orange sauce as a condiment.

Nutritional Values: Calories: 400-450 kcal, Protein: 20-25 g, Fat: 25-30 g, Carbohydrates: 10-15 g, Fiber: 1-2 g

34.Pork Curry with Pumpkin

Ingredients:

For the Quinoa Meatballs: 1 cup cooked quinoa, 1/2 cup canned black beans, 1/4 cup grated carrots, 1/4 cup grated zucchini, 1/4 cup breadcrumbs, 1/4 cup grated Parmesan cheese, 1 egg, 1 clove garlic (minced), 1/2 teaspoon ground cumin, 1/2 teaspoon paprika, Salt and black pepper to taste, Olive oil for cooking.

For the Tomato Sauce: 1 can (14 oz) crushed tomatoes, 1/4 cup diced onions, 2 cloves garlic (minced), 1/2 teaspoon dried oregano, 1/2 teaspoon dried basil, Salt and black pepper to taste.

Preparation:
- Over medium-high heat, place the chopped garlic and onion in a large skillet.
- Sauté until golden and aromatic. Add the pork cubes and cook until browned on all sides. Add the curry powder and the diced pumpkin.
- Mix well to cover everything with the curry. Pour the chicken broth and coconut milk into the pot.
- Bring everything to the boil, then reduce the heat and simmer until the pork is tender and the squash is soft, this may take about 20-25 minutes.
- Add pepper and salt to taste after tasting. Serve the pumpkin curry pork hot as a main course.
- You can accompany it with basmati rice or naan bread if you wish.

Nutritional Values: Calories: 350-400 kcal, Protein: 20-25 g, Fat: 20-25 g, Carbohydrates: 15-20 g, Fiber: 3-4 g

35.Beef Steak with Red Wine Sauce

Ingredients:

For the Beef Steak: 4 beef steak cuts (such as ribeye or sirloin), 2 tablespoons olive oil, Salt and black pepper to taste

For the Red Wine Sauce: 1 cup red wine, 1/2 cup beef broth, 2 shallots, finely chopped, 2 cloves garlic, minced, 2 tablespoons butter, 1 tablespoon all-purpose flour, Fresh thyme sprigs, Salt and black pepper to taste

Preparation:
- Heat a heatproof skillet over medium-high heat with a little olive oil. Sprinkle pepper and salt on the steak to taste.
- Once the pan is hot, add the steak and cook to your preferred doneness. Cook 3-4 minutes per side for medium doneness.
- Set the steak aside after removing it from the pan. In the same pan, add the chopped onion and cook until translucent and starting to brown.
- Pour the red wine into the pan and scrape the bottom to incorporate all the cooking juices.
- Add the beef broth and cook over medium heat until the sauce reduces and thickens slightly. Add the butter to the sauce, stir until completely melted and the sauce is glossy
- Pour the sauce over the sliced steak and serve hot.

Nutritional Values: Calories: 350-400 kcal, Protein: 25-30 g, Fat: 20-25 g, Carbohydrates: 5-10 g, Fiber: 2-3 g

36.Chilli Chicken with Peppers and Onions

Ingredients:

For the Chili Chicken: 1 pound boneless, skinless chicken breasts, cut into cubes, 2 tablespoons vegetable oil, 2 cloves

garlic, minced, 1 tablespoon chili powder, 1 teaspoon cumin, 1 teaspoon paprika, Salt and black pepper to taste
For the Peppers and Onions: 1 red bell pepper, sliced, 1 green bell pepper, sliced, 1 yellow onion, sliced, 1 tablespoon vegetable oil, Salt and black pepper to taste

Preparation:
- Cut the chicken breast into thin strips. Heat a pan or wok over medium-high heat with a little olive oil.
- Add chopped garlic and thinly sliced fresh red chilli.
- Cook for a minute until fragrant. Cook until chicken is golden brown.
- Arrange the chicken after removing it from the pan. In the same pan, add the onions and mixed peppers cut into strips.
- Cook until tender. Add the chicken back to the pan.
- Add the soy sauce and grated fresh ginger. To distribute the flavors evenly, mix well.
- Another 2-3 minutes of cooking to get everything hot.
- Serve hot chilli chicken as a main course.

Nutritional Values: Calories: 300-350 kcal, Protein: 20-25 g, Fat: 10-15 g, Carbohydrates: 15-20 g, Fiber: 2-3 g

37. Grilled Salmon with Basil Sauce
Ingredients:
For the Grilled Salmon: 4 salmon fillets, 2 tablespoons olive oil, Salt and black pepper to taste, 2 cloves garlic, minced, Zest of 1 lemon
For the Basil Sauce: 1 cup fresh basil leaves, 1/4 cup grated Parmesan cheese, 1/4 cup pine nuts, 2 cloves garlic, 1/2 cup olive oil, Juice of 1 lemon, Salt and black pepper to taste

Preparation:
- Preheat the grill to medium-high heat and brush the grill lightly with olive oil to prevent the fish from sticking.
- Season the salmon fillet with salt and pepper to taste. Grill the salmon skin side down for about 3-4 minutes, until the skin is crispy and comes off the grill easily.
- Using a large spatula, flip the salmon and continue grilling for another 2-3 minutes or until cooked to your liking.
- Meanwhile, prepare the basil sauce. In a blender, combine fresh basil leaves, garlic, lemon juice, olive oil, salt, and pepper.
- Blend until smooth. Once the salmon is cooked, remove from the grill and pour the basil sauce over the top. Serve the grilled salmon with the basil sauce as a condiment.

Nutritional Values: Calories: 350-400 kcal, Protein: 25-30 g, Fat: 20-25 g, Carbohydrates: 5-10 g, Fiber: 2-3 g

38. Chicken Tacos with Avocado and Tomato Sauce
Ingredients:
For the Chicken Tacos: 1 pound boneless, skinless chicken breast, diced, 1 tablespoon olive oil, 1 packet (1.25 ounces) taco seasoning, 8 small tortillas, Shredded lettuce, Diced tomatoes, Sliced red onion, Grated cheese (optional), Sliced jalapeños (optional)
For the Avocado and Tomato Sauce: 1 ripe avocado, mashed, 1 cup diced tomatoes, 1/4 cup diced red onion, 1/4 cup fresh cilantro, chopped, 1 lime, juiced, Salt and black pepper to taste

Preparation:
- Cut the chicken breast into thin strips and season with salt, cayenne pepper, cumin powder and sweet paprika.
- Heat a nonstick pan with a little olive oil over medium-high heat.
- Cook the chicken until golden brown and fully cooked.
- While the chicken is cooking, make the tomato sauce: finely chop the tomatoes, red onion and garlic.
- Add lemon, pepper and salt to your liking. Cut the avocado into thin slices.
- To reheat the tortillas, use the microwave or a pan.
- Assemble the tacos: Place a portion of cooked chicken on each tortilla, top with avocado slices and tomato sauce. Garnish with fresh coriander leaves.
- Roll up tortillas and serve hot chicken tacos. You can accompany with additional lime wedges if desired.

Nutritional Values: Calories: 300-350 kcal, Protein: 20-25 g, Fat: 10-15 g, Carbohydrates: 25-30 g, Fiber: 4-5 g

39. Quinoa Meatballs with Tzatziki Sauce
Ingredients:
For the Quinoa Meatballs: 1 cup cooked quinoa, 1 cup canned chickpeas, drained and rinsed, 1/4 cup breadcrumbs, 1/4 cup grated Parmesan cheese, 1/4 cup fresh parsley, chopped, 1 clove garlic, minced, 1/2 teaspoon ground cumin, Salt and black pepper to taste, Olive oil for cooking
For the Tzatziki Sauce: 1 cup Greek yogurt, 1/2 cucumber, grated and drained, 1 clove garlic, minced, 1 tablespoon fresh dill, chopped, 1 tablespoon lemon juice, Salt and black pepper to taste

Preparation:
- Prepare the tzatziki sauce: grate the cucumber and squeeze it to remove excess water.
- Mix the grated cucumber with the Greek yogurt, minced garlic, lemon juice, chopped fresh mint, chopped fresh parsley, salt and pepper.
- Cool the sauce in the fridge. In a bowl, combine the cooked quinoa with chopped parsley, salt, and pepper. Form small meatballs with the quinoa mixture.
- Over medium-high heat, heat a drizzle of olive oil in a pan.
- Cook the meatballs until golden brown on all sides. Serve the quinoa meatballs hot, accompanied by the tzatziki sauce as a condiment.

Nutritional Values: Calories: 300-350 kcal, Protein: 15-20 g, Fat: 10-15 g, Carbohydrates: 20-25 g, Fiber: 3-4 g

40. Baked trout fillet with lemon and garlic
Ingredients:
For the Baked Trout Fillet: 4 trout fillets, 2 tablespoons olive oil, 2 cloves garlic, minced, Zest of 1 lemon, Salt and black pepper to taste
For the Lemon and Garlic Sauce: Juice of 1 lemon, 2 tablespoons melted butter, 2 cloves garlic, minced, 1 tablespoon fresh parsley, chopped, Salt and black pepper to taste

Preparation:
- Preheat the oven to 180°C. Peel and finely chop the garlic. Cut the lemons into thin slices.
- Prepare aluminum foil and place the trout fillets on top.
- Season the trout fillets with salt, pepper, minced garlic and a drizzle of olive oil. Place lemon slices on top of the fish.
- Close the aluminum foil over the fish, creating a "pochette".
- Bake in the preheated oven for about 15-20 minutes or until the fish is cooked through and flakes easily with a fork.
- Serve the baked trout fillet hot, garnished with chopped fresh parsley and additional lemon wedges if desired.

Nutritional Values: Calories: 250-300 kcal, Protein: 20-25 g, Fat: 15-20 g, Carbohydrates: 5-10 g, Fiber: 1-2 g

41.Cotechino with Lentils and Carrots

Ingredients:

For the Cotechino: 1 Cotechino sausage (about 1 pound), Water (enough to cover the Cotechino)

For the Lentils and Carrots: 1 cup dried green or brown lentils, 2 cups water, 2 carrots, diced, 2 cloves garlic, minced, 1 onion, chopped, 2 tablespoons olive oil, Salt and black pepper to taste, Fresh parsley for garnish (optional)

Preparation:

- In a large pot, heat some olive oil over medium heat.
- Add chopped onion, celery and garlic and sauté until translucent.
- Add the lentils, diced carrots and fresh rosemary.
- Mix well. Add the cotechino to the pan and place it on top of the vegetables.
- The chicken or vegetable broth should now be poured onto the mixture. Make sure the broth completely covers the ingredients.
- Bring everything to the boil, then reduce the heat, cover the pan and leave to simmer for about 1 hour or until the lentils and carrots are soft and the cotechino is fully cooked.
- Serve the sliced cotechino with lentils and carrots as a side dish. Add salt and pepper to taste.

Nutritional Values: Calories: 350-400 kcal, Protein: 15-20 g, Fat: 10-15 g, Carbohydrates: 40-45 g, Fiber: 10-12 g

42.Grilled Salmon with Citrus Sauce

Ingredients:

For the Grilled Salmon: 4 salmon fillets, 2 tablespoons olive oil, Salt and black pepper to taste, Zest of 1 lemon, Zest of 1 orange

For the Citrus Sauce: Juice of 1 lemon, Juice of 1 orange, 2 tablespoons honey, 1 teaspoon Dijon mustard, 1 clove garlic, minced, Salt and black pepper to taste

Preparation:

- Prepare the citrus sauce: grate the zest of oranges, lemons and limes and squeeze their juice. In a bowl, mix the grated zest and citrus juice with minced garlic, olive oil, chopped fresh parsley, salt and pepper.
- This will be the marinade and sauce for the salmon. Place the salmon fillet in a bowl and pour the citrus marinade over the fish.
- Cover and leave to marinate in the refrigerator for at least 30 minutes.
- Preheat grill to medium-high heat and brush lightly with oil to prevent fish from sticking.
- Grill the salmon for about 4-5 minutes per side or until the fish flakes easily with a fork and the outside is slightly crispy.
- Serve the grilled salmon with a generous dollop of citrus sauce on top.

Nutritional Values: Calories: 350-400 kcal, Protein: 25-30 g, Fat: 20-25 g, Carbohydrates: 5-10 g, Fiber: 2-3 g

43.Chicken Curry with Coconut and Spinach

Ingredients:

For the Chicken Curry: 1.5 pounds boneless, skinless chicken thighs, cut into cubes, 2 tablespoons vegetable oil, 1 onion, finely chopped, 3 cloves garlic, minced, 1-inch piece of fresh ginger, minced, 2 tablespoons curry powder, 1 teaspoon ground turmeric, 1 can (14 ounces) coconut milk, 2 cups fresh spinach, Salt and black pepper to taste

Preparation:

- Cut the chicken breast into cubes. Over medium-high heat, heat a drizzle of olive oil in a pan.
- Add and sauté the onion until it becomes translucent. Add the chopped garlic and grated ginger and cook for a minute or until they release their aroma.
- Add and cook until chicken is golden brown. Add curry powder and chili powder (if desired) and mix well to coat the chicken in the spices.
- Pour the coconut milk and the peeled tomatoes (previously crushed with your hands or chopped) into the pan.
- Mix well and let simmer for about 10-15 minutes or until the chicken is cooked.
- Add and cook the spinach until tender.
- Serve the chicken curry with rice or naan bread, if desired. Add salt and pepper to taste.

Nutritional Values: Calories: 350-400 kcal, Protein: 20-25 g, Fat: 15-20 g, Carbohydrates: 20-25 g, Fiber: 5-6 g

44.Grilled Tofu with Peanut Sauce

Ingredients:

For the Grilled Tofu: 1 block of extra-firm tofu, drained and pressed, 2 tablespoons soy sauce, 2 tablespoons olive oil, 1 teaspoon garlic powder, 1 teaspoon ginger powder, Salt and black pepper to taste

For the Peanut Sauce: 1/4 cup peanut butter, 2 tablespoons soy sauce, 2 tablespoons rice vinegar, 1 tablespoon honey, 1 teaspoon sesame oil, 1/2 teaspoon red pepper flakes (adjust to taste), Water (as needed for desired consistency)

Preparation:

- Cut the tofu into thick slices and press gently with a tea towel to remove excess water.
- In a bowl, mix soy sauce, sesame oil, minced garlic and grated ginger to create a marinade.
- Place the tofu in the marinade and let it rest for at least 15-20 minutes.
- While the marinated tofu rests, prepare the peanut sauce. In a bowl, mix peanut sauce, lemon juice, brown sugar, red pepper flakes (if desired), and a little water to achieve desired consistency.
- Preheat a grill or nonstick pan over medium-high heat and brush with a little oil. Grill the tofu for 2 to 3 minutes per side or until nicely grilled.
- Serve the grilled tofu with the peanut sauce and garnish with fresh cilantro. You can serve it with rice or vegetables of your choice.

Nutritional Values: Calories: 250-300 kcal, Protein: 15-20 g, Fat: 12-15 g, Carbohydrates: 15-20 g, Fiber: 3-4 g

45.Tuna Steak with Lime and Coriander Sauce

Ingredients:

For the Tuna Steak: 4 tuna steak fillets, 2 tablespoons olive oil, Salt and black pepper to taste, Zest and juice of 1 lime, 1 tablespoon fresh coriander, chopped

For the Lime and Coriander Sauce: 1/4 cup mayonnaise, Zest and juice of 1 lime, 2 tablespoons fresh coriander, chopped, 1 clove garlic, minced, Salt and black pepper to taste

Preparation:

- Prepare the lime and coriander sauce: grate the lime zest and squeeze the juice.
- Mix with chopped fresh coriander, olive oil, salt and pepper. This will be the sauce for the steak.
- Brush the tuna steak with a little olive oil and sprinkle with salt and pepper.
- Preheat a grill to high heat.

- Grill the tuna steak for about 2-3 minutes per side or until pink on the inside but still slightly pink in the center.
- Serve the tuna steak with the cilantro lime sauce on top.

Nutritional Values: Calories: 350-400 kcal, Protein: 25-30 g, Fat: 10-15 g, Carbohydrates: 15-20 g, Fiber: 2-3 g

46. Duck Breast with Blackcurrant Sauce

Ingredients:

For the Duck Breast: 4 duck breast fillets, Salt and black pepper to taste

For the Blackcurrant Sauce: 1/2 cup blackcurrant preserves or jelly, 1/4 cup red wine, 2 tablespoons balsamic vinegar, 1 shallot, finely chopped, 2 cloves garlic, minced, 1 tablespoon butter, Salt and black pepper to taste

Preparation:

- Make the blackcurrant sauce: In a small saucepan, melt the sugar over medium heat until golden and starting to caramelize.
- Add the balsamic vinegar and blackcurrants and bring to the boil.
- Reduce the heat and simmer the sauce until the blackcurrants break down and the sauce thickens.
- This should take approximately 10-15 minutes. Add salt and pepper to taste.
- Meanwhile, make shallow cuts in the skin of the duck breast and sprinkle it with salt and pepper.
- Melt the butter in a skillet with a nonstick coating over medium-high heat.
- Add the duck breast skin side down and cook for 3-4 minutes until the skin is crispy.
- Turn the duck breast and cook for an additional 2-3 minutes for medium-rare, but you can extend the cooking time if you prefer your duck breast cooked more.
- Cut the duck breast into thin slices and serve with the blackcurrant sauce on top.

Nutritional Values: Calories: 400-450 kcal, Protein: 20-25 g, Fat: 25-30 g, Carbohydrates: 10-15 g, Fiber: 1-2 g

47. Turkey Meatballs with Tomato and Basil Sauce

Ingredients:

For the Turkey Meatballs: 1 pound ground turkey, 1/2 cup breadcrumbs, 1/4 cup grated Parmesan cheese, 1/4 cup fresh parsley, chopped, 1 egg, 1/2 teaspoon garlic powder, Salt and black pepper to taste, Olive oil for cooking

For the Tomato and Basil Sauce: 1 can (14 ounces) crushed tomatoes, 1/4 cup fresh basil, chopped, 2 cloves garlic, minced, Salt and black pepper to taste

Preparation:

- In a bowl, mix the ground turkey, breadcrumbs, beaten egg, chopped onion, chopped garlic, chopped fresh basil, salt and pepper.
- With slightly damp hands, form meatballs of the desired size. In a skillet, heat the olive oil over medium-high heat and brown the meatballs until well browned on all sides.
- Add the peeled tomatoes and tomato puree to the pan.
- Bring to the boil, then reduce the heat and simmer for about 20-25 minutes or until the meatballs are cooked and the sauce has thickened.
- Serve the turkey meatballs with the tomato and basil sauce, garnished with fresh basil.

Nutritional Values: Calories: 300-350 kcal, Protein: 20-25 g, Fat: 10-15 g, Carbohydrates: 15-20 g, Fiber: 3-4 g

48. Beef Steak with Green Pepper Sauce

Ingredients:

For the Beef Steak: 4 beef steak fillets (e.g., sirloin or ribeye), Salt and black pepper to taste, 2 tablespoons olive oil

For the Green Pepper Sauce: 1 green bell pepper, finely chopped, 1/2 cup heavy cream, 1/4 cup beef broth, 2 cloves garlic, minced, 1 tablespoon butter, 1 tablespoon olive oil, Salt and black pepper to taste

Preparation:

- Heat a nonstick pan over medium-high heat. Place the beef steak in the pan and cook for the desired time on both sides to achieve the desired doneness.
- Adjust the cooking time based on the thickness of the steak and your preferences.
- When the steak is cooked to your liking, transfer it to a plate and cover it with aluminum foil to rest while you prepare the sauce.
- In the same pan where you cooked the steak, pour the brandy and let it evaporate over medium heat.
- Then add the pickled green pepper and mix.
- Pour the cream into the pan and continue stirring until the sauce thickens slightly.
- This should take approximately 2-3 minutes. Add the butter, salt and pepper to taste, stirring until the butter has completely melted and the sauce is well combined.
- Pour the green pepper sauce over the sirloin steak and serve.

Nutritional Values: Calories: 350-400 kcal, Protein: 25-30 g, Fat: 20-25 g, Carbohydrates: 5-10 g, Fiber: 2-3 g

49. Mustard Chicken with Asparagus

Ingredients:

For the Mustard Chicken: 4 boneless, skinless chicken breasts, 2 tablespoons Dijon mustard, 2 tablespoons honey, 2 cloves garlic, minced, Salt and black pepper to taste, 1 tablespoon olive oil

For the Asparagus: 1 bunch of asparagus, tough ends trimmed, 1 tablespoon olive oil, Salt and black pepper to taste, Zest of 1 lemon, Juice of 1 lemon

Preparation:

- In a bowl, mix Dijon mustard, crushed mustard seeds, minced garlic, fresh thyme leaves, olive oil, salt and pepper.
- Spread this mixture on the surface of the chicken breasts and leave to marinate for at least 15-20 minutes.
- In a nonstick pan, heat some olive oil over medium-high heat.
- Cook chicken breasts until golden brown and cooked through, about 6-7 minutes per side, depending on thickness.
- While the chicken is cooking, also cook the asparagus in a separate pan with a little olive oil, salt and pepper until tender but crunchy.
- Remove the chicken from the pan and let it rest for a few minutes before cutting it into thin slices.
- Serve the chicken with the asparagus and garnish with a little extra mustard sauce, if desired.

Nutritional Values: Calories: 300-350 kcal, Protein: 20-25 g, Fat: 15-20 g, Carbohydrates: 10-15 g, Fiber: 4-5 g

50. Grilled Pork with Apple Sauce

Ingredients:

For the Grilled Pork: 4 pork chops, 2 tablespoons olive oil, Salt and black pepper to taste, 1 teaspoon dried thyme, 1 teaspoon dried rosemary
For the Apple Sauce: 2 apples, peeled, cored, and chopped, 1/4 cup water, 2 tablespoons brown sugar, 1/2 teaspoon cinnamon, 1/4 teaspoon nutmeg
Preparation:
- In a bowl, mix the pork slices with olive oil, chopped fresh rosemary, salt and pepper.
- Cut the apples into slices and finely slice the onion. Preheat grill to medium-high heat.
- Grill the pork until cooked through and has nice streaks from the grill, about 4-5 minutes per side depending on thickness.
- Meanwhile, in a pan, heat some olive oil and cook the apple slices and onion until soft and slightly caramelised.
- Serve the grilled pork with caramelized apples and onion as a side dish.

Nutritional Values: Calories: 350-400 kcal, Protein: 20-25 g, Fat: 20-25 g, Carbohydrates: 15-20 g, Fiber: 3-4 g

51. Baked Salmon with Dill and Lemon Sauce
Ingredients:
- For the Baked Salmon: 4 salmon fillets, 2 tablespoons olive oil, Salt and black pepper to taste, 1 lemon, thinly sliced, Fresh dill sprigs for garnish
- For the Dill and Lemon Sauce: 1/2 cup mayonnaise, 2 tablespoons fresh dill, chopped, Juice and zest of 1 lemon, 1 clove garlic, minced, Salt and black pepper to taste
- Preparation:
- Preheat the oven to 180°C. In a bowl, mix the lemon juice, minced garlic, chopped fresh dill, olive oil, salt and pepper to create the sauce.
- Place the salmon on a baking tray lined with baking paper.
- Spread the lemon dill sauce evenly over the salmon.
- Cook the salmon for 15-20 minutes in an oven that has been preheated, or until it flakes easily with a fork.
- Serve the salmon hot, garnished with lemon slices and sprigs of fresh dill.

Nutritional Values: Calories: 350-400 kcal, Protein: 25-30 g, Fat: 20-25 g, Carbohydrates: 5-10 g, Fiber: 2-3 g

52.Quinoa Meatballs with Spinach and Feta
Ingredients:
For the Quinoa Meatballs: 1 cup cooked quinoa, 1 cup fresh spinach, finely chopped, 1/2 cup crumbled feta cheese, 1/4 cup breadcrumbs, 1/4 cup grated Parmesan cheese, 1/4 cup red onion, finely chopped, 2 cloves garlic, minced, 1 large egg, 1 teaspoon dried oregano, Salt and black pepper to taste, Olive oil for cooking.
For the Tomato and Basil Sauce: 1 can (14 ounces) crushed tomatoes, 1/4 cup fresh basil, chopped, 2 cloves garlic, minced, Salt and black pepper to taste.
Preparation:
- Cook the quinoa following the instructions on the package and let it cool.
- In a pan, sauté the chopped red onion and the chopped garlic with a little olive oil.
- Add the spinach and cook until wilted. In a bowl, mix the cooked quinoa, cooked spinach, crumbled feta, beaten egg, breadcrumbs, chopped fresh parsley, salt and pepper.

- With slightly damp hands, form meatballs with the quinoa mixture.
- In a nonstick pan, heat some olive oil over medium-high heat.
- Cook the quinoa balls until golden on all sides and cooked through.
- Serve the meatballs hot, perhaps with a lime sauce or yogurt as a condiment.

Nutritional Values: Calories: 300-350 kcal, Protein: 15-20 g, Fat: 10-15 g, Carbohydrates: 20-25 g, Fiber: 3-4 g

53.Duck Breast with Cranberry Sauce
Ingredients:
For the Duck Breast: 4 duck breast fillets, Salt and black pepper to taste
For the Cranberry Sauce: 1 cup fresh or frozen cranberries, 1/2 cup orange juice, 1/4 cup sugar, 1/4 cup water, Zest of 1 orange, 1 cinnamon stick (optional)
Preparation:
- Start by making the cranberry sauce. In a saucepan, cook the cranberries, sugar, balsamic vinegar and onion over medium heat until the cranberries are soft and the sauce thickens slightly.
- In the meantime, lightly score the skin of the duck breast with a sharp knife without cutting the meat.
- Preheat a nonstick skillet over a medium-high flame.
- Place the duck breast in the pan, skin side down, and cook for about 6-8 minutes or until the skin is golden and crispy.
- Turn the duck breast and cook on the other side for another 4-6 minutes for medium rare.
- Adjust the cooking times according to the desired degree of doneness. Cut the duck breast into thin slices and serve with the cranberry sauce on top.

Nutritional Values: Calories: 400-450 kcal, Protein: 20-25 g, Fat: 25-30 g, Carbohydrates: 10-15 g, Fiber: 1-2 g

54.Trout fillet with toasted almonds
Ingredients:
For the Trout Fillet: 4 trout fillets, 2 tablespoons olive oil, Salt and black pepper to taste, Juice of 1 lemon
For the Toasted Almonds: 1/2 cup sliced almonds, 1 tablespoon butter, 1 tablespoon fresh parsley, chopped, Salt and black pepper to taste
Preparation:
- Melt the butter in a nonstick skillet over a medium-high flame. Add the sliced almonds and cook, stirring frequently, until golden and fragrant. Put them on a platter and put away.
- In the same pan, place the trout fillets skin side down.
- Cook the trout fillets for 3-4 minutes on one side and then turn them gently.
- Continue cooking for another 2-3 minutes or until fish flakes easily with a fork.
- Sprinkle the lemon juice over the trout fillets, add the chopped fresh parsley and sprinkle the toasted almonds over the fish.
- Serve the trout fillet hot with a slice of lemon as decoration.

Nutritional Values: Calories: 250-300 kcal, Protein: 20-25 g, Fat: 15-20 g, Carbohydrates: 5-10 g, Fiber: 1-2 g

55.Grilled Tofu with Ginger Sauce
Ingredients:
For the Grilled Tofu: 1 block of firm tofu, sliced into rectangles, 2 tablespoons soy sauce, 1 tablespoon sesame oil, 1 tablespoon

fresh ginger, minced, 2 cloves garlic, minced, Salt and black pepper to taste
For the Ginger Sauce: 2 tablespoons soy sauce, 1 tablespoon rice vinegar, 1 tablespoon fresh ginger, minced, 1 tablespoon honey or maple syrup, 1 clove garlic, minced, Red pepper flakes, to taste (optional)
Preparation:

- Prepare the marinade by mixing grated ginger, minced garlic, soy sauce, honey, sesame oil, rice vinegar, salt and pepper in a bowl.
- Cut the tofu into thick slices and place it in the marinade. Let rest for at least 15-20 minutes to allow the tofu to absorb the flavors.
- Heat a grill or a nonstick skillet on medium to high.
- Grill the marinated tofu for about 2-3 minutes per side or until grilled and lightly browned.
- Serve the grilled tofu hot, sprinkling the chopped scallions, sesame seeds and a generous amount of the marinade sauce over the tofu.

Nutritional Values: Calories: 250-300 kcal, Protein: 15-20 g, Fat: 12-15 g, Carbohydrates: 15-20 g, Fiber: 3-4 g

56.Cotechino with Quinoa Salad
Ingredients:
For the Cotechino: 2 cotechino sausages, Water for cooking
For the Quinoa Salad: 1 cup quinoa, 2 cups water, 1 cup cherry tomatoes (halved), 1 cucumber (diced), 1/4 cup red onion (finely chopped), 1/4 cup fresh parsley (chopped), 2 tbsp olive oil, 2 tbsp lemon juice, to taste salt and black pepper.
Preparation:

- Cook the cotechino according to the package directions. Usually, cotechino requires long cooking in boiling water.
- While the cotechino is cooking, prepare the quinoa salad. Wash the quinoa well under cold running water to remove the starch.
- Cook the quinoa in line with the package guidelines. Usually, it is cooked in lightly salted boiling water for about 15-20 minutes or until tender and the outer shoots separate.
- Rinse the quinoa and set it aside to cool.
- In a large bowl, mix the cooked quinoa, chopped sun-dried tomatoes, chopped red onion and chopped fresh parsley.
- Squeeze the lemon juice over the salad, add a drizzle of olive oil, salt and pepper to taste. Mix well.
- Once cooked, cut the cotechino into thick slices. Serve the hot cotechino slices on a bed of quinoa salad.

Nutritional Values: Calories: 350-400 kcal, Protein: 15-20 g, Fat: 10-15 g, Carbohydrates: 40-45 g, Fiber: 10-12 g

57.Tuna Steak with Chilli Sauce
Ingredients:
For the Tuna Steak: 4 tuna steak fillets, 2 tablespoons olive oil, Salt and black pepper to taste, Lime wedges for serving
For the Chili Sauce: 2 tablespoons soy sauce, 2 tablespoons sweet chili sauce, 1 tablespoon lime juice, 1 clove garlic, minced
Preparation:

- Start by preparing the chili sauce. Cut the fresh red chili pepper into thin slices and mince the garlic.
- In a pan, heat some olive oil over medium heat and add the chilli and garlic. Fry for a couple of minutes or until fragrant but not burning.
- Pour in the lemon juice and stir well. Wait for one minute of simmering before withdrawing from heat.
- Heat a grill or a nonstick skillet on medium to high.

- Brush both sides of the tuna steak with a little olive oil and season with salt and pepper.
- Cook the tuna steak on the grill for about 2-3 minutes per side or until grill marked on the outside but still pink on the inside.
- Serve the tuna steak with the chili sauce on top.

Nutritional Values: Calories: 350-400 kcal, Protein: 25-30 g, Fat: 10-15 g, Carbohydrates: 15-20 g, Fiber: 2-3 g

58.Lemon Chicken with Olives and Parsley
Ingredients:
For the Lemon Chicken: 4 boneless, skinless chicken breasts, 2 tablespoons olive oil, Salt and black pepper to taste, Juice of 2 lemons, 2 cloves garlic, minced
For the Olives and Parsley Topping: 1/2 cup green olives, pitted and chopped, 1/2 cup fresh parsley, chopped, Zest of 1 lemon, 2 tablespoons olive oil, Salt and black pepper to taste
Preparation:

- In a bowl, prepare a marinade by mixing the lemon juice, minced garlic, olive oil, salt and pepper.
- Cut the chicken breast into thin slices and place it in the marinade.
- Set aside for a minimum of 20-30 minutes to marinate.
- In a pan over medium-high heat, heat some olive oil.
- Add the marinated chicken breast and cook for approximately 3-4 minutes per side or until well cooked and golden brown.
- During the last few minutes of cooking, add the black olives to the chicken in the pan to heat them.
- Serve the lemon chicken breast with the olives on top, sprinkling fresh chopped parsley as decoration.

Nutritional Values: Calories: 350-400 kcal, Protein: 20-25 g, Fat: 15-20 g, Carbohydrates: 20-25 g, Fiber: 4-5 g

59.Pork Curry with Mango
Ingredients:
For the Pork Curry: 1 pound pork, cut into bite-sized pieces, 2 tablespoons vegetable oil, 1 onion, finely chopped, 2 cloves garlic, minced, 1-inch piece of fresh ginger, minced, 2 tablespoons curry powder, 1 can (14 ounces) diced tomatoes, 1 cup coconut milk, 1 ripe mango, peeled and diced, Salt and black pepper to taste, Fresh cilantro leaves for garnish.
Preparation:

- Start by preparing the mango salsa. Peel the ripe mango and cut it into pieces. Gently slice the onion, garlic, and ginger.
- Heat some olive oil in a pan over medium heat and add onion, garlic and ginger. Fry until soft and golden.
- Add the mango pieces to the pan and cook for a few minutes until softened.
- Add curry powder and mix well. Cook for a minute to allow the spices to activate.
- Pour the coconut milk into the pan and mix everything well.
- Cook over medium-low heat for about 10-15 minutes or until the sauce thickens and the mango is well cooked.
- Sprinkle using salt and pepper according to preference.
- In the meantime, chop the pork into thin strips.
- In another pan, heat some olive oil and cook the pork until fully cooked and browned.
- Pour the mango salsa over the cooked pork and mix well. Allow for a few minutes of flavoring before serving.

Nutritional Values: Calories: 350-400 kcal, Protein: 20-25 g, Fat: 20-25 g, Carbohydrates: 15-20 g, Fiber: 3-4 g

60. Grilled Salmon with Avocado and Cucumber Sauce

Ingredients:

For the Grilled Salmon: 4 salmon fillets, 2 tablespoons olive oil, Salt and black pepper to taste, Lemon wedges for serving

For the Avocado and Cucumber Sauce: 2 ripe avocados (peeled and pitted), 1 cucumber (peeled and diced), 1/4 cup Greek yogurt, 2 cloves garlic (minced), 2 tablespoons fresh dill (chopped), Juice of 1 lemon, Salt and black pepper to taste

Preparation:
- Start by preparing the avocado salsa. Get rid of the stone from the ripe the avocado and peel it. Cut it into pieces.
- Cut the cucumber into small pieces and finely chop the garlic and red pepper.
- Place the avocado, cucumber, garlic, chili pepper, lime juice, and some fresh cilantro in a blender or immersion blender.
- Blend everything until you obtain a smooth and creamy sauce. Sprinkle with pepper and salt to taste as wanted.
- Preheat grill to medium-high heat. Brush the salmon with a little olive oil and season with salt and pepper.
- Cook the salmon on the grill for about 4-5 minutes per side or until well-cooked but still juicy inside.
- Serve the grilled salmon with the avocado sauce on top, decorating with fresh coriander leaves.

Nutritional Values: Calories: 350-400 kcal, Protein: 25-30 g, Fat: 20-25 g, Carbohydrates: 5-10 g, Fiber: 2-3 g

61. Turkey Meatballs with Tzatziki Sauce

Ingredients:

For the Turkey Meatballs: 1 pound ground turkey, 1/2 cup breadcrumbs, 1/4 cup finely chopped red onion, 2 cloves garlic (minced), 1 egg, Salt and black pepper to taste, Olive oil for cooking.

For the Tzatziki Sauce: 1 cup Greek yogurt, 1 cucumber (peeled and grated), 2 cloves garlic (minced), 2 tablespoons lemon juice, 1 tablespoon chopped fresh mint, Salt and black pepper to taste.

Preparation:
- Start by preparing the tzatziki sauce. Peel and grate the cucumber, then squeeze it to remove excess water.
- In a bowl, mix the grated cucumber, Greek yogurt, chopped garlic, chopped fresh mint, lemon juice, a little olive oil, salt and pepper.
- Mix well and place the sauce in the refrigerator to cool.
- For the turkey meatballs, in a large bowl, combine the ground turkey, chopped onion, minced garlic, chopped fresh parsley, ground cumin, paprika, eggs, and breadcrumbs.
- Sprinkle according to preference with salt and pepper.
- With wet hands, form small meatballs with the mixture.
- Heat some olive oil in a nonstick pan over medium-high heat.
- Cook the turkey meatballs in the pan for about 4-5 minutes per side or until cooked through and golden brown on the outside.
- Serve the meatballs hot with the tzatziki sauce as a side dish or condiment.

Nutritional Values: Calories: 300-350 kcal, Protein: 20-25 g, Fat: 10-15 g, Carbohydrates: 15-20 g, Fiber: 3-4 g

62. Duck breast with red grape sauce

Ingredients:

For the Duck Breast: 4 duck breast fillets, Salt and black pepper to taste

For the Red Grape Sauce: 2 cups red grapes, 1/4 cup red wine, 1/4 cup chicken or beef broth, 2 tablespoons butter, 1 shallot (finely chopped), 2 cloves garlic (minced), Salt and black pepper to taste

Preparation:
- Start by preparing the red grape sauce. In a saucepan, melt some sugar over medium heat until golden.
- Add the halved red grapes to the saucepan and stir well to caramelize the grapes.
- Pour in the red wine and cook until the wine is reduced by half.
- Add the chicken broth and rosemary and cook over medium-low heat for about 15-20 minutes or until the sauce thickens.
- Be sure to lightly crush the grapes as they cook to extract their flavor.
- Meanwhile, score the skin of the duck breast with a sharp blade to form a diamond pattern, being careful not to cut the meat.
- Sprinkle both sides of the duck breast with pepper and salt.
- Heat a non-stick pan over medium-high heat and add the duck breast, skin side down.
- Cook for 4-5 minutes, so that the skin becomes crispy and brown.
- Turn the duck breast and cook for a further 2-3 minutes for medium-rare, or longer if you prefer your meat rarer.
- Allow it to rest for a few minutes until slicing it thinly.
- Serve the duck breast with the red grape sauce on top.

Nutritional Values: Calories: 400-450 kcal, Protein: 20-25 g, Fat: 25-30 g, Carbohydrates: 10-15 g, Fiber: 1-2 g

63. Beef Steak with Mushroom Sauce

Ingredients:

For the Beef Steak: 4 beef steak fillets (such as sirloin or ribeye), 2 tablespoons olive oil, Salt and black pepper to taste, Fresh thyme or rosemary sprigs for garnish

For the Mushroom Sauce: 2 cups sliced mushrooms (such as cremini or button mushrooms), 2 tablespoons butter, 1/4 cup diced onion, 2 cloves garlic (minced), 1 cup beef broth, 1/2 cup heavy cream, according to preference, salt and black pepper

Preparation:
- Start by preparing the mushroom sauce. Finely chop the shallot and garlic. Heat a pan with a little olive oil over medium heat and add the shallots and garlic. Fry until soft and translucent.
- Add the sliced mixed mushrooms to the pan and cook until they start to brown.
- Pour in the red wine and cook until the wine is reduced by half.
- Add the meat broth, rosemary and thyme. Let cook over medium low heat for about 15-20 minutes or until the sauce thickens. Sprinkle according to preference with salt and pepper.
- Meanwhile, preheat a grill or nonstick skillet over high heat. Sprinkle the sirloin steak liberally with salt and pepper.

- Cook the steak on the grill or in the pan for the desired time depending on your preferred doneness (for example, 3-4 minutes per side for medium-rare).
- Allow it to cool down for a few minutes before slicing it thinly. Serve the steak with the mushroom sauce on top.

Nutritional Values: Calories: 350-400 kcal, Protein: 25-30 g, Fat: 20-25 g, Carbohydrates: 5-10 g, Fiber: 2-3 g

64.Fish Tacos with Coleslaw

Ingredients:

For the Fish Tacos: 1 pound white fish fillets (such as cod or tilapia), 1 cup cornmeal, 1 cup breadcrumbs, 2 eggs, Vegetable oil for frying, Salt and black pepper (to taste), 8 small corn or flour tortillas, Shredded lettuce or cabbage for garnish, Lemon or lime wedges for serving

For the Coleslaw: 4 cups finely chopped green cabbage, 1 cup grated carrots, 1/2 cup mayonnaise, 2 tablespoons apple cider vinegar, 1 tablespoon sugar, Salt and black pepper (to taste)

Preparation:

- Start by preparing the coleslaw. Cut the cabbage into thin strips and the carrots into julienne strips.
- Finely chop the fresh coriander and jalapeño pepper, being careful to remove the seeds if you want a less spicy dish.
- Mix the cabbage, carrots, coriander and chili pepper in a bowl. Season with lime juice, some minced garlic, salt and black pepper to taste. Mix well and set aside.
- Prepare the fish seasoning by mixing the paprika, cumin powder, black pepper, minced garlic and olive oil in a bowl.
- Brush the fish fillets with the prepared seasoning on both sides.
- Heat a non-stick pan over medium-high heat and cook the fish fillets for about 2-3 minutes per side or until cooked through and flakes easily with a fork.
- Heat the tortillas in a hot pan or in the oven.
- Fill each tortilla with cooked fish fillets and dressed coleslaw. To create tacos, split the tortillas in half.
- Serve fish tacos hot with extra lime wedges and garnishes such as avocado, jalapeño or salsa of your choice.

Nutritional Values: Calories: 300-350 kcal, Protein: 15-20 g, Fat: 10-15 g, Carbohydrates: 30-35 g, Fiber: 4-5 g

65. Mustard Chicken with Sweet Potatoes

Ingredients:

For the Mustard Chicken: 4 boneless, skinless chicken breasts, 2 tablespoons Dijon mustard, 2 tablespoons honey, 2 cloves garlic (minced), 2 tablespoons olive oil, Salt and black pepper to taste.

For the Sweet Potatoes: 4 sweet potatoes (peeled and cubed), 2 tablespoons olive oil, 1 teaspoon dried rosemary, Salt and black pepper to taste

Preparation:

- Start by preparing a marinade for the chicken. In a bowl, mix the Dijon mustard, minced garlic, chopped fresh rosemary, olive oil, salt and pepper.
- Cut the chicken into desired size pieces and place in the marinade.
- Make certain the chicken is thoroughly coated in the marinade.
- Cover the bowl with cling film and leave to marinate in the fridge for at least 30 minutes, or even overnight for a more intense flavour.

- Warm up the oven's temperature to 200 degrees Celsius and line a baking sheet with baking parchment. Cut sweet potatoes to cubes after peeling them.
- Place the sweet potatoes in the baking dish and season with a little olive oil, salt and pepper. Mix well.
- Place the marinated chicken on top of the sweet potatoes in the baking dish.
- Place in the oven and cook for about 25-30 minutes or until the chicken is cooked through and the sweet potatoes are soft and lightly browned.
- Serve the mustard chicken with sweet potatoes on the side.

Nutritional Values: Calories: 350-400 kcal, Protein: 20-25 g, Fat: 15-20 g, Carbohydrates: 30-35 g, Fiber: 5-6 g

66.Tuna Steak with Mango Sauce

Ingredients:

For the Tuna Steak: 4 tuna steak fillets, 2 tablespoons olive oil, Salt and black pepper to taste, Lime wedges for serving

For the Mango Sauce: 2 ripe mangoes (peeled and diced), 1/4 cup red onion (finely chopped), 2 tablespoons fresh cilantro (chopped), 2 tablespoons lime juice, 1 teaspoon honey (optional, adjust to taste), Season with salt and black pepper according to preference.

Preparation:

- Start by preparing the mango salsa. Peel and cut the mango into cubes and place it in a bowl.
- Finely chop the red onion and jalapeño pepper, being careful to remove the seeds if you want a less spicy dish.
- Also, chop the fresh coriander and add it to the mango.
- Squeeze the lemon juice over the bowl's contents.
- Add a little olive oil, salt and pepper. Mix the mango sauce well and set aside.
- Preheat a grill or a nonstick skillet to medium-high. Season the tuna steak with salt and pepper.
- Cook the tuna steak on the grill or in the pan for about 2-3 minutes per side or until cooked through on the outside but still pink on the inside.
- Make thin slices of tuna steak. Serve the tuna steak with the mango sauce on top.

Nutritional Values: Calories: 350-400 kcal, Protein: 25-30 g, Fat: 10-15 g, Carbohydrates: 15-20 g, Fiber: 2-3 g

67.Grilled Pork with Pineapple Sauce

Ingredients:

For the Grilled Pork: 4 pork chops or pork tenderloin pieces, 2 tablespoons olive oil, Salt and black pepper to taste

For the Pineapple Sauce: 2 cups fresh pineapple (diced), 1/4 cup soy sauce, 1/4 cup brown sugar, 2 cloves garlic (minced), 1 teaspoon grated fresh ginger, 1/2 teaspoon red pepper flakes (adjust to taste)

Preparation:

- Start by preparing the marinade for the pork. In a bowl, combine the lime juice, brown sugar, soy sauce, minced garlic, chopped jalapeño pepper (seeded if you want less heat), olive oil, salt and pepper.
- Cut the pork into pieces or slices and immerse it in the marinade.
- Cover the bowl with cling film and leave to marinate in the refrigerator for at least 30 minutes, or even several hours for a better infusion of flavors.
- In the meantime, prepare the pineapple skewers by cutting the fresh pineapple into cubes.

- Thread the marinated pork pieces and the pineapple cubes alternately onto the skewers.
- Preheat an outdoor grill or indoor grill over medium-high heat.
- Cook the pork and pineapple skewers on the grill for about 2-3 minutes per side or until the pork is cooked through and the pineapple is lightly caramelized.
- Serve the grilled pork with the pineapple skewers and garnish to taste.

Nutritional Values: Calories: 350-400 kcal, Protein: 20-25 g, Fat: 20-25 g, Carbohydrates: 15-20 g, Fiber: 3-4 g

68.Quinoa Meatballs with Tomato Sauce

Ingredients:

For the Quinoa Meatballs: 1 cup cooked quinoa, 1 cup breadcrumbs, 1/2 cup grated Parmesan cheese, 1/4 cup finely chopped onion, 2 cloves garlic (minced), 2 eggs, 2 tablespoons fresh parsley (chopped), Salt and black pepper to taste, Olive oil for cooking.

For the Tomato Sauce: 1 can (14 ounces) crushed tomatoes, 2 cloves garlic (minced), 1 teaspoon dried basil, Salt and black pepper to taste

Preparation:

- In a saucepan, cook the quinoa following the instructions on the package. Once cooked, let it cool.
- In a bowl, mix the cooked quinoa, eggs, breadcrumbs, grated cheese, finely chopped red onion, minced garlic, chopped fresh parsley, salt and pepper.
- Mix well until you obtain a homogeneous mixture.
- With wet hands, form the quinoa mixture into meatballs.
- Heat some olive oil in a non-stick pan and cook the meatballs until they are golden brown on all sides.
- In the meantime, prepare the tomato sauce. In another pan, heat some olive oil and add the peeled tomatoes, fresh basil, sugar, salt and pepper.
- Cook over medium heat for about 15-20 minutes or until the sauce has thickened.
- Serve the quinoa meatballs hot with the tomato sauce on top.

Nutritional Values: Calories: 300-350 kcal, Protein: 15-20 g, Fat: 10-15 g, Carbohydrates: 20-25 g, Fiber: 3-4 g

69.Grilled Tofu with Garlic Sauce

Ingredients: 1 block of tofu, 2 cloves of garlic, minced, 2 tablespoons soy sauce, 1 tablespoon olive oil, 1 teaspoon sesame oil,1 teaspoon rice vinegar, 1 teaspoon honey or maple syrup (for a vegan version), Salt and pepper to taste Garnish with freshly chopped cilantro or green onions (optional).

Preparation:

- Cut the tofu into thick slices.
- In a bowl, mix the minced garlic, olive oil, lemon juice, salt, pepper and chopped fresh parsley to make the marinade.
- Dip the tofu slices in the marinade and let them marinate for at least 30 minutes.
- Warm up a grill or a nonstick skillet to medium to high. Cook the tofu on the grill or in the pan for about 3-4 minutes per side or until golden brown.
- Serve the grilled tofu hot with a generous amount of garlic sauce on top.

Nutritional Values: Calories: 250-300 kcal, Protein: 15-20 g, Fat: 12-15 g, Carbohydrates: 15-20 g, Fiber: 3-4 g

70.Trout fillet with lemon and caper sauce

Ingredients: 1 trout fillet, Juice of 1/2 lemon,1 teaspoon capers,1 teaspoon butter or olive oil, Salt and pepper to taste Fresh parsley for garnish (optional)

Preparation:

- Start by preparing the lemon and caper sauce. Warm the butter in a skillet over a moderate flame.
- Add the capers, freshly squeezed lemon juice, chopped fresh parsley, salt and pepper.
- Cook the sauce for a few minutes until the capers are soft and the sauce has thickened slightly. Keep warm.
- Heat a non-stick pan over medium-high heat and add a little butter.
- Cook the trout fillets in the pan for about 2-3 minutes per side or until cooked through and lightly browned.
- Serve the trout fillets hot with the lemon and caper sauce on top.

Nutritional Values: Calories: 250-300 kcal, Protein: 20-25 g, Fat: 15-20 g, Carbohydrates: 5-10 g, Fiber: 1-2 g

71. Baked Salmon with Rosemary Sauce

Ingredients: For the Baked Salmon: 4 salmon fillets,2 tablespoons olive oil, 2 cloves garlic, minced, 2 teaspoons fresh rosemary, chopped, Salt and black pepper to taste.

For the Rosemary Sauce:1/2 cup sour cream
1 tablespoon fresh rosemary, finely chopped,1 tablespoon lemon juice,1 teaspoon Dijon mustard, Salt and black pepper to taste.

Preparation:

- Take some salmon fillets and place them on a baking tray lined with baking paper.
- In a bowl, mix olive oil, finely chopped garlic, fresh rosemary leaves, lemon juice, salt and pepper to create the marinade.
- Spread the marinade generously over the salmon fillets.
- Preheat the oven to 180°C and cook the salmon for about 15-20 minutes or until evenly cooked and the top is lightly browned.
- Serve the baked salmon hot with a squeeze of fresh lemon juice on top.

Nutritional Values: Calories, 350-400 kcal. Protein, 25-30 g. Fat, 20-25 g. Carbohydrates, 5-10 g. Fiber, 2-3 g.

72.Chicken Curry with Mixed Vegetables

Ingredients:

For the Chicken Curry: 1.5 pounds boneless, skinless chicken breasts or thighs (cut into bite-sized pieces), 2 tablespoons vegetable oil, 1 onion (finely chopped), 3 cloves garlic (minced), 1-inch piece of fresh ginger (minced), 2 tablespoons curry powder, 1 can (14 ounces) diced tomatoes, 1 can (14 ounces) coconut milk, 2 cups mixed vegetables (e.g., bell peppers, peas, carrots), Salt and black pepper to taste, Fresh cilantro leaves for garnish

Preparation:

- Cut the chicken breast into cubes and season with curry powder, salt and pepper.
- Heat some olive oil in a pan over medium-high heat and cook the chicken until browned on all sides.
- Set it away after removing it from the pan.
- In the same pan, add a little oil if necessary and fry the chopped onion, garlic and ginger until fragrant.
- Add the peppers, carrots and courgettes cut into cubes and cook for a few minutes until they become tender but crunchy.
- Put in the coconut milk and stir properly.

- Add the previously cooked chicken to the pan with the vegetables and coconut milk.
- Cook everything over medium-low heat for about 10-15 minutes or until the chicken is fully cooked and the vegetables are tender.
- Serve the chicken curry hot with basmati rice or naan.

Nutritional Values: Calories, 350-400 kcal. Protein, 25-30 g. Fat, 15-20 g. Carbohydrates, 20-25 g. Fiber, 5-6 g.

73.Duck Breast in Port

Ingredients:

For the Duck Breast: 4 duck breast fillets, Salt and black pepper to taste

For the Port Sauce: 1 cup port wine, 1/4 cup chicken or beef broth, 2 tablespoons butter, 1 shallot (finely chopped), 2 cloves garlic (minced), Salt and black pepper to taste.

Preparation:

- Start by lightly scoring the skin of the duck breast with a sharp knife. This will aid in the release of fat while cooking.
- Heat a nonstick pan over medium-high heat and place the duck breast skin-side down in the pan.
- Cook the duck breast for a few minutes until the skin is crispy and golden. Turn it over and cook the other side for a few minutes.
- Remove the duck breast from the pan and set aside.
- In the same pan, pour the port wine and let it reduce by half.
- Add the chicken broth, sugar, salt and pepper. Let the sauce cook for a few minutes until it has thickened slightly.
- Add the duck breast to the pan with the sauce and cook over medium heat for about 5-7 minutes or until the duck breast is cooked to perfection.
- Serve the port duck breast with the sauce on top as a condiment.

Nutritional Values: Calories, 350-400 kcal. Protein, 20-25 g. Fat, 25-30 g. Carbohydrates, 5-10 g. Fiber, 1-2 g.

74.Beef Steak with White Wine Sauce

Ingredients:

For the Beef Steak: 4 beef steaks (such as sirloin or ribeye), 2 tablespoons olive oil, Salt and black pepper to taste, Fresh thyme or rosemary sprigs for garnish

For the White Wine Sauce: 1 cup white wine (such as Chardonnay or Sauvignon Blanc), 1/2 cup heavy cream, 2 tablespoons butter, 1 shallot (finely chopped), 2 cloves garlic (minced), Salt and black pepper to taste

Preparation:

- Start by heating a nonstick pan over medium-high heat and add a small amount of butter.
- Season the sirloin steak with salt and pepper and place in the hot skillet.
- Cook the steak for the desired time, turning it halfway through cooking to obtain even cooking.
- Take away the steak from the pan and set aside for a few minutes to rest. In the same pan, add the chopped onion and garlic and fry until golden and fragrant.
- Pour the white wine into the deglaze pan, scraping the bottom to release all the juices and meat residue.
- Add the beef broth and rosemary and cook over medium-low heat until the sauce has reduced and thickened.
- Serve the sirloin steak hot with the white wine sauce on top.

Nutritional Values: Calories, 350-400 kcal. Protein, 25-30 g. Fat, 15-20 g. Carbohydrates, 5-10 g. Fiber, 2-3 g.

75.Turkey Meatballs with Mustard and Honey Sauce

Ingredients:

For the Turkey Meatballs: 1 pound ground turkey, 1/2 cup breadcrumbs, 1/4 cup finely chopped onion, 1 egg, Salt and black pepper to taste, Olive oil for cooking

For the Mustard and Honey Sauce: 2 tablespoons Dijon mustard, 2 tablespoons honey, 1/4 cup chicken broth, 2 tablespoons fresh parsley (chopped), Salt and black pepper to taste

Preparation:

- In a large bowl, mix the ground turkey, breadcrumbs, finely chopped onion, egg, mustard, honey, salt and pepper. Mix thoroughly until the mixture is homogeneous.
- Take small portions of the dough and form round meatballs.
- Heat some olive oil in a nonstick pan over medium-high heat.
- Cook the turkey meatballs in the pan until golden brown and evenly cooked, turning occasionally.
- While the meatballs are cooking, mix the mustard and honey in a small bowl to make the sauce.
- Once cooked, serve the meatballs hot with the mustard and honey sauce as a condiment.

Nutritional Values: Calories, 300-350 kcal. Protein, 15-20 g. Fat, 10-15 g. Carbohydrates, 15-20 g. Fiber, 3-4 g.

76.Fish Tacos with Avocado and Tomato Sauce

Ingredients:

For the Fish Tacos: 1 pound white fish fillets (such as cod or tilapia), 1 cup all-purpose flour, 1 teaspoon chili powder, 1 teaspoon cumin, Salt and black pepper to taste, 8 small corn or flour tortillas, Shredded cabbage or lettuce, Sliced tomatoes, Sliced avocados, Fresh cilantro for garnish, Lime wedges for serving.

For the Avocado and Tomato Sauce: 2 ripe avocados (peeled and pitted), 2 tomatoes (diced), 1/4 cup sour cream or Greek yogurt, Juice of 2 limes, 1/4 cup fresh cilantro (chopped), Salt and black pepper to taste

Preparation:

- Start by preparing the avocado and tomato sauce. In a bowl, mash ripe avocados and mix with diced tomato, chopped red onion, lime juice, fresh cilantro, salt and pepper. Mix well and set aside.
- Cook the fish fillets on a grill or in a non-stick pan with a drizzle of oil until they are cooked and golden on both sides.
- Heat the tortillas in a small pan or in the microwave until warm and soft.
- Fill each tortilla with a grilled fish fillet and a generous portion of avocado-tomato salsa.
- Roll the tortillas around the filling to form your tacos.
- Serve the fish tacos hot, perhaps with an extra sprinkle of fresh cilantro and lime slices for garnish.

Nutritional Values: Calories, 300-350 kcal. Protein, 15-20 g. Fat, 10-15 g. Carbohydrates, 30-35 g. Fiber, 4-5 g.

77.Grilled Chicken with Ginger and Lime Sauce

Ingredients:

For the Grilled Chicken: 4 boneless, skinless chicken breasts, 2 tablespoons olive oil, 1 teaspoon ground ginger, 1 teaspoon garlic powder, Salt and black pepper to taste

For the Ginger and Lime Sauce: Juice of 2 limes, 1 tablespoon fresh ginger (minced), 2 cloves garlic (minced), 2 tablespoons soy sauce, 1 tablespoon honey, Salt and black pepper to taste

Preparation:

- Start by preparing the marinade. In a bowl, grate the fresh
- ginger and add the finely chopped garlic, lime juice and zest, soy sauce, honey, olive oil, salt and pepper. Mix all the ingredients well.
- Place the chicken breasts in an airtight bag or bowl, then pour the marinade over them.
- Seal the bag or cover the bowl and place the chicken in the refrigerator for at least 30 minutes (better if you leave to marinate for several hours or overnight for a more intense flavor).
- Preheat the grill to medium-high heat and brush the grates with a little oil to prevent the chicken from sticking.
- Remove the chicken from the marinade and grill for 6-8 minutes per side or until well cooked and has nice streaks from the grill.
- While the chicken is grilling, bring the remaining marinade to the boil in a small saucepan and boil for a few minutes until reduced and thickened slightly.
- Serve the grilled chicken hot with the ginger-lime sauce on top.

Nutritional Values: Calories, 350-400 kcal. Protein, 20-25 g. Fat, 15-20 g. Carbohydrates, 15-20 g. Fiber, 3-4 g.

78. Turmeric Tofu with Spinach and Carrots

Ingredients: For the Turmeric Tofu: 1 block of firm tofu, cubed, 2 tablespoons olive oil, 1 teaspoon ground turmeric, 1 teaspoon ground cumin, Salt and black pepper to taste

For the Spinach and Carrots: 2 cups fresh spinach leaves, 2 carrots (thinly sliced), 1 onion (finely chopped), 2 cloves garlic (minced), 2 tablespoons olive oil, 1 teaspoon ground turmeric, 1/2 teaspoon ground cumin seeds, Salt and black pepper according to preference.

Preparation:

- Start by preparing the tofu. Cut the tofu into cubes or thick slices, then place it in a bowl.
- Mix the turmeric powder with sesame oil, soy sauce, minced garlic, grated ginger, salt and pepper. This will be the marinade.
- Pour the marinade over the tofu and let it marinate for at least 30 minutes, so that it absorbs the flavors.
- In the meantime, cut the carrots into thin slices and prepare the spinach by washing them carefully.
- Heat a large skillet or wok over medium-high heat and add the marinated tofu. Cook until golden on all sides, turning gently.
- Add the carrots to the pan and cook for a few minutes until tender.
- Finally, add the spinach and cook until wilted and reduced in volume.
- Before serving, sprinkle the tofu, vegetables and dish with toasted sesame seeds for a touch of crunch and flavor.

Nutritional Values: Calories, 300-350 kcal. Protein, 15-20 g. Fat, 10-15 g. Carbohydrates, 20-25 g. Fiber, 4-5 g.

79. Grilled Tuna Steak with Basil Sauce

Ingredients:

For the Grilled Tuna Steak: 4 tuna steak fillets, 2 tablespoons olive oil, Salt and black pepper to taste, 1 lemon (cut into wedges), Fresh basil leaves for garnish

For the Basil Sauce: 1 cup fresh basil leaves, 1/2 cup olive oil, 1/4 cup grated Parmesan cheese, 2 cloves garlic (minced), Juice of 1 lemon, Salt and black pepper to taste

Preparation:

- Start by preparing the basil sauce. In a blender, place fresh basil leaves, squeezed lemon juice, garlic, olive oil, salt and pepper.
- Blend all that until it's smooth and creamy. Preheat the grill to medium-high heat and brush the grates with a little oil to prevent the tuna from sticking.
- Sprinkle both sides of the steak of tuna with pepper and salt.
- Place the steak on the hot grill and cook for 2-3 minutes per side to obtain rare doneness or longer if you prefer your tuna cooked more.
- When the tuna is ready, transfer it to a serving plate and pour the basil sauce over it.
- Serve the grilled tuna immediately with the delicious basil sauce.

Nutritional Values: Calories, 350-400 kcal. Protein, 25-30 g. Fat, 15-20 g. Carbohydrates, 5-10 g. Fiber, 2-3 g.

80. Mustard Pork with Mashed Potatoes

Ingredients: For the Mustard Pork: 4 boneless pork chops, 2 tablespoons Dijon mustard, 2 tablespoons olive oil, 2 cloves garlic (minced), 1 teaspoon dried thyme, Salt and black pepper to taste

For the Mashed Potatoes: 4 large potatoes (peeled and cubed), 4 tablespoons butter, 1/4 cup milk, Salt and black pepper to taste, Chopped chives for garnish (optional)

Preparation:

- Start by preparing the mashed potatoes. Peel the potatoes, cut them into cubes and boil them in lightly salted water until soft.
- Place the potatoes in a bowl after draining them. Add the hot milk, butter, salt and pepper, then mash the potatoes with a potato masher or fork until you get a creamy puree.
- Cover the bowl with a lid to keep the puree warm.
- Take the pork fillet and spread plenty of mustard on both sides.
- Heat an ovenproof pan with a little olive oil and brown the pork on both sides until golden brown.
- Add rosemary sprigs to the pan and transfer to a preheated oven at 180°C.
- Cook the pork in the oven for about 15-20 minutes or until it has reached the desired doneness.
- Once cooked, remove the pork from the pan and let it rest for a few minutes before slicing.
- Serve the mustard pork on a bed of hot mashed potatoes. You can decorate with a few fresh rosemary leaves, if you wish.

Nutritional Values: Calories, 350-400 kcal. Protein, 20-25 g. Fat, 15-20 g. Carbohydrates, 30-35 g. Fiber, 3-4 g.

81. Baked Salmon with Pink Pepper Sauce

Ingredients:

For the Baked Salmon: 4 salmon fillets, 2 tablespoons olive oil, Salt and black pepper to taste, 1 lemon (thinly sliced), Fresh dill for garnish

For the Pink Pepper Sauce: 1/4 cup pink peppercorns, 1/4 cup heavy cream, 2 tablespoons butter, 2 tablespoons lemon juice, 1 shallot (finely chopped), Salt to taste

Preparation:

- Start by preparing the pink pepper sauce. In a pan, melt butter and add garlic that has been minced. Sauté the garlic until fragrant.
- Add the cream and pink peppercorns to the pan. Cook over medium-low heat until the sauce thickens slightly, stirring occasionally.
- Season with salt and pepper to taste.
- Take the salmon fillet, squeeze the lemon juice over it and season it with salt and pepper on both sides.
- Heat a non-stick pan, add a little olive oil and place the salmon in the pan skin side down.
- Cook for just a few minutes, or until the skin crisps up. Transfer the salmon to a baking tray and cook it in a preheated oven at 180°C for approximately 10-12 minutes or until the salmon is cooked to perfection.
- Serve the salmon hot with the pink pepper sauce on top, decorated with fresh parsley and lemon slices.

Nutritional Values: Calories, 350-400 kcal. Protein, 25-30 g. Fat, 20-25 g. Carbohydrates, 5-10 g. Fiber, 2-3 g.

82.Quinoa Meatballs with Chili Sauce

Ingredients:

For the Quinoa Meatballs: 1 cup quinoa, 2 cups water, 1 cup dry red lentils, 1 onion (finely chopped), 2 garlic cloves (finely chopped), 1 teaspoon extra virgin olive oil, 1 teaspoon ground cumin, 1 teaspoon sweet paprika, Salt and black pepper to taste, 2 tablespoons fresh parsley (chopped), 1 egg (optional, as a binder)

For the Chili Sauce: 1 can (14 ounces) diced tomatoes, 1/4 cup tomato paste, 1/4 cup honey or maple syrup (adjust to taste), 2 tablespoons soy sauce, 1 teaspoon chili powder (adjust to taste), 1/2 teaspoon garlic powder, Salt to taste

Preparation:

- Start by cooking the quinoa according to the instructions on the package. Once cooked, let it cool.
- In a bowl, mix the cooked quinoa with beaten eggs, grated cheese, breadcrumbs, finely chopped fresh chili pepper, minced garlic, chopped fresh parsley, salt and pepper.
- The consistency of the mixture should allow it to form compact meatballs.
- Form the dough into meatballs and place them on a lightly floured tray.
- Heat a non-stick pan with a little olive oil over medium-high heat.
- Cook the meatballs until they are golden and crispy on all sides, turning them carefully.
- Drain the meatballs on absorbent paper to remove excess oil.
- Serve the quinoa meatballs hot with a spicy fresh chili sauce or your favorite sauce. They are also excellent on their own as a snack or appetizer.

Nutritional Values: Calories, 300-350 kcal. Protein, 15-20 g. Fat, 10-15 g. Carbohydrates, 30-35 g. Fiber, 4-5 g.

83.Duck Breast with Honey and Lemon Sauce

Ingredients: For the Duck Breast: 4 duck breast fillets, Salt and black pepper to taste

For the Honey and Lemon Sauce: Juice of 2 lemons, Zest of 1 lemon, 1/4 cup honey, 2 tablespoons butter, 2 cloves garlic (minced), Salt and black pepper to taste

Preparation:

- Start by preparing the honey and lemon sauce. In a small
- bowl, mix honey, freshly squeezed lemon juice and a little grated ginger. Add salt and pepper to taste. This sauce will be used to season the duck breast after cooking.
- Before cooking the duck breast, be sure to lightly score the fat (without cutting the meat) to allow the excess fat to melt during cooking.
- Heat a nonstick pan over medium-high heat. There is no need to add oil, as the duck breast will release enough fat during cooking.
- Place the duck breast in the pan, fat side down, and cook for about 6-8 minutes or until the skin is crisp and golden.
- Turn the duck breast and cook for a further 2-3 minutes on the opposite side, or until it reaches the desired doneness (usually medium-rare or rare).
- Place the duck breast on a cutting board and set aside for some minutes to rest. After resting, cut the duck breast into thin slices and season them with the honey and lemon sauce prepared previously.
- Serve the duck breast with rice, potatoes or vegetables of your choice and garnish with grated lemon zest and fresh parsley, if desired.

Nutritional Values: Calories, 350-400 kcal. Protein, 20-25 g. Fat, 25-30 g. Carbohydrates, 5-10 g. Fiber, 1-2 g.

84.Beef Steak with Porcini Sauce

Ingredients:

For the Beef Steak: 4 beef steaks (such as sirloin or ribeye), 2 tablespoons olive oil, Salt and black pepper to taste, Fresh thyme or rosemary sprigs for garnish

For the Porcini Sauce: 1/2 cup dried porcini mushrooms (rehydrated and chopped), 1 cup beef broth, 2 tablespoons butter, 1 shallot (finely chopped), 2 cloves garlic (minced), 1/2 cup dry red wine, according to preference, salt and black pepper

Preparation:

- Start by preparing the porcini sauce. If you use dried porcini mushrooms, soak them in hot water for about 20-30 minutes, then squeeze them well and chop them finely. If you use fresh porcini mushrooms, clean them and cut them into thin slices.
- Heat a pan with a little butter and olive oil over medium-high heat. Cook up until the onion is transparent, about 5 minutes.
- Add the porcini mushrooms (both dried and fresh, if you have them) to the pan and cook until golden.
- Pour the red wine into the pan and let the alcohol evaporate.
- Add the beef broth and cook over medium-low heat until the sauce reduces and thickens slightly.
- Add the cream, mix well and cook for a few minutes. Season according to preference with pepper and salt.
- Meanwhile, prepare the beef steak. Over a medium-high flame, heat a grill or a nonstick skillet.
- Lightly brush the steak with olive oil, then cook for the desired time on both sides, adding salt and pepper to taste.
- Once the steak is cooked, let it rest for a few minutes, then cut it into thin slices.
- Serve the steak slices with the porcini sauce on top and garnish with chopped fresh parsley if desired.

Nutritional Values: Calories, 350-400 kcal. Protein, 25-30 g. Fat, 15-20 g. Carbohydrates, 5-10 g. Fiber, 2-3 g.

85.Chicken Curry with Coconut and Peppers

Ingredients:

For the Chicken Curry: 1.5 pounds boneless, skinless chicken breasts or thighs (cut into bite-sized pieces), 2 tablespoons vegetable oil, 1 onion (finely chopped), 3 cloves garlic (minced), 1-inch piece of fresh ginger (minced), 2 tablespoons curry powder, 1 can (14 ounces) diced tomatoes, 1 can (14 ounces) coconut milk, 2 bell peppers (red, green, or yellow, sliced), Salt and black pepper to taste, Fresh cilantro leaves for garnish

Preparation:

- Start by cutting the chicken breast into cubes and set aside.
- Heat a small amount of olive oil in a pan over medium-high heat. Add the chopped onion and minced garlic and cook until golden and fragrant.
- Cook the chicken in the pan until golden brown on every side.
- Add the peppers cut into strips and cook for a few minutes until tender.
- Add curry powder and mix well.
- Pour in the coconut milk and mix to combine.
- Cook over medium-low heat for about 10-15 minutes or until the chicken is fully cooked and the sauce has thickened slightly.
- Season according to preference with pepper and salt.
- Serve the chicken curry with basmati rice or any other side dish you like. If wanted, garnish with new coriander leaves.

Nutritional Values: Calories, 350-400 kcal. Protein, 20-25 g. Fat, 15-20 g. Carbohydrates, 20-25 g. Fiber, 3-4 g.

86.Chicken Tacos with Lime and Coriander Sauce

Ingredients:

For the Chicken Tacos: 1 pound boneless, skinless chicken breasts or thighs (cut into strips), 1 tablespoon olive oil, 2 teaspoons chili powder, 1 teaspoon ground cumin, 1/2 teaspoon paprika, Salt and black pepper to taste, 8 small flour or corn tortillas, Shredded lettuce, Diced tomatoes, Sliced red onion, Grated cheddar cheese (optional), Lime wedges for serving

For the Lime and Coriander Sauce: 1/2 cup Greek yogurt, Juice of 2 limes, 2 tablespoons fresh coriander (cilantro, chopped), 1 minced garlic clove, salt and black pepper according to preference

Preparation:

- Start by preparing the seasoning for the chicken. In a bowl, mix freshly squeezed lime juice, chopped fresh coriander leaves, chopped chili pepper (adjust amount to your preferred spiciness level), chopped red onion and minced garlic. This seasoning will give the chicken a fresh, spicy flavor.
- Cut the chicken breast into thin strips and season them with salt and pepper.
- Heat a pan with a drizzle of olive oil over medium-high heat. Add the chicken and cook until fully cooked and a nice golden color.
- Reheat tortillas in a skillet or microwave until hot and pliable.
- Fill each tortilla with grilled chicken and cilantro-lime dressing. Fold the tortillas in half to create your tacos.
- Serve the chicken tacos with additional lime slices and fresh cilantro leaves for garnish. You can also add avocado pieces if you wish.

Nutritional Values: Calories, 350-400 kcal. Protein, 20-25 g. Fat, 10-15 g. Carbohydrates, 30-35 g. Fiber, 4-5 g.

87.Grilled Salmon with Mango and Chili Sauce

Ingredients:

For the Grilled Salmon: 4 salmon fillets, 2 tablespoons olive oil, Salt and black pepper to taste, 1 lemon (sliced), Fresh dill for garnish.

For the Mango and Chili Sauce: 2 ripe mangoes (peeled, pitted, and chopped), 1 red chili pepper (finely chopped, adjust to taste), Juice of 1 lime, 2 tablespoons honey, 2 cloves garlic (minced), Salt to taste.

Preparation:

- Start by preparing the mango salsa. Peel and cut the mango into cubes. Finely chop the red chilli, red onion and fresh coriander. Mix all these ingredients in a bowl.
- Add the lime juice to the mango sauce and mix well. This sauce will be fresh, sweet and tangy, the perfect complement to the salmon.
- Preheat a grill or a nonstick skillet to medium-high flame.
- Brush the salmon fillet lightly with olive oil and cook on the grill or in the pan for about 3-4 minutes per side or until cooked through but still soft on the inside.
- Season the salmon according to preference with pepper and salt.
- Serve the grilled salmon with plenty of mango sauce on top. Garnish with additional fresh cilantro if desired.

Nutritional Values: Calories, 350-400 kcal. Protein, 25-30 g. Fat, 15-20 g. Carbohydrates, 20-25 g. Fiber, 3-4 g.

88.Turkey Meatballs with Tzatziki Sauce and Cucumbers

Ingredients:

For the Turkey Meatballs: 1 pound ground turkey, 1/2 cup breadcrumbs, 1/4 cup grated Parmesan cheese, 1/4 cup finely chopped onion, 1 clove garlic (minced), 1 teaspoon dried oregano, Salt and black pepper to taste, 1 egg, 2 tablespoons olive oil for cooking

For the Tzatziki Sauce: 1 cup Greek yogurt, 1/2 cucumber (peeled, seeded, and finely grated), 2 cloves garlic (minced), 1 tablespoon fresh dill (chopped), 1 tablespoon fresh lemon juice, Salt and black pepper to taste

Preparation:

- Start by preparing the tzatziki sauce. Peel and grate the cucumbers, then squeeze them well to remove excess water.
- In a bowl, mix the grated cucumbers with the Greek yogurt, minced garlic, freshly squeezed lemon juice, chopped fresh mint leaves and chopped fresh parsley.
- Add a pinch of cumin powder, salt and pepper to taste. Mix well and place the tzatziki sauce in the refrigerator until ready to serve.
- In a bowl, mix the ground turkey with salt, pepper and chopped fresh mint leaves. Form meatballs with wet hands to prevent the mixture from sticking to your hands.
- Heat a nonstick skillet over a medium-high flame with a small amount of olive oil.
- Cook turkey meatballs until golden brown and cooked through, turning occasionally to ensure even cooking.
- Serve the turkey meatballs with the tzatziki sauce and fresh cucumber slices as a garnish.
- You can also prepare tacos using meatballs, pitas or tortillas and fresh salad if you prefer.

Nutritional Values: Calories, 300-350 kcal. Protein, 15-20 g. Fat, 10-15 g. Carbohydrates, 20-25 g. Fiber, 3-4 g.

89. Grilled Tofu with Peanut and Ginger Sauce
Ingredients:

For the Grilled Tofu: 1 block of firm tofu (sliced into 1-inch thick pieces), 2 tablespoons soy sauce, 1 tablespoon sesame oil, 1 clove garlic (minced), Salt and black pepper to taste, Fresh cilantro for garnish

For the Peanut and Ginger Sauce: 1/4 cup peanut butter, 2 tablespoons soy sauce, 1 tablespoon rice vinegar, 1 tablespoon fresh ginger (grated), 1 tablespoon honey or maple syrup (adjust to taste), 1 clove garlic (minced), Water to thin the sauce to your desired consistency

Preparation:
- Begin by making the tofu marinade. In a bowl, mix the soy sauce, sesame oil, grated fresh ginger, minced garlic and crumbled dried red chili pepper (adjust the amount according to your preferred level of spiciness).
- Cut the tofu into thick slices and place them in the marinade.
- Let the tofu marinate for at least 30 minutes, but it's even better if you let it sit for a few hours or overnight in the refrigerator.
- While the tofu marinates, prepare the peanut sauce. In a small bowl, mix the peanut sauce, lemon juice, brown sugar, salt and pepper.
- The sauce will be creamy and tasty.
- Heating a grill or a nonstick skillet on medium-high flame.
- When hot, grill the marinated tofu for about 3-4 minutes per side or until it has golden grill marks.
- Serve the grilled tofu with the peanut sauce on top as a condiment. You can garnish with pieces of fresh ginger and additional crushed dried chilli if you wish.

Nutritional Values: Calories, 350-400 kcal. Protein, 15-20 g. Fat, 20-25 g. Carbohydrates, 15-20 g. Fiber, 4-5 g.

90. Tuna steak with lemon and parsley sauce
Ingredients:

For the Tuna Steak: 4 tuna steak fillets, 2 tablespoons olive oil, Salt and black pepper to taste, 1 lemon (cut into wedges), Fresh parsley for garnish.

For the Lemon and Parsley Sauce: Juice of 2 lemons, Zest of 1 lemon, 1/4 cup fresh parsley (finely chopped), 2 cloves garlic (minced), 2 tablespoons olive oil, Salt and black pepper to taste.

Preparation:
- Start by preparing the lemon and parsley sauce. In a bowl, mix freshly squeezed lemon juice, chopped fresh parsley, olive oil, salt and pepper.
- This sauce will be fresh and citrusy, the
- perfect complement to tuna.
- Preheat a grill or nonstick skillet over medium-high heat. Brush the tuna steak lightly with olive oil and season with salt and pepper.
- Cook the tuna on the grill or in the pan for about 2-3 minutes per side to obtain rare doneness or until it reaches the desired level of doneness.
- Serve the tuna steak with the lemon and parsley sauce on top as a condiment. You can garnish with thin slices of lemon and sprigs of fresh parsley if desired.

Nutritional Values: Calories, 350-400 kcal. Protein, 25-30 g. Fat, 15-20 g. Carbohydrates, 5-10 g. Fiber, 2-3 g.

91. Mustard Pork with Sweet Potatoes and Onions
Ingredients:

For the Mustard Pork: 4 boneless pork chops, 2 tablespoons Dijon mustard, 2 tablespoons olive oil, 2 cloves garlic (minced), 1 teaspoon dried thyme, Salt and black pepper to taste.

For the Sweet Potatoes and Onions: 2 large sweet potatoes (peeled and cut into chunks), 2 onions (thinly sliced), 2 tablespoons olive oil, 1 teaspoon dried rosemary, Salt and black pepper to taste.

Preparation:
- Start by preparing the marinade for the pork. In a bowl, mix the mustard, honey, chopped garlic, chopped fresh rosemary, olive oil, salt and pepper. This marinade will give the pork a rich, aromatic flavor.
- Cut the pork fillet into smaller pieces and place them in the marinade. Let the pork marinate for at least 30 minutes, if possible, or longer for a more intense flavor.
- Meanwhile, peel the sweet potatoes and cut them into cubes. Also, cut the red onions into thin slices.
- Preheat the oven to 180°C. Place the sweet potatoes and onions on a baking sheet, season with olive oil, salt and pepper, and mix well.
- Place the marinated pork on the baking tray with the potatoes and onions.
- Cook everything in the preheated oven for about 25-30 minutes or until the pork is cooked through and the potatoes are tender.
- Serve mustard pork with sweet potatoes and onions as a main course. You can garnish with fresh rosemary leaves if you wish.

Nutritional Values: Calories, 350-400 kcal. Protein, 20-25 g. Fat, 15-20 g. Carbohydrates, 30-35 g. Fiber, 3-4 g.

92. Baked Trout Fillet with Citrus Sauce
Ingredients:

For the Baked Trout Fillet: 4 trout fillets, 2 tablespoons olive oil, Salt and black pepper to taste, 1 lemon (thinly sliced), Fresh dill for garnish.

For the Citrus Sauce: Juice of 2 oranges, Juice of 1 lemon, 2 tablespoons honey, 1 tablespoon Dijon mustard, 1 tablespoon olive oil, Salt and black pepper to taste, Zest of 1 orange for garnish.

Preparation:
- Preheat the oven to 180°C.
- Wash and dry the trout fillets, then place them on a baking tray lightly greased with butter or lined with baking paper.
- Squeeze the juice from oranges, lemons and limes. In a small bowl, mix the resulting juices.
- Pour the citrus juice over the trout fillets.
- Sprinkle the fillets with minced garlic, chopped fresh parsley, salt and pepper to taste.
- Cover the pan with foil and bake for about 15-20 minutes or until the trout is cooked and flakes easily with a fork.
- Serve the baked trout fillet with hot citrus sauce, garnished with fresh citrus slices and sprigs of parsley, if desired.

Nutritional Values: Calories, 350-400 kcal. Protein, 25-30 g. Fat, 15-20 g. Carbohydrates, 5-10 g. Fiber, 2-3 g.

93. Chicken Curry with Lentils and Spinach
Ingredients:

For the Chicken Curry: 4 boneless, skinless chicken breasts or thighs (cut into bite-sized pieces), 2 tablespoons vegetable oil, 1 onion (finely chopped), 2 cloves garlic (minced), 1-inch piece of fresh ginger (minced), 2 tablespoons curry powder, 1 teaspoon ground cumin, 1 teaspoon ground coriander, 1/2 teaspoon turmeric, 1/2 teaspoon cayenne pepper (adjust to taste), 1 can (14 ounces) diced tomatoes, 1 can (14 ounces) coconut milk, Salt and black pepper to taste, Fresh cilantro leaves for garnish.

For the Lentils and Spinach: 1 cup dried red or green lentils (rinsed and drained), 2 cups water, 4 cups fresh spinach leaves, Salt to taste.

Preparation:

- Start by preparing the lentils. Rinse them under cold water and let them drain.
- In a large pot, heat some vegetable oil and add chopped onion, chopped garlic and grated ginger. Fry until the onion becomes transparent.
- Add the curry powder and mix well for a minute to develop its flavour.
- Add the drained lentils and chicken broth. Bring everything to the boil, then reduce the heat, cover and cook for about 20-25 minutes or until the lentils are tender.
- In the meantime, cut the chicken breast into cubes. In a separate pan, heat some oil and cook the chicken until golden brown and fully cooked.
- When the lentils are done, add the cooked chicken and fresh spinach to the pot. Stir until the spinach is wilted.
- Pour the coconut milk into the pan and simmer for a further 5 minutes or until the curry is hot and well mixed. Season with salt and pepper to taste.
- Serve the chicken curry with lentils and spinach hot, perhaps accompanied with basmati rice.

Nutritional Values: Calories, 350-400 kcal. Protein, 20-25 g. Fat, 15-20 g. Carbohydrates, 20-25 g. Fiber, 3-4 g.

94.Duck Breast with Green Pepper

Ingredients: For the Duck Breast: 4 duck breast fillets, Salt and black pepper to taste.

For the Green Pepper Sauce: 2 green bell peppers (seeded and thinly sliced), 1 tablespoon olive oil, 2 cloves garlic (minced), 1 cup chicken or vegetable broth, 1/4 cup heavy cream, 2 tablespoons butter, Salt and black pepper to taste, Fresh parsley for garnish.

Preparation:

- Start by preparing the duck breast. Score the skin of the duck breast with a sharp blade to create a square pattern, being careful not to cut the meat.
- In a non-stick pan, heat the duck breast skin side over medium-high heat. Cook up until the skin is crispy and golden, between five and seven minutes.
- Turn the duck breast and cook it on the other side for another 3-5 minutes, depending on the desired degree of doneness. For rare cooking, cook for a shorter time.
- Take away the duck breast from the pan and place it on a cutting board to rest.
- In the same pan, add the green peppercorns and toast them for a couple of minutes.
- Add the fresh cream and chicken broth to the pan with the green pepper. Bring to the boil and cook for about 5 minutes or until the sauce thickens slightly.
- Cut the duck breast into thin slices and serve with the hot green pepper sauce on top. Depending on your preference, season with salt and black pepper.

Nutritional Values: Calories, 350-400 kcal. Protein, 20-25 g. Fat, 25-30 g. Carbohydrates, 5-10 g. Fiber, 1-2 g.

95. Baked Trout Fillet with Citrus Sauce

Ingredients:

For the Baked Trout Fillet: 4 trout fillets, 2 tablespoons olive oil, Salt and black pepper to taste, 1 lemon (thinly sliced), Fresh dill for garnish.

For the Citrus Sauce: Juice of 2 oranges, Juice of 1 lemon, 2 tablespoons honey, 1 tablespoon Dijon mustard, 1 tablespoon olive oil, Salt and black pepper to taste, Zest of 1 orange for garnish.

Preparation:

- Preheat the oven to 180°C.
- Wash and dry the trout fillet, then place it on a baking tray lightly greased with butter or lined with baking paper.
- Squeeze the juice from oranges, lemons and limes. In a small bowl, mix the resulting juices.
- Pour the citrus juice over the trout fillet.
- Sprinkle the fillet with minced garlic, chopped fresh parsley, salt and pepper to taste.
- Cover the pan with foil and bake for about 15-20 minutes or until the trout is cooked and flakes easily with a fork.
- Serve the baked trout fillet with hot citrus sauce, garnished with fresh citrus slices and sprigs of parsley, if desired.

Nutritional Values : Calories, 350-400 kcal. Protein, 25-30 g. Fat, 15-20 g. Carbohydrates, 5-10 g. Fiber, 2-3 g.

96.Chicken Curry with Lentils and Spinach

Ingredients:

For the Chicken Curry: 4 boneless, skinless chicken breasts or thighs (cut into bite-sized pieces), 2 tablespoons vegetable oil, 1 onion (finely chopped), 2 cloves garlic (minced), 1-inch piece of fresh ginger (minced), 2 tablespoons curry powder, 1 teaspoon ground cumin, 1 teaspoon ground coriander, 1/2 teaspoon turmeric, 1/2 teaspoon cayenne pepper (adjust to taste), 1 can (14 ounces) diced tomatoes, 1 can (14 ounces) coconut milk, Salt and black pepper to taste, Fresh cilantro leaves for garnish.

For the Lentils and Spinach: 1 cup dried red or green lentils (rinsed and drained), 2 cups water, 4 cups fresh spinach leaves, Salt to taste.

Preparation:

- Start by preparing the lentils. Allow them to drain after rinsing them in cold water.
- In a large pot, heat some vegetable oil and add chopped onion, chopped garlic and grated ginger. Fry until the onion becomes transparent.
- Add the curry powder and mix well for a minute to develop its flavour.
- Add the drained lentils and chicken broth. Bring everything to the boil, then reduce the heat, cover and cook for about 20-25 minutes or until the lentils are tender.
- While you're waiting the meanwhile, cut the chicken breast into cubes.
- In a separate pan, heat some oil and cook the chicken until golden brown and fully cooked.
- When the lentils are done, add the cooked chicken and fresh spinach to the pot. Stir until the spinach is wilted.
- Pour the coconut milk into the pan and simmer for a further 5 minutes or until the curry is hot and well mixed. Season according to preference with pepper and salt.

- Serve the chicken curry with lentils and spinach hot, perhaps accompanied with basmati rice.

Nutritional Values: Calories, 350-400 kcal. Protein, 20-25 g. Fat, 15-20 g. Carbohydrates, 20-25 g. Fiber, 3-4 g.

97.Duck Breast with Green Pepper

Ingredients: For the Duck Breast: 4 duck breast fillets, Salt and black pepper to taste.

For the Green Pepper Sauce: 2 green bell peppers (seeded and thinly sliced), 1 tablespoon olive oil, 2 cloves garlic (minced), 1 cup chicken or vegetable broth, 1/4 cup heavy cream, 2 tablespoons butter, Salt and black pepper to taste, Fresh parsley for garnish.

Preparation:
- Start by preparing the duck breast. Score the skin of the duck breast with a sharp blade to create a square pattern, being careful not to cut the meat.
- In a non-stick pan, heat the duck breast skin side over medium-high heat. Cook till the skin is crispy and golden, between five and seven minutes.
- Turn the duck breast and cook it on the other side for another 3-5 minutes, depending on the desired degree of doneness. For rare cooking, cook for a shorter time.
- Take away the duck breast from the pan and place it on a cutting board to rest.
- In the same pan, add the green peppercorns and toast them for a couple of minutes.
- Add the fresh cream and chicken broth to the pan with the green pepper. Bring to the boil and cook for about 5 minutes or until the sauce thickens slightly.
- Cut the duck breast into thin slices and serve with the hot green pepper sauce on top. Sprinkle to taste using salt and freshly ground black pepper.

Nutritional Values: Calories, 350-400 kcal. Protein, 20-25 g. Fat, 25-30 g. Carbohydrates, 5-10 g. Fiber, 1-2 g.

98.Beef Steak with Chilli Sauce

Ingredients: For the Beef Steak: 4 beef steaks (such as sirloin or ribeye), 2 tablespoons olive oil, Salt and black pepper to taste.

For the Chili Sauce: 2 red chili peppers (finely chopped, adjust the amount for desired spiciness), 2 cloves garlic (minced), 1/4 cup soy sauce, 2 tablespoons honey or brown sugar (adjust to taste), 1 tablespoon rice vinegar, 1 teaspoon sesame oil, 1 teaspoon grated fresh ginger, 2 green onions (chopped for garnish).

Preparation:
- Start by preparing the chilli sauce. Finely chop the fresh red chili pepper (remove the seeds if you prefer a less spicy sauce) and the garlic.
- In a pan, heat some olive oil over medium heat and add the chopped chilli and garlic. Sauté for approximately 2-3 minutes, until it's fragrant.
- Add the chopped fresh parsley and cook for another minute. Season according to preference with salt and black pepper.
- Set aside the chilli sauce.
- Prepare the sirloin steak: Heat a grill or nonstick skillet over medium-high heat. Lightly brush the steak with olive oil and sprinkle with salt and black pepper.
- Cook the steak for the desired time on both sides, depending on the desired doneness (for rare, about 3-4 minutes per side).
- When the steak is done, transfer it to a cutting board and set it aside for a few minutes to rest.

- Cut the steak into thin slices and serve with the chilli sauce on top. You can add a squeeze of lemon juice if you wish.

Nutritional Values: Calories, 350-400 kcal. Protein, 25-30 g. Fat, 15-20 g. Carbohydrates, 5-10 g. Fiber, 2-3 g.

99. Baked Salmon with Basil and Tomato Sauce

Ingredients:

For the Baked Salmon: 4 salmon fillets, 2 tablespoons olive oil, Salt and black pepper to taste, 1 lemon (sliced), Fresh basil leaves for garnish.

For the Basil and Tomato Sauce: 2 cups cherry tomatoes (halved), 2 cloves garlic (minced), 1/4 cup fresh basil (chopped), 1/4 cup balsamic vinegar, 2 tablespoons olive oil, Salt and black pepper to taste.

Preparation:
- Preheat the oven to 180°C.
- Start by preparing the basil and tomato sauce. Cube the tomatoes and mince the garlic.
- In a pan, heat some olive oil over medium heat and add the minced garlic. Cook for about 1 minute, or until fragrant.
- Add the diced tomatoes and cook for 5-7 minutes or until they soften and release their juice.
- Add the chopped fresh basil and cook for another 2 minutes. Season according to preference with salt and black pepper. Set the sauce aside.
- Place the salmon fillet on a baking tray lightly greased with olive oil. Sprinkle the salmon with salt and black pepper.
- Pour the basil and tomato sauce over the salmon.
- Place the salmon in the oven and cook for about 15-20 minutes or until the salmon flakes easily with a fork.
- Serve the baked salmon with the basil and tomato sauce on top. It goes well with rice or steamed vegetables.

Nutritional Values: Calories, 350-400 kcal. Protein, 25-30 g. Fat, 15-20 g. Carbohydrates, 5-10 g. Fiber, 2-3 g.

100.Quinoa Meatballs with Tomato and Basil Sauce

Ingredients:

For the Quinoa Meatballs: 1 cup quinoa, 2 cups water, 1 cup dry red lentils, 1 onion (finely chopped), 2 garlic cloves (finely chopped), 1 teaspoon extra virgin olive oil, 1 teaspoon ground cumin, 1 teaspoon sweet paprika, Salt and black pepper to taste, 2 tablespoons fresh parsley (chopped), 1 egg (optional, as a binder)

For the Tomato and Basil Sauce: 2 cans of whole peeled tomatoes (approximately 800g), 2 garlic cloves (finely chopped), 1 teaspoon extra virgin olive oil, 1 bunch of fresh basil, Salt and black pepper to taste

Preparation:
- In a large bowl, mix the cooked quinoa, eggs, grated cheese, chopped fresh parsley, breadcrumbs, minced garlic, salt and black pepper.
- •
- Mix thoroughly until the mixture is homogeneous. With wet hands, shape the quinoa mixture into round meatballs.
- • Heat some of the olive oil in a pan over a medium-high flame.
- Cook the quinoa balls for about 3-4 minutes per side or until golden and crispy.
- In the meantime, prepare the tomato and basil sauce. Chop the tomatoes and fresh basil.

- In a pan, heat some olive oil and add the chopped tomatoes and basil.
- Cook for 5-7 minutes, or until the sauce is slightly thickened.
- Season with salt and black pepper to taste.
- Serve the quinoa meatballs with the tomato and basil sauce on top. You can add extra grated cheese and fresh basil leaves for garnish if desired.

Nutritional Values: Calories, 300-350 kcal. Protein, 15-20 g. Fat, 10-15 g. Carbohydrates, 30-35 g. Fiber, 4-5 g.

Chapter 9: Side dishes and salads

50 recipes for anti-inflammatory side dishes and salads

1. Beetroot Salad with Toasted Almonds and Parsley

Ingredients: Beetroot (2 medium), Almonds (1/4 cup, toasted), Fresh Parsley (1/4 cup, chopped), Olive Oil (2 tablespoons), Balsamic Vinegar (1 tablespoon), Salt (1/2 teaspoon), Black Pepper (1/4 teaspoon).

Preparation:

- Boil or steam beets until tender. Then peel them and cut them into small slices. Lightly toast the almonds in a pan until fragrant.
- Mix the beets with the toasted almonds and chopped parsley.
- Make a vinaigrette by mixing olive oil, balsamic vinegar, salt and pepper. Pour this vinaigrette over the beetroot salad.

Nutritional Values: Calories, 120-150 kcal. Protein, 3-4 g. Fat, 8-10 g. Carbohydrates, 12-15 g. Fiber, 3-4 g.

2. Quinoa with Cucumbers, Tomatoes and Black Olives

Ingredients: Quinoa (1 cup, cooked), Cucumbers (1 medium, diced), Tomatoes (2 medium, diced), Black Olives (1/2 cup, sliced), Olive Oil (2 tablespoons), Lemon Juice (2 tablespoons), Fresh Parsley (1/4 cup, chopped), Salt (1/2 teaspoon), Black Pepper (1/4 teaspoon).

Preparation:

- Follow the package guidelines for preparing the quinoa. While the quinoa cooks, dice the cucumbers, tomatoes and black olives.
- In a large bowl, mix the cooked quinoa with the cucumbers, tomatoes and black olives.
- Make a simple vinaigrette by mixing olive oil, lemon juice, dried oregano, salt and pepper. Pour this vinaigrette over the quinoa and mix well.

Nutritional Values: Calories, 200-250 kcal. Protein, 6-8 g. Fat, 8-10 g. Carbohydrates, 25-30 g. Fiber, 4-6 g.

3. Avocado and Mango Salad with Lime and Coriander

Ingredients: Avocado (2 ripe, diced), Mango (1 ripe, diced), Lime Juice (2 tablespoons), Fresh Coriander (1/4 cup, chopped), Red Onion (1/4 cup, finely chopped), Salt (1/4 teaspoon), Black Pepper (1/4 teaspoon).

Preparation:

- Peel and dice the avocado and mango.
- Finely chop the fresh coriander and red chili pepper (the amount depends on your preference for spiciness).
- In a large bowl, combine the avocado, mango, cilantro, red pepper, lime juice, salt and pepper.
- Stir gently to avoid mashing the avocado too much.

Nutritional Values: Calories, 150-180 kcal. Protein, 2-3 g. Fat, 10-12 g. Carbohydrates, 15-18 g. Fiber, 4-5 g.

4. Stir-fried Chinese Cabbage with Ginger and Garlic

Ingredients: Chinese Cabbage (1 small head, thinly sliced), Ginger (1 tablespoon, minced), Garlic (2 cloves, minced), Vegetable Oil (2 tablespoons), Soy Sauce (2 tablespoons), Sesame Oil (1 teaspoon), Salt (1/4 teaspoon), Black Pepper (1/4 teaspoon).

Preparation:

- Cut the bok choy into thin strips, chop the fresh ginger and garlic.
- In a large skillet, heat the sesame oil and sauté the ginger and garlic until fragrant.
- Add the bok choy to the pan and sauté until tender but still crunchy.
- Sprinkle with soy sauce, salt, and pepper before serving.

Nutritional Values: Calories, 50-70 kcal. Protein, 2-3 g. Fat, 3-4 g. Carbohydrates, 5-7 g. Fiber, 2-3 g.

5. Lentil Salad with Carrots and Spinach

Ingredients: Lentils (1 cup, cooked), Carrots (2, finely chopped), Spinach (2 cups, fresh and chopped), Red Onion (1/2, finely chopped), Olive Oil (2 tablespoons), Lemon Juice (2 tablespoons), Dijon Mustard (1 teaspoon), Salt (1/2 teaspoon), Black Pepper (1/4 teaspoon), Feta Cheese (1/2 cup, crumbled, optional).

Preparation:

- Cook the lentils in accordance with the package directions. Drain them and let them cool.
- Cut the carrots into thin slices and chop the fresh spinach. In a large bowl, combine the lentils, carrots, and spinach.
- Make a simple vinaigrette by mixing olive oil, balsamic vinegar, salt and pepper. Pour this vinaigrette over the salad and mix well.

Nutritional Values: Calories, 150-180 kcal. Protein, 6-8 g. Fat, 4-6 g. Carbohydrates, 20-25 g. Fiber, 5-7 g.

6. Cucumbers Marinated with Apple Cider Vinegar and Cumin Seeds

Ingredients: Cucumbers (2, thinly sliced), Apple Cider Vinegar (1/4 cup), Cumin Seeds (1 teaspoon), Sugar (1 tablespoon), Salt (1/2 teaspoon), Black Pepper (1/4 teaspoon), Red Onion (1/4, thinly sliced, optional).

Preparation:

- Cut the cucumbers into thin slices. In a bowl, pour some apple cider vinegar over the cucumbers and add the cumin seeds. Mix well.
- Let the cucumbers marinate in the refrigerator for at least 30 minutes to absorb the flavors.

For serving, season with pepper and salt according to preference.

Nutritional Values: Calories, 20-30 kcal. Protein, 1-2 g. Fat, 0-1 g. Carbohydrates, 3-5 g. Fiber, 1-2 g.

7. Melon Salad with Fresh Mint and Lemon

Ingredients: Melon (1/2, diced), Fresh Mint Leaves (2 tablespoons, chopped), Lemon Juice (2 tablespoons), Honey (1 tablespoon, optional).

Preparation:

- Discard the seeds from the melon and chop it into cubes. Chop the fresh mint and grate the lemon zest to obtain its peel.
- In a bowl, combine the melon cubes with the fresh mint and lemon zest.
- If you want a touch of sweetness, you can add a little honey to taste.

Nutritional Values: Calories, 30-40 kcal. Protein, 1-2 g. Fat, 0-1 g. Carbohydrates, 7-9 g. Fiber, 1-2 g.

8. Roasted Cauliflower with Olive Oil and Paprika

Ingredients: Cauliflower (1 head, cut into florets), Olive Oil (2 tablespoons), Paprika (1 teaspoon), Salt (1/2 teaspoon), Black Pepper (1/4 teaspoon).

Preparation:
- Remove the leaves off the cauliflower and chop it into florets.
- In a bowl, season the cauliflower with plenty of olive oil, sweet paprika, salt and pepper.
- Spread the cauliflower florets on a baking tray and cook in a preheated oven at 200°C until tender and lightly golden.

Nutritional Values: Calories, 50-70 kcal. Protein, 2-3 g. Fat, 3-4 g. Carbohydrates, 5-7 g. Fiber, 2-3 g.

9. Spinach Salad with Strawberries and Sliced Almonds

Ingredients: Spinach (6 cups), Strawberries (1 cup, sliced), Sliced Almonds (1/2 cup), Red Onion (1/4 cup, thinly sliced), Balsamic Vinaigrette Dressing (1/4 cup), Feta Cheese (1/4 cup, crumbled), Salt (1/4 teaspoon), Black Pepper (1/8 teaspoon).

Preparation:
- Chop the fresh spinach coarsely and slice the strawberries.
- Combine the spinach, strawberries, and sliced almonds in a large mixing bowl.
- Make a vinaigrette by mixing olive oil, balsamic vinegar, honey (if desired), salt and pepper.
- Pour this vinaigrette over the salad and mix well.

Nutritional Values: Calories, 100-120 kcal. Protein, 3-4 g. Fat, 6-8 g. Carbohydrates, 10-12 g. Fiber, 3-4 g.

10. Grilled Red Beets with Goat Cheese and Walnuts

Ingredients: Red Beets (4 medium-sized), Goat Cheese (1/2 cup, crumbled), Walnuts (1/4 cup, chopped), Olive Oil (2 tablespoons), Balsamic Vinegar (2 tablespoons), Honey (1 tablespoon), Salt (1/4 teaspoon), Black Pepper (1/8 teaspoon), Fresh Thyme Leaves (1 teaspoon, optional for garnish).

Preparation:
- Prepare the red beets by grilling them until tender and the skin begins to peel. Peel and cut them into slices.
- In a bowl, mix the beets with the shredded goat cheese and chopped walnuts.
- Make a vinaigrette by mixing olive oil, balsamic vinegar, salt and pepper. Pour this vinaigrette over the salad and mix well.

Nutritional Values: Calories, 150-180 kcal. Protein, 6-8 g. Fat, 10-12 g. Carbohydrates, 10-12 g. Fiber, 3-4 g.

11. Quinoa with Roasted Peppers and Lime Sauce

Ingredients: Quinoa (1 cup, uncooked), Red Bell Pepper (1, roasted and diced), Yellow Bell Pepper (1, roasted and diced), Lime Juice (2 tablespoons), Olive Oil (3 tablespoons), Fresh Cilantro (1/4 cup, chopped), Salt (1/2 teaspoon), Black Pepper (1/4 teaspoon).

Preparation:
- Follow the package guidelines for preparing the quinoa. Drain it and let it cool.
- While the quinoa cools, grill the peppers until the skin is browned and peels away easily.
- Peel the peppers, remove the seeds and cut them into strips.
- In a large bowl, combine the quinoa with the grilled pepper strips.
- Make a lime sauce by mixing lime juice, olive oil, chopped fresh cilantro, salt and pepper. Pour this sauce over the quinoa and mix well.

Nutritional Values: Calories, 180-220 kcal. Protein, 5-7 g. Fat, 5-7 g. Carbohydrates, 30-35 g. Fiber, 3-4 g.

12. Avocado, Cucumber and Cherry Tomato Salad

Ingredients: Avocado (1, diced), Cucumber (1, diced), Cherry Tomatoes (1 cup, halved), Olive Oil (2 tablespoons), Fresh Lemon Juice (2 tablespoons), Fresh Basil Leaves (2 tablespoons, chopped), Salt (1/2 teaspoon), Black Pepper (1/4 teaspoon).

Preparation:
- Dice the avocado, cucumber and cherry tomatoes. Finely chop the red onion and fresh parsley.
- In a bowl, combine the avocado, cucumber, cherry tomatoes, red onion and parsley.
- Make a simple vinaigrette by mixing olive oil, lemon juice, salt and pepper. Pour this vinaigrette over the salad and mix well.

Nutritional Values: Calories, 120-150 kcal. Protein, 2-3 g. Fat, 10-12 g. Carbohydrates, 8-10 g. Fiber, 3-4 g.

13. Steamed Green Beans with Mustard and Lemon Sauce

Ingredients: Green Beans (1 pound, trimmed), Dijon Mustard (1 tablespoon), Fresh Lemon Juice (2 tablespoons), Olive Oil (2 tablespoons), Garlic (1 clove, minced), Salt (1/2 teaspoon), Black Pepper (1/4 teaspoon), Lemon Zest (1 teaspoon).

Preparation:
- Steam green beans until tender but crunchy. Drain them and let them cool.
- While the green beans cool, prepare the sauce. Mix the mustard, lemon juice, olive oil, minced garlic, salt and pepper in a bowl.
- Pour the mustard-lemon sauce over the green beans and mix well.

Nutritional Values: Calories, 60-80 kcal. Protein, 2-3 g. Fat, 2-3 g. Carbohydrates, 10-12 g. Fiber, 4-5 g.

14. Chickpea Salad with Parsley and Lemon

Ingredients: Chickpeas (1 can, drained and rinsed), Fresh Parsley (1/2 cup, chopped), Lemon Juice (2 tablespoons), Olive Oil (2 tablespoons), Garlic (1 clove, minced), Salt (1/2 teaspoon), Black Pepper (1/4 teaspoon).

Preparation:
- Rinse and drain the canned chickpeas.
- In a bowl, combine the chickpeas with chopped fresh parsley, grated lemon zest, lemon juice, olive oil, minced garlic, salt and pepper.
- Mix all the ingredients well and make sure the chickpeas are well seasoned with the lemon and parsley sauce.

Nutritional Values: Calories, 150-180 kcal. Protein, 5-7 g. Fat, 7-9 g. Carbohydrates, 15-18 g. Fiber, 4-5 g.

15. Grilled Eggplant with Peppers and Red Onions

Ingredients: Eggplant (1 large, sliced), Red Bell Peppers (2, sliced), Red Onions (2, sliced), Olive Oil (3 tablespoons), Balsamic Vinegar (2 tablespoons), Fresh Basil (1/4 cup, chopped), Salt (1/2 teaspoon), Black Pepper (1/4 teaspoon).

Preparation:
- Cut the aubergines into thin slices and the peppers into strips. Also slice the red onions.

- Light the grill or barbecue. Brush the eggplant slices, pepper strips and red onions with olive oil and season with salt and pepper.
- Grill vegetables until soft and lightly charred.
- Serve grilled eggplant with peppers and red onions as a side dish or as an appetizer.

Nutritional Values: Calories, 120-150 kcal. Protein, 2-3 g. Fat, 6-8 g. Carbohydrates, 15-18 g. Fiber, 4-5 g.

16. Avocado and Cherry Tomato Salad with Basil

Ingredients: Avocado (2, diced), Cherry Tomatoes (1 pint, halved), Fresh Basil (1/4 cup, chopped), Olive Oil (2 tablespoons), Balsamic Vinegar (1 tablespoon), Salt (1/2 teaspoon), Black Pepper (1/4 teaspoon).

Preparation:
- Dice the avocado and cherry tomatoes. Chop the fresh basil.
- In a bowl, combine the avocado, cherry tomatoes and basil.
- Make a simple vinaigrette by mixing olive oil, lemon juice, salt and pepper. Pour this vinaigrette over the salad and mix well.
- Serve the salad as a side dish or as a light dish.

Nutritional Values: Calories, 160-190 kcal. Protein, 2-3 g. Fat, 14-16 g. Carbohydrates, 8-10 g. Fiber, 5-6 g.

17. Roasted Red Turnip with Olive Oil and Rosemary

Ingredients: Red Turnip (2, peeled and diced), Olive Oil (2 tablespoons), Fresh Rosemary (1 tablespoon, chopped), Salt (1/2 teaspoon), Black Pepper (1/4 teaspoon).

Preparation:
- Preheat the oven to 200°C.
- Peel the red turnips and cut them into slices or cubes.
- Place the turnips on a baking tray. Sprinkle them with olive oil, salt, pepper and fresh rosemary.
- Bake for about 25-30 minutes or until the turnips are tender and slightly crispy on the outside.
- Serve roasted red beets as a side dish or as part of a main course.

Nutritional Values: Calories, 40-50 kcal. Protein, 1-2 g. Fat, 2-3 g. Carbohydrates, 6-8 g. Fiber, 2-3 g.

18. Carrot Salad with Ginger and Sesame Seeds

Ingredients: Carrots (4, grated), Fresh Ginger (1 tablespoon, minced), Sesame Seeds (2 tablespoons), Rice Vinegar (2 tablespoons), Soy Sauce (1 tablespoon), Honey (1 tablespoon), Sesame Oil (1 tablespoon), Salt (1/2 teaspoon), Black Pepper (1/4 teaspoon).

Preparation:
- Peel and grate the carrots. Finely chop the fresh ginger.
- In a bowl, combine the grated carrots, fresh ginger and sesame seeds.
- Make a vinaigrette by mixing olive oil, lemon juice, honey, salt and pepper. Pour this vinaigrette over the salad and mix well.
- Enable the salad to chill for at least 30 minutes before dishing to enable the flavors to meld.

Nutritional Values: Calories, 60-80 kcal. Protein, 1-2 g. Fat, 3-4 g. Carbohydrates, 8-10 g. Fiber, 2-3 g.

19. Pan-fried Spinach with Pine Nuts and Raisins

Ingredients: Spinach (8 cups, fresh), Pine Nuts (1/4 cup), Raisins (1/4 cup), Olive Oil (2 tablespoons), Garlic (2 cloves, minced), Lemon Juice (2 tablespoons), Salt (1/2 teaspoon), Black Pepper (1/4 teaspoon).

Preparation:
- Heat the olive oil in a big skillet over a moderate flame.
- Cook until the minced garlic is brown.
- Add fresh spinach to the pan and sauté until wilted and reduced in volume.
- Add the pine nuts and raisins to the pan and continue to sauté for a couple of minutes, until the pine nuts are lightly browned.
- Sprinkle according to preference with pepper and salt.
- Serve the sautéed spinach as a side dish or as a light dish.

Nutritional Values: Calories, 90-110 kcal. Protein, 2-3 g. Fat, 7-9 g. Carbohydrates, 6-8 g. Fiber, 2-3 g.

20. Baked Pumpkin with Cinnamon and Nutmeg

Ingredients: Pumpkin (1 small, about 2-3 pounds), Cinnamon (1 teaspoon), Nutmeg (1/2 teaspoon), Olive Oil (2 tablespoons), Salt (1/2 teaspoon), Black Pepper (1/4 teaspoon).

Preparation:
- Preheat the oven to 200°C.
- Peel and cut the pumpkin into pieces or slices.
- Spread the pumpkin chunks out on a baking sheet.
- Sprinkle them with olive oil, cinnamon, nutmeg, salt and pepper.
- Bake for 25-30 minutes, or until the squash is soft and golden brown.
- Serve baked squash as a side dish or as part of a main course.

Nutritional Values: Calories, 60-80 kcal. Protein, 1-2 g. Fat, 0-1 g. Carbohydrates, 15-20 g. Fiber, 2-3 g.

21. Napa Cabbage Salad with Mandarins and Almonds

Ingredients: Napa Cabbage (1 small head), Mandarins (2, peeled and segmented), Almonds (1/2 cup, sliced), Rice Vinegar (2 tablespoons), Soy Sauce (1 tablespoon), Sesame Oil (1 tablespoon), Honey (1 tablespoon), Sesame Seeds (1 tablespoon, toasted), Salt (1/4 teaspoon), Black Pepper (1/4 teaspoon).

Preparation:
- Finely chop the Napa cabbage and place in a large bowl.
- Peel the mandarins and cut them into segments.
- In a nonstick pan, lightly toast the almonds.
- In a small bowl, make a vinaigrette by mixing olive oil, lemon juice, honey, salt and pepper.
- Pour the vinaigrette over the Napa coleslaw and mix well.
- Add tangerines and toasted almonds to the salad.
- Let the salad rest in the refrigerator for at least 30 minutes before serving.

Nutritional Values: Calories, 120-140 kcal. Protein, 2-4 g. Fat, 7-9 g. Carbohydrates, 12-15 g. Fiber, 3-4 g.

22. Steamed Asparagus with Lemon Butter and Thyme

Ingredients: Asparagus (1 bunch), Butter (2 tablespoons), Lemon Zest (1 teaspoon), Lemon Juice (1 tablespoon), Fresh Thyme (1 tablespoon, chopped), Salt (1/2 teaspoon), Black Pepper (1/4 teaspoon).

Preparation:
- Wash them and cut off the tough bottom part of the asparagus.
- Prepare a steamer and cook the asparagus until tender but still crunchy, usually 3 to 5 minutes.

- Meanwhile, in a tiny saucepan, melt the butter. Add lemon juice, fresh thyme, salt and pepper.
- Drain the asparagus and transfer them to a serving dish. Pour the lemon-thyme butter over the asparagus.
- Serve steamed asparagus as a side dish.

Nutritional Values: Calories, 60-80 kcal. Protein, 2-4 g. Fat, 5-7 g. Carbohydrates, 4-6 g. Fiber, 2-3 g.

23. Green Bean Salad with Yogurt and Garlic Dressing

Ingredients: Green Beans (1 pound), Greek Yogurt (1/2 cup), Garlic (2 cloves, minced), Lemon Juice (2 tablespoons), Olive Oil (2 tablespoons), Dill (2 tablespoons, chopped), Salt (1/2 teaspoon), Black Pepper (1/4 teaspoon).

Preparation:
- Boil mung beans in boiling water until tender but still crunchy, usually 2-3 minutes. Then immediately cool them in cold water to stop cooking.
- In a bowl, mix the Greek yogurt with minced garlic, lemon juice, chopped fresh parsley, salt and pepper.
- Add the boiled green beans to the yogurt sauce and mix well.
- Let the salad rest in the refrigerator for at least 30 minutes before serving.

Nutritional Values: Calories, 70-90 kcal. Protein, 2-4 g. Fat, 4-6 g. Carbohydrates, 7-9 g. Fiber, 3-4 g.

24. Fresh Fennel with Oranges and Green Olives

Ingredients: Fresh Fennel (2 bulbs), Oranges (2), Green Olives (1/2 cup, pitted), Extra Virgin Olive Oil (2 tablespoons), Fresh Lemon Juice (2 tablespoons), Fresh Mint Leaves (2 tablespoons, chopped), Salt (1/2 teaspoon), Black Pepper (1/4 teaspoon).

Preparation:
- Cut the fennel into thin slices.
- Peel the oranges and cut them into slices or wedges.
- Arrange the fennel, oranges and green olives on a serving platter.
- Sprinkle with olive oil, salt and pepper.
- Serve fresh fennel with oranges and green olives as a side dish or as part of an appetizer.

Nutritional Values: Calories, 60-80 kcal. Protein, 1-2 g. Fat, 3-5 g. Carbohydrates, 8-10 g. Fiber, 3-4 g.

25. Cucumber Salad with Balsamic Vinegar and Mint

Ingredients: Cucumbers (2), Balsamic Vinegar (2 tablespoons), Fresh Mint Leaves (2 tablespoons, chopped), Extra Virgin Olive Oil (1 tablespoon), Salt (1/2 teaspoon), Black Pepper (1/4 teaspoon).

Preparation:
- Cucumbers should be cut into small slices or circles.
- In a bowl, mix the vinaigrette ingredients: balsamic vinegar, olive oil, salt and pepper.
- Finely chop the fresh mint leaves.
- Pour the vinaigrette over the cucumbers and add the chopped mint. Mix well.
- Refrigerate the salad for at least 30 minutes prior to serving.

Nutritional Values: Calories, 15-25 kcal. Protein, 1-2 g. Fat, 0 g. Carbohydrates, 3-5 g. Fiber, 1-2 g.

26. Dried Tomatoes Stuffed with Olives and Basil

Ingredients: Dried tomatoes, pitted black olives, fresh basil, olive oil.

Preparation:
- Prepare the sun-dried tomatoes by gently opening them and shaking out any excess seeds.
- Finely chop the black olives and basil leaves.
- In a small bowl, mix the chopped black olives with the basil and a little olive oil.
- Fill the dried tomatoes with the olive and basil mixture.
- Keep refrigerated until ready to serve.

Nutritional Values: Calories, 45-60 kcal. Protein, 1-2 g. Fat, 4-5 g. Carbohydrates, 2-3 g. Fiber, 1-2 g.

27. Brussels Sprouts Salad with Bacon and Walnuts

Ingredients: Brussels Sprouts (1 pound), Bacon (4 slices, cooked and crumbled), Walnuts (1/2 cup, toasted and chopped), Olive Oil (2 tablespoons), Apple Cider Vinegar (1 tablespoon), Honey (1 tablespoon), Dijon Mustard (1 tsp), Salt (1/2 tsp), Black Pepper (1/4 tsp).

Preparation:
- Cut the Brussels sprouts in half and remove the outer leaves if they are damaged.
- Cook the bacon in a pan until crispy, then drain on absorbent paper.
- In a pan, heat some olive oil and add the halved Brussels sprouts.
- Cook them until golden and tender.
- Coarsely chop the walnuts and crispy bacon.
- In a large bowl, combine the cooked Brussels sprouts, walnuts, bacon, salt and pepper.
- Let the salad rest in the refrigerator for a while before serving.

Nutritional Values: Calories, 150-200 kcal. Protein, 3-5 g. Fat, 10-15 g. Carbohydrates, 10-15 g. Fiber, 3-5 g.

28. Baked Celeriac with Olive Oil and Rosemary

Ingredients: Celeriac (1 medium-sized), Olive Oil (2 tablespoons), Fresh Rosemary (2-3 sprigs), Salt (to taste), Black Pepper (to taste).

Preparation:
- Preheat the oven to 200°C.
- Peel the celeriac and cut it into cubes or slices.
- Arrange the celeriac pieces on a baking tray. Sprinkle them with olive oil, chopped fresh rosemary, salt and pepper.
- Bake for about 25-30 minutes or until the celeriac is tender and golden.
- Serve baked celeriac as a side dish or as part of a main course.

Nutritional Values: Calories, 100-150 kcal. Protein, 1-2 g. Fat, 7-10 g. Carbohydrates, 10-15 g. Fiber, 2-4 g.

29. Cabbage Salad with Apple and Sunflower Seeds

Ingredients: Cabbage (1 small head), Apple (1, preferably a sweet variety like Fuji or Honeycrisp), Sunflower Seeds (1/4 cup), Lemon Juice (2 tablespoons), Olive Oil (2 tablespoons), Honey (1 tablespoon), Salt (to taste), Black Pepper (to taste).

Preparation:
- Finely chop the cabbage or cut it into thin slices.
- Cut the apple into thin slices or cubes.
- In a pan, gently toast the sunflower seeds.
- In a small bowl, make a vinaigrette by mixing olive oil, lemon juice, honey, salt and pepper.
- Mix the cabbage, apples and sunflower seeds in a bowl. Pour the vinaigrette over the salad and mix well.
- Refrigerate the salad for at least 30 minutes prior to serving.

Nutritional Values: Calories, 100-150 kcal. Protein, 1-2 g. Fat, 6-8 g. Carbohydrates, 10-15 g. Fiber, 2-4 g.

30. Steamed Peas with Mint and Pecorino

Ingredients: Peas (2 cups), Fresh Mint Leaves (2 tablespoons, chopped), Pecorino Cheese (1/4 cup, grated), Olive Oil (1 tablespoon), Salt (to taste), Black Pepper (to taste).

Preparation:
- Steam the peas until tender but still crunchy.
- In a skillet over a medium-high flame, melt the butter.
- Add the cooked peas and season with salt and pepper.
- Finely chop the fresh mint and sprinkle it over the peas.
- Sprinkle with grated pecorino and mix well before serving.

Nutritional Values: Calories, 100-150 kcal. Protein, 5-7 g. Fat, 4-6 g. Carbohydrates, 10-12 g. Fiber, 4-6 g.

31. Sweet Potato Salad with Red Onion and Parsley

Ingredients: Sweet Potatoes (2 cups, diced), Red Onion (1/2 cup, finely chopped), Fresh Parsley (1/4 cup, chopped), Olive Oil (2 tablespoons), Lemon Juice (1 tablespoon), Salt (to taste), Black Pepper (to taste).

Preparation:
- Peel and dice the sweet potatoes.
- Steam or boil them until they are tender but not too soft.
- While the potatoes cool, thinly slice the red onion and finely chop the fresh parsley.
- In a large bowl, combine the sweet potatoes, red onion and parsley.
- Toss with olive oil, lemon juice, salt, and pepper to taste.
- Mix well and let rest in the refrigerator before serving.

Nutritional Values: Calories, 150-200 kcal. Protein, 2-4 g. Fat, 2-3 g. Carbohydrates, 25-30 g. Fiber, 4-6 g.

32. Marinated Cucumbers with Red Wine Vinegar and Dill

Ingredients: Cucumbers (2 cups, thinly sliced), Red Wine Vinegar (1/4 cup), Fresh Dill (2 tablespoons, chopped), Sugar (1 teaspoon), Salt (1/2 teaspoon), Black Pepper (to taste).

Preparation:
- Cut the cucumbers into thin slices. In a bowl, mix the red wine vinegar, sugar and salt until the sugar dissolves completely.
- Finely chop the fresh dill. Add the cucumbers and dill to the vinegar mixture.
- Mix well. Put the container in the freezer for no less than an hour before serving.

Nutritional Values: Calories, 20-30 kcal. Protein, 1-2 g. Fat, 0 g. Carbohydrates, 3-4 g. Fiber, 1-2 g.

33. Radicchio Salad with Oranges and Pecans

Ingredients: Radicchio (2 cups, chopped), Oranges (2, peeled and segmented), Pecans (1/2 cup, chopped), Olive Oil (2 tablespoons), Balsamic Vinegar (1 tablespoon), Honey (1 tablespoon), Dijon Mustard (1 teaspoon), Salt (1/2 teaspoon), Black Pepper (to taste).

Preparation:
- Cut the radicchio into thin strips. Peel the oranges and cut them into thin slices or cubes.
- Lightly toast the pecans in a pan. In a large bowl, mix the radicchio, oranges, and toasted pecans.
- In a smaller bowl, make a vinaigrette by mixing olive oil, balsamic vinegar, honey, salt and pepper.
- Put the vinaigrette over the salad and toss to combine.

- Let the salad rest in the refrigerator for a while before serving.

Nutritional Values: Calories, 50-80 kcal. Protein, 1-2 g. Fat, 4-6 g. Carbohydrates, 5-10 g. Fiber, 2-4 g.

34. Roasted Turnip with Olive Oil and Black Pepper

Ingredients: Turnip (2 medium-sized, peeled and cubed), Olive Oil (2 tablespoons), Black Pepper (to taste), Salt (to taste).

Preparation:
- Preheat the oven to 200°C. Turnips should be peeled and cut into cubes or slices. Place the turnip pieces on a baking tray.
- Sprinkle them with olive oil, freshly ground black pepper and salt.
- Bake for about 25-30 minutes or until turnips are tender and lightly browned. Serve it as an additional dish or as part of a meal.

Nutritional Values: Calories, 50-70 kcal. Protein, 1-2 g. Fat, 3-5 g. Carbohydrates, 5-7 g. Fiber, 2-3 g.

35. Pomegranate Salad with Avocado and Almonds

Ingredients: Pomegranate Seeds (1 cup), Avocado (1, diced), Almonds (1/2 cup, sliced), Olive Oil (2 tablespoons), Lemon Juice (1 tablespoon), Honey (1 tablespoon), Salt (to taste), Black Pepper (to taste).

Preparation:
- Peel and cut the avocado into cubes and place it in a bowl.
- Toss the avocado with the pomegranate seeds. Toast the almonds in a dry pan until lightly browned and then roughly chop them.
- In a separate bowl, combine lemon juice, olive oil, chopped fresh parsley, salt and pepper to make a vinaigrette.
- Pour the vinaigrette over the avocado and pomegranate. Add the toasted almonds and mix well. Serve the salad cold.

Nutritional Values: Calories, 250-350 kcal. Protein, 3-5 g. Fat, 20-25 g. Carbohydrates, 15-20 g. Fiber, 7-9 g.

36. Grilled Beets with Goat Cheese and Parsley

Ingredients: Beets (4, medium-sized), Goat Cheese (1/2 cup, crumbled), Fresh Parsley (1/4 cup, chopped), Olive Oil (2 tablespoons), Balsamic Vinegar (1 tablespoon), Salt (to taste), Black Pepper (to taste).

Preparation:
- Preheat grill to medium-high heat.
- Peel and cut the beets into thin slices.
- Brush the beetroot slices with olive oil and grill until tender and have grill marks.
- Set up the cooked slices on a platter to serve.
- Crumble goat cheese over grilled beets.
- Sprinkle fresh chopped parsley and season with salt, pepper and an additional drizzle of olive oil, if desired.

Nutritional Values: Calories, 150-200 kcal. Protein, 7-10 g. Fat, 10-15 g. Carbohydrates, 15-20 g. Fiber, 4-6 g.

37. Baked courgettes with garlic and chilli

Ingredients: Courgettes (4, medium-sized), Garlic (4 cloves, minced), Red Chilli (1, finely chopped), Olive Oil (2 tablespoons), Salt (to taste), Black Pepper (to taste).

Preparation:
- Preheat the oven to 200°C.
- Cut the courgettes into rounds or sticks.
- In a bowl, mix the courgettes with minced garlic, red chili pepper (to taste), olive oil, salt and pepper.

- Place the seasoned courgettes on a baking tray.
- Bake for about 15-20 minutes or until the courgettes are tender and lightly browned.

Nutritional Values: Calories, 50-80 kcal. Protein, 1-3 g. Fat, 2-4 g. Carbohydrates, 7-12 g. Fiber, 2-4 g.

38. Avocado and Cherry Tomato Salad with Parsley

Ingredients: Avocado (2, ripe), Cherry Tomatoes (1 cup), Fresh Parsley (1/2 cup, chopped), Olive Oil (2 tablespoons), Lemon Juice (1 tablespoon), Salt (to taste), Black Pepper (to taste).

Preparation:

- Cube the avocado and reduce the cherry tomatoes in half. In a bowl, combine the avocado and cherry tomatoes.
- Finely chop the fresh parsley and add it to the avocado and tomatoes.
- Squeeze lemon juice over the salad and season with olive oil, salt and pepper. Mix gently and serve.

Nutritional Values: Calories, 150-180 kcal. Protein, 2-3 g. Fat, 13-15 g. Carbohydrates, 9-12 g. Fiber, 5-7 g.

39. Steamed Broccoli with Lemon and Almonds

Ingredients: Broccoli (1 pound, steamed), Lemon Zest (1 lemon, grated), Almonds (1/4 cup, sliced and toasted), Olive Oil (2 tablespoons), Lemon Juice (2 tablespoons), Salt (to taste), Black Pepper (to taste).

Preparation:

- Steam broccoli up until tender but not mushy. Lightly toast the almonds in a dry pan and then chop them coarsely.
- Squeeze lemon juice over the steamed broccoli and sprinkle with the toasted almonds.
- Sprinkle with olive oil and season according to preference with salt and pepper. Mix well and serve.

Nutritional Values: Calories, 50-70 kcal. Protein, 2-4 g. Fat, 2-4 g. Carbohydrates, 5-8 g. Fiber, 3-4 g.

40. Chickpea Salad with Dried Tomatoes and Kalamata Olives

Ingredients: Chickpeas (1 can, drained and rinsed), Dried Tomatoes (1/2 cup, chopped), Kalamata Olives (1/4 cup, pitted and sliced), Red Onion (1/4 cup, finely chopped), Fresh Parsley (1/4 cup, chopped), Olive Oil (3 tablespoons), Red Wine Vinegar (2 tablespoons), Garlic (1 clove, minced), Dried Oregano (1 teaspoon), Salt (to taste), Black Pepper (to taste).

Preparation:

- Rinse and drain the canned chickpeas.
- Cut the dried tomatoes and kalamata olives into small pieces.
- In a large bowl, combine the chickpeas, sun-dried tomatoes and olives.
- Make a vinaigrette by mixing olive oil, lemon juice, salt and pepper. Put the vinaigrette over the salad and toss to combine.
- You can add chopped fresh parsley as a garnish if desired.

Nutritional Values: Calories, 180-220 kcal. Protein, 5-7 g. Fat, 12-14 g. Carbohydrates, 15-18 g. Fiber, 4-6 g.

41. Steamed Baby Carrots with Butter and Fresh Thyme

Ingredients: Baby Carrots (1 pound), Butter (2 tablespoons), Fresh Thyme Leaves (1 tablespoon), Salt (to taste), Black Pepper (to taste).

Preparation:

- Peel the baby carrots if necessary and steam them until tender.
- Melt the butter in a skillet over a medium-low flame. Add the carrots to the melted butter and add the fresh thyme.
- Season with salt and pepper to taste. Cook for a few minutes to absorb the flavor of the butter and thyme.
- Serve hot as a side dish.

Nutritional Values: Calories, 80-100 kcal. Protein, 1-2 g. Fat, 6-8 g. Carbohydrates, 6-10 g. Fiber, 2-4 g.

42. Spinach Salad with Strawberries and Toasted Walnuts

Ingredients: Spinach (6 cups), Strawberries (1 cup, sliced), Walnuts (1/2 cup, toasted), Balsamic Vinaigrette (1/4 cup), Feta Cheese (1/4 cup, crumbled), Red Onion (1/4 cup, thinly sliced), Salt (to taste), Black Pepper (to taste).

Preparation:

- Wash and dry fresh spinach.
- Cut the strawberries into slices.
- Toast the walnuts in a dry pan and then chop them coarsely.
- In a large bowl, combine the spinach, strawberries and toasted walnuts. Add goat cheese if desired.
- Make the vinaigrette by mixing olive oil, balsamic vinegar, honey, salt and pepper. Put the vinaigrette over the salad and toss to combine.

Nutritional Values: Calories, 150-200 kcal. Protein, 3-5 g. Fat, 10-15 g. Carbohydrates, 15-20 g. Fiber, 4-6 g.

43. Roasted Champignon Mushrooms with Olive Oil and Rosemary

Ingredients: Champignon Mushrooms (8 oz), Olive Oil (2 tablespoons), Fresh Rosemary (1-2 sprigs), Salt (to taste), Black Pepper (to taste).

Preparation:

- Clean the button mushrooms and cut them into slices or quarters, depending on their size.
- In a bowl, mix the mushrooms with olive oil, fresh rosemary leaves, salt and pepper.
- Place the mushrooms on a baking tray and cook in a preheated 200°C oven until golden and tender, stirring occasionally.

Nutritional Values: Calories, 70-90 kcal. Protein, 1-3 g. Fat, 5-7 g. Carbohydrates, 4-6 g. Fiber, 1-2 g.

44. Avocado, Cucumber and Tomato Salad with Fresh Mint

Ingredients: Avocado (1, diced), Cucumber (1, diced), Tomato (1, diced), Fresh Mint Leaves (2 tablespoons, chopped), Olive Oil (2 tablespoons), Lime Juice (1 tablespoon), Salt (to taste), Black Pepper (to taste).

Preparation:

- Peel and dice the avocado, cucumber and tomato.
- Finely chop the fresh mint leaves.
- In a large bowl, combine the avocado, cucumber and tomato. Add the chopped mint.
- Make a vinaigrette by mixing olive oil, lemon juice, salt and pepper.
- Put the vinaigrette over the salad and toss to combine.

Nutritional Values: Calories, 120-150 kcal. Protein, 2-3 g. Fat, 10-12 g. Carbohydrates, 8-10 g. Fiber, 4-5 g.

45. Baked Red Turnip with Ginger and Rosemary

Ingredients: Red Turnip (1, sliced), Fresh Ginger (1 tablespoon, minced), Rosemary (1 teaspoon, chopped), Olive Oil (2 tablespoons), Salt (to taste), Black Pepper (to taste).

Preparation:
- Preheat the oven to 200°C.
- Peel and dice the red turnips.
- Grate some fresh ginger and chop the rosemary.
- In a bowl, mix the red turnips with the olive oil, grated ginger, fresh rosemary, salt and pepper to taste.
- Spread the turnips onto a baking tray and cook in the preheated oven until tender and lightly browned.

Nutritional Values: Calories, 45-60 kcal. Protein, 1-2 g. Fat, 0-1 g. Carbohydrates, 10-12 g. Fiber, 2-3 g.

46. Black Bean Salad with Corn and Chilli

Ingredients: Black Beans (1 can, drained and rinsed), Corn Kernels (1 cup, fresh or frozen), Red Chilli (1, finely chopped), Red Onion (1/2, finely chopped), Fresh Cilantro (1/4 cup, chopped), Lime Juice (2 tablespoons), Olive Oil (2 tablespoons), Salt (to taste), Black Pepper (to taste).

Preparation:
- Wash and drain canned black beans and corn.
- Chop fresh chili pepper if desired.
- Finely slice the red onion and chop the fresh coriander.
- In a large bowl, combine the black beans, corn, chili pepper (if using), red onion and cilantro.
- Make a vinaigrette by mixing olive oil, lime juice, salt and pepper. Put the vinaigrette over the salad and toss to combine.

Nutritional Values: Calories, 150-200 kcal. Protein, 6-8 g. Fat, 2-4 g. Carbohydrates, 30-35 g. Fiber, 6-8 g.

47. Grilled Eggplant with Peppers and Red Onion

Ingredients: Eggplants (2, sliced), Red Bell Peppers (2, sliced), Red Onion (1, sliced), Olive Oil (3 tablespoons), Balsamic Vinegar (2 tablespoons), Garlic (2 cloves, minced), Fresh Basil (2 tablespoons, chopped), Salt (to taste), Black Pepper (to taste).

Preparation:
- Cut the aubergines into slices and the peppers into strips.
- Thinly slice the red onion.
- In a bowl, toss the eggplant, peppers and onion with olive oil, salt and pepper.
- Heat a grill or nonstick skillet and grill vegetables until soft and lightly smoky.

Nutritional Values: Calories, 80-100 kcal. Protein, 2-3 g. Fat, 4-5 g. Carbohydrates, 10-15 g. Fiber, 3-4 g.

48. Avocado and Cherry Tomato Salad with Basil and Black Olives

Ingredients: Avocados (2, diced), Cherry Tomatoes (1 cup, halved), Black Olives (1/2 cup, pitted and sliced), Fresh Basil Leaves (1/4 cup, chopped), Extra Virgin Olive Oil (2 tablespoons), Balsamic Vinegar (1 tablespoon), Salt (to taste), Black Pepper (to taste).

Preparation:
- Dice the avocado and cherry tomatoes.
- Chop the fresh basil and cut the black olives into slices.
- In a bowl, combine the avocado, cherry tomatoes, basil and black olives.
- Make a vinaigrette by mixing olive oil, lemon juice, salt and pepper. Put the vinaigrette over the salad and toss to combine.

Nutritional Values: Calories, 150-180 kcal. Protein, 2-3 g. Fat, 12-14 g. Carbohydrates, 8-10 g. Fiber, 4-5 g.

49. Pan-fried courgettes with garlic and parsley

Ingredients: Courgettes (2, thinly sliced), Garlic Cloves (2, minced), Fresh Parsley (2 tablespoons, chopped), Olive Oil (2 tablespoons), Salt (to taste), Black Pepper (to taste).

Preparation:
- Cut the courgettes into thin slices.
- Finely chop the garlic and fresh parsley.
- In a pan, heat the olive oil and fry the garlic until golden.
- Add the courgettes to the pan and cook until tender and lightly browned.
- Add chopped fresh parsley, salt and pepper to taste before serving.

Nutritional Values: Calories, 60-80 kcal. Protein, 1-2 g. Fat, 4-6 g. Carbohydrates, 5-7 g. Fiber, 2-3 g.

50. Lentil Salad with Carrots and Baby Spinach

Ingredients: Green Lentils (1 cup, cooked and drained), Carrots (2, finely diced), Baby Spinach (2 cups, fresh), Red Onion (1/2, finely chopped), Olive Oil (3 tablespoons), Balsamic Vinegar (2 tablespoons), Dijon Mustard (1 teaspoon), Salt (1/2 teaspoon), Black Pepper (1/4 teaspoon).

Preparation:
- Cook the lentils according to the instructions on the package, then drain them and let them cool.
- Peel and grate the carrots, then cut them into thin slices.
- In a large bowl, combine the cooked lentils, carrots and baby spinach.
- Make a vinaigrette by mixing olive oil, balsamic vinegar, salt and pepper. Put the vinaigrette over the salad and toss to combine.

Nutritional Values: Calories, 180-220 kcal. Protein, 10-12 g. Fat, 2-4 g. Carbohydrates, 30-35 g. Fiber, 7-9 g.

51. Baked Brussels Sprouts with Olive Oil and Black Pepper

Ingredients: Brussels Sprouts (1 pound, trimmed and halved), Olive Oil (2 tablespoons), Black Pepper (1/2 teaspoon), Salt (1/2 teaspoon).

Preparation:
- Preheat the oven to 200°C.
- Clean and divide the Brussels sprouts in half.
- Arrange the sprouts on a baking sheet and season them with olive oil, salt and black pepper.
- Cook in the preheated oven until the sprouts are golden brown and tender.

Nutritional Values: Calories, 70-90 kcal. Protein, 3-4 g. Fat, 3-4 g. Carbohydrates, 10-12 g. Fiber, 3-4 g.

Chapter 10: Main Dishes-Dinner

100 Anti-Inflammatory Main Dish Recipes for Dinner

Welcome to the chapter dedicated to 100 anti-inflammatory dinner recipes. In this section of our book, we will explore a wide range of delicious and healthy dishes, specially designed to help you maintain a fit and healthy body by reducing inflammation in your body. On the next few pages, you'll find an assortment of recipes that use fresh, nutritious ingredients known for their anti-inflammatory properties. These dishes will not only help reduce inflammation in your body, but they are also tasty and satisfying. It will be a pleasure for your taste buds to discover how ingredients such as omega-3-rich salmon, aromatic spices and nutritious vegetables can be combined in delicious and health-promoting ways.

Each recipe has been carefully selected and prepared to help you create balanced, nutritious meals for you and your family. Whether you are a cooking enthusiast or a beginner, you are sure to find something here that will inspire you to experiment in the kitchen and enjoy the process of preparing meals.

1. Baked salmon with lemon and rosemary sauce

Ingredients: Salmon Fillets (4, about 6 ounces each), Lemon Juice (3 tablespoons), Olive Oil (2 tablespoons), Fresh Rosemary (1 tablespoon, chopped), Garlic (2 cloves, minced), Salt (1/2 teaspoon), Black Pepper (1/4 teaspoon), Lemon Zest (1 tablespoon), Lemon Slices (for garnish).

Preparation:

- Preheat the oven to 180°C (350°F).
- Prepare the salmon fillets, making sure they are clean and free of bones.
- In a small bowl, combine the lemon juice, olive oil, chopped rosemary, salt and pepper. This is going to be the salmon marinade.
- Place the salmon fillets on a lightly greased baking tray or one lined with baking paper.
- Brush the lemon-rosemary marinade evenly over the salmon fillets.
- Place the pan in the preheated oven and cook for about 15-20 minutes or until the salmon is soft and flakes easily with a fork.
- While cooking, you can additionally brush the salmon with the marinade to keep it juicy.
- Remove the salmon from the heated oven and set aside for a few minutes before being served.
- You can decorate with lemon slices and sprigs of fresh rosemary if desired.

Nutritional Values (per serving): Calories: 280 kcal, Protein: 28g, Fat: 18g, Carbohydrates: 2g, Fiber: 1g

2. Beef steak with red wine sauce and mushrooms

Ingredients: Beef steak (200g each), fresh mushrooms (200g, sliced), olive oil (1 tablespoon), onion (1/2, finely chopped), garlic (1 clove, finely chopped), dry red wine (1 cup), meat broth (1/2 cup), butter (2 tablespoons), salt and black pepper (to taste), chopped fresh parsley (for garnish).

Preparation:

- Bring the beef steaks to room temperature by leaving them out of the refrigerator for about 30 minutes before cooking. This allows for uniform cooking.
- Heat the olive oil in a large skillet over a medium-high flame and cook the steaks for three to four minutes per side (for medium rare).
- Adjust the cooking time as desired.
- Remove the steaks from the pan and keep warm by covering them with aluminum foil.
- Melt the butter in the same pan. Add chopped onion and garlic and cook for 2-3 minutes until golden brown.
- Add the sliced mushrooms and cook for a further 5 minutes until soft and have released their juices.
- Bring the red wine to boiling point in a small saucepan. Reduce the heat and cook for about 10 minutes until the wine is reduced by half.
- Add the beef broth and cook for a further 5 minutes until the sauce has thickened slightly.
- Return the steaks to the pan for a few minutes to reheat and coat with the sauce.
- Serve the beef steaks with the red wine and mushroom sauce on top, garnished with chopped fresh parsley. Change the seasoning with salt and freshly ground black pepper to taste.

Nutritional Values (per serving): Calories: 450kcal, Protein: 30g, Fat: 28g, Carbohydrates: 12g, Fiber: 2g.

3. Grilled tilapia with basil and tomato sauce

Ingredients: Tilapia (4 fillets), ripe tomatoes (2 large, diced), fresh basil leaves (1 cup, chopped), garlic (2 cloves, chopped), lemon juice (2 tablespoons), olive oil (2 tablespoons), salt and black pepper (to taste).

Preparation:

- Preheat the grill to medium-high heat and lightly brush the grill with a little olive oil to prevent the fish from sticking.
- In a bowl, combine diced tomatoes, chopped basil leaves, minced garlic, lemon juice, olive oil, salt and black pepper to make the sauce.
- Brush the tilapia fillets on both sides with a little olive oil and season with salt and black pepper to taste.
- Place the tilapia fillets on the preheated grill and cook for about 3 to 4 minutes per side or until the fish flakes easily with a fork and has dark streaks from the grill.
- While the fish cooks, heat the tomato basil sauce in a saucepan over medium-low heat for a few minutes until hot.
- Once cooked, transfer the grilled tilapia to a serving platter and cover with the hot tomato basil sauce.
- Garnish with fresh basil leaves and serve the grilled tilapia with the sauce as a condiment.

Nutritional Values (per serving): Calories: 200kcal, Protein: 30g, Fat: 8g, Carbohydrates: 6g, Fiber: 2g.

4. Chicken tacos with avocado and corn

Ingredients:

Skinless chicken breast (2 breasts, cut into thin strips), Ripe avocado (1, peeled, pitted and sliced), Canned corn (1 cup, drained), Cherry tomatoes (1 cup, halved), Onion red lettuce (1/2, chopped), Jalapeño pepper (1, seeded and chopped), Iceberg lettuce leaves (4 leaves, washed and dried), Corn or flour tortillas (8 pieces, reheated), Olive oil (2 tablespoons),Lime juice (1 lime, squeezed),Fresh coriander (2 tablespoons, chopped),Black pepper (to taste),Salt (to taste)

Preparation:

- In a nonstick skillet, heat the olive oil over medium-high heat. Add the chicken breast strips and cook until golden brown and cooked through, about 5 to 7 minutes per side. Season the chicken with salt and black pepper to taste.

- While the chicken cooks, make the sauce by mixing the cherry tomatoes, red onion, jalapeño pepper, lime juice and chopped cilantro in a bowl. If desired, season with salt.
- Once the chicken is cooked, remove from the heat and cut it into thin slices.
- To assemble the tacos, heat the tortillas and spread the chicken evenly on each tortilla.
- Add the avocado slices, corn and lettuce leaves.
- Pour the prepared sauce over each taco.
- Fold the tortillas to close the tacos and serve hot.

Nutritional Values (per serving, excluding tortilla values): Calories: 250kcal, Protein: 20g, Fat: 10g, Carbohydrates: 20g, Fiber: 6g.

5. Grilled pork with mango and chili sauce

Ingredients: 4 pork steaks (approximately 150 g each), 2 ripe mangoes, peeled, pitted and diced, 1 finely chopped red chili pepper, 2 tablespoons olive oil, Juice of 2 limes, 2 tablespoons honey, 1 teaspoon of fresh grated ginger, salt and black pepper to taste.

For the side dish: 2 cups of cooked quinoa, 1 cup of green beans cut into pieces, 1 teaspoon of olive oil, Salt and black pepper to taste.

Preparation:

- In a bowl, mix the diced mango, chopped red chili pepper, juice of 1 lime, honey and grated ginger. Adjust the seasoning with salt and freshly ground black pepper to taste.
- This will be the mango and chili sauce. Leave it aside.
- Heat an outdoor grill or indoor kitchen grill to medium-high heat.
- Brush the pork steaks with a little olive oil and sprinkle with salt and black pepper.
- Grill the pork steaks for about 4-5 minutes per side or until they are cooked through and have nice streaks from the grill.
- The duration of cooking will depend on the thickness of the steaks. An internal temperature of 70-75°C is a good indicator of safe cooking for pork.
- While the pork steaks are grilling, bring a pan of lightly salted water to a boil. Add the green beans and cook for 2-3 minutes or until tender but crunchy.
- Drain them and rinse them under cold water to stop the cooking process. Season the green beans with a teaspoon of olive oil, salt and pepper.
- When the pork steaks are done, remove them from the grill and let them rest for a few minutes before cutting them into thin slices.
- To serve, portion the cooked quinoa onto plates and place the pork slices on top of the quinoa.
- Serve with seasoned green beans and generously pour the mango and chili sauce over the pork. Top with remaining lime juice.

Nutritional Values (per serving): Calories: 450 kcal, Protein: 32 g, Fat: 14 g, Carbohydrates: 50 g, Fiber: 6 g

6. Grilled salmon with cilantro-lime sauce

Ingredients: 4 salmon fillets (about 150 g each), Juice and zest of 1 lime, 2 tablespoons of olive oil, 2 finely chopped garlic cloves, 1 teaspoon of powdered coriander, Salt and black pepper to taste, 1 /4 cup chopped fresh coriander leaves, 2 cups cooked quinoa, 2 cups steamed broccoli

Preparation:

- In a bowl, mix the lime juice and zest, olive oil, minced garlic, coriander powder, salt and black pepper. This will serve as the marinade for the salmon.
- Place the salmon fillets in a shallow baking dish and pour the marinade over them. Make sure the salmon is well covered in the marinade. Cover the pan and leave to marinate in the refrigerator for at least 30 minutes.
- Meanwhile, light an outdoor grill or indoor kitchen grill over medium-high heat. Brush the grill with a little olive oil to prevent the salmon from sticking.
- When the salmon is finished marinating, grill the fillets for about 3-4 minutes per side or until the salmon is cooked through and has nice streaks from the grill. The amount of time needed to cook will depend on the thickness of the fillets.
- While the salmon is grilling, you can reheat the cooked quinoa and steamed broccoli.
- To serve, portion the quinoa and broccoli onto plates. Place the grilled salmon on top of the bed of quinoa and broccoli. Complete the dish with a generous sprinkling of fresh coriander leaves.

Nutritional Values (per serving): Calories: 350 kcal, Protein: 30 g, Fat: 18 g, Carbohydrates: 20 g, Fiber: 4 g

7. Quinoa meatballs with tomato and basil sauce

Ingredients: 1 cup quinoa, 2 cups water, 1 egg, 1/4 cup shredded cheese (of your choice), 1/4 cup breadcrumbs, 2 tablespoons chopped fresh basil, 1 clove minced garlic finely, Salt and black pepper to taste, 2 cups of tomato sauce, Fresh basil leaves for garnish.

Preparation:

- Start by rinsing the quinoa well under running water.
- In a saucepan, bring 2 cups of water to a boil and add the rinsed quinoa.
- Reduce the heat, cover and simmer for about 15-20 minutes or until the quinoa is cooked and has absorbed the water. Let cool.
- In a bowl, mix the cooked quinoa with the egg, grated cheese, breadcrumbs, chopped fresh basil and garlic.
- Taste and adjust the amount of seasoning with pepper and salt. Shape meatballs with wet hands and arrange them on a tray.
- Heating some olive oil in a nonstick skillet over a medium-high flame. Cook the meatballs until golden brown on all sides, turning them gently.
- Meanwhile, reheat the tomato sauce in another saucepan over medium-low heat.
- Once cooked, transfer the meatballs to the hot tomato sauce.
- Simmer for about 10-15 minutes or until meatballs are heated through.
- Serve the quinoa meatballs with plenty of tomato sauce and fresh basil as a garnish.

Nutritional Values (per serving): Calories: 280 kcal, Protein: 10 g, Fat: 7 g, Carbohydrates: 45 g, Fiber: 6 g.

8. Duck breast with pomegranate

Ingredients: Duck Breasts (2), Pomegranate Juice (1 cup), Pomegranate Seeds (from 1 pomegranate), Honey (2 tablespoons), Balsamic Vinegar (2 tablespoons), Olive Oil (2 tablespoons), Salt (1 teaspoon), Black Pepper (1/2 teaspoon), Fresh Thyme (1 tablespoon, chopped).

Preparation:

- Start by preparing the duck breast. Make light cuts in the breast skin to form a checkered pattern, without cutting into the meat. This will help make it crispy while cooking.
- Heat a nonstick pan over medium-high heat. There is no need to add oil as the duck breast will release its fat.
- Put the side with the skin down duck breast in the pan. Cook for about 5-6 minutes or until the skin is golden brown and crispy.
- Turn the duck breast and cook on the other side for another 3-4 minutes to obtain rare doneness or for longer if you prefer it more done.
- Take the duck breast out of the pan and set aside for a few minutes before slicing.
- Meanwhile, prepare the pomegranate sauce. Eliminate the seeds from the pomegranate by cutting it in half.
- In a small pot, heat a drizzle of olive oil over medium-low heat. Add the pomegranate seeds and cook them for a couple of minutes.
- Lightly crush the seeds with a spoon to extract the juice and flavor.
- Add a pinch of brown sugar, salt and black pepper to the pomegranate seeds. Cook for another 2-3 minutes until the sauce is slightly thick.
- Make thin slices of the duck breast.
- Serve the duck breast slices with the pomegranate sauce poured over the top.

Nutritional Values (per serving): Calories: 300 kcal, Proteins: 25g, Fats: 20g, Carbohydrates: 8g, Sugars: 6g

9. Tuna steak with mint sauce

Ingredients: Tuna Steaks (2), Fresh Mint Leaves (1/4 cup, chopped), Olive Oil (2 tablespoons), Lemon Juice (2 tablespoons), Garlic (2 cloves, minced), Salt (1/2 teaspoon), Black Pepper (1/4 teaspoon).

Preparation:

- Start by making the mint sauce. Finely chop the fresh mint leaves and place them in a bowl.
- Add the minced garlic, lemon juice, extra virgin olive oil, sea salt and black pepper to the bowl with the mint.
- Mix all the sauce ingredients well until you obtain a smooth mixture. Let the sauce sit while you prepare the tuna.
- Heat a nonstick skillet or grill over medium-high heat.
- Brush both sides of the tuna steak with a drizzle of olive oil and season with a pinch of salt and black pepper.
- When the pan or grill is hot, cook the tuna steak for about 2-3 minutes per side. The tuna should be pink in the center for rare. Cook for longer if you prefer it less raw.
- Remove the tuna steak from the pan or grill and let rest for a minute.
- Serve the tuna steak with a generous dollop of the mint sauce on top.

Nutritional Values (per serving): Calories: 300 kcal, Protein: 40g, Fat: 15g, Carbohydrates: 2g, Fibre: 1g

10. Turkey meatballs with yogurt and cucumber sauce

Ingredients: Ground Turkey (1 pound), Bread Crumbs (1/2 cup), Onion (1 small, finely chopped), Garlic (2 cloves, minced), Egg (1), Fresh Parsley (2 tablespoons, chopped), Salt (1/2 teaspoon), Black Pepper (1/4 teaspoon), Greek Yogurt (1 cup), Cucumber (1/2, grated and squeezed dry), Lemon Juice (2 tablespoons), Dill (1 tablespoon, fresh and chopped), Olive Oil (2 tablespoons).

Preparation:

- In a large bowl, combine the ground turkey, chopped red onion, minced garlic, breadcrumbs, chopped fresh parsley and egg. Add a generous amount of salt and black pepper.
- Mix the ingredients well until you obtain a homogeneous mixture.
- Take small portions of dough and shape round meatballs with your hands. Arrange them on a tray lightly greased with olive oil.
- Heat a non-stick pan over medium-high heat with a drizzle of extra virgin olive oil.
- Once the pan is hot, add the meatballs and cook for about 4-5 minutes per side or until golden brown and fully cooked.
- Meanwhile, prepare the yogurt and cucumber sauce. Grate the cucumber and squeeze it to remove excess water.
- In a bowl, mix Greek yogurt, grated cucumber, lemon juice and chopped fresh mint. Add salt and pepper to taste.
- Serve the turkey meatballs hot with the yogurt and cucumber sauce on the side.

Nutritional Values (per serving): Calories: 280 kcal, Protein: 25g, Fat: 12g, Carbohydrates: 18g, Fiber: 2g

11. Fish tacos with cabbage slaw

Ingredients: White Fish Fillets (e.g., cod or tilapia, 1 pound), Flour Tortillas (8 small-sized), Green Cabbage (3 cups, shredded), Carrots (2, grated), Fresh Cilantro (1/2 cup, chopped), Lime Juice (2 limes), Sour Cream (1/2 cup), Mayonnaise (1/2 cup), Ground Cumin (1 teaspoon), Ground Paprika (1 teaspoon), Ground Cayenne Pepper (1/2 teaspoon), Salt (1/2 teaspoon), Black Pepper (1/4 teaspoon), Olive Oil (2 tablespoons).

Preparation:

- Start by making the cabbage slaw. Finely chop the green cabbage, carrots and red onion. Mix together all of this in a large mixing a bowl.
- In another bowl, prepare the sauce by mixing light mayonnaise, lime juice, chopped fresh cilantro, black pepper, sweet paprika, cumin powder, garlic powder and salt to taste.
- Pour the sauce over the cabbage, carrot and onion mix. Mix well so that all the ingredients are well coated with the sauce. Set the slaw aside.
- Cook the fish fillets. You can make this by grilling, pan-frying with a little olive oil, or baking until the fish flakes easily with a fork.
- While the fish cooks, heat the corn or flour tortillas in a hot skillet or in the microwave.
- Assemble the tacos: Take a tortilla, top with a portion of cooked fish and a layer of cabbage slaw. You can add extras like avocado pieces, hot sauce or lime slices, to taste.
- Repeat for the other tacos.
- Serve fish tacos with cabbage slaw and enjoy your meal!

Nutritional Values (per serving, excluding extras such as avocado or hot sauce): Calories: 300 kcal, Protein: 20g, Fat: 10g, Carbohydrates: 30g, Fiber: 4g

12. Beef steak with green pepper sauce

Ingredients: Beef steak (200g), olive oil, salt, black pepper, butter, red onion (1/2), garlic (2 cloves), cooking cream, green peppercorns, brandy (optional).

Preparation:

- Start by bringing the sirloin steak to room temperature at least 30 minutes before cooking. This will allow for even cooking.
- Using a nonstick skillet, heat a drizzle of olive oil over medium to high heat. While the pan heats, rub the steak with salt and plenty of black pepper. Lightly press the pepper into the meat to help it stick.
- When the pan is warm, add the steak to it. Cook for desired doneness (for medium-rare, about 3-4 minutes per side). Remember to turn the steak only once during cooking.
- Remove the steak from the pan and set aside to rest, covered with aluminum foil to keep warm.
- In the same pan, reduce the heat to medium-low and add the butter, finely chopped red onion and crushed garlic. Cook until the onions are tender.
- Add the green peppercorns and brandy (if using). Let the alcohol evaporate.
- Pour the cooking cream into the pan and mix well. Allow to cook until the sauce thickens slightly. Cut the steak into thin slices and arrange on a serving plate.
- Pour the green pepper sauce over the steak slices.
- Serve the sirloin steak with hot green pepper sauce.

Nutritional Values (per serving): Calories: 400 kcal, Protein: 30g, Fat: 28g, Carbohydrates: 6g, Fiber: 1g

13. Grilled chicken with orange and rosemary sauce

Ingredients: Chicken breast (2 pieces), oranges (2), fresh rosemary (2 tablespoons, chopped), garlic (2 cloves, chopped), olive oil, salt, black pepper.

Preparation:

- Prepare the marinade: grate the zest of the oranges and squeeze the juice from both.
- In a bowl, mix the juice and grated zest of the oranges with the chopped rosemary, chopped garlic, 2 tablespoons of olive oil, salt and black pepper to taste.
- Pour the marinade over the chicken breasts and cover them tightly. Leave to marinate in the fridge for at least 30 minutes or ideally for up to 4 hours.
- Preheat the grill to medium-high heat and brush the grates with a little oil to prevent the chicken from sticking.
- Drain the chicken from the marinade and place it on the grill. Cook for about 6-8 minutes per side or until the chicken is fully cooked and has nice streaks from the grill.
- Make sure the chicken is an internal temperature of 165°F. While the chicken cooks, bring the marinade to a boil in a small saucepan. Boil for a few minutes until the sauce reduces slightly and becomes thicker.
- Once cooked, transfer the grilled chicken to a serving platter and pour the orange-rosemary sauce over the top.
- Serve the grilled chicken with hot orange and rosemary sauce.

Nutritional Values (per serving): Calories: 300 kcal, Protein: 30g, Fat: 10g, Carbohydrates: 20g, Fiber: 4g

14. Turmeric tofu with peppers and onions

Ingredients: Tofu (350g, diced), peppers (2, cut into strips), onion (1, thinly sliced), olive oil, turmeric powder (1 teaspoon), smoked paprika (1/2 teaspoon), salt, black pepper, fresh parsley (optional, for garnish).

Preparation:

- In a bowl, mix the cubed tofu with the turmeric powder, smoked paprika, salt and black pepper. Make sure the tofu is well coated in the spices. Leave to marinate for at least 15-20 minutes.
- In a large nonstick skillet, heat a couple tablespoons of olive oil over medium-high heat.
- Add the marinated tofu and fry until golden brown on all sides, turning occasionally. It will take about 5-7 minutes.
- Take the tofu out of the pan and set it aside.In the same pan, add a little olive oil if necessary and add the onion slices and pepper strips.
- Cook for 5 to 7 minutes or until the vegetables are soft and lightly browned. Return the tofu to the pan with the vegetables and mix well.
- Cook for an additional 2-3 minutes to let the flavors meld.
- Serve the turmeric tofu with peppers and onions hot, garnished with fresh parsley if desired.

Nutritional Values (per serving): Calories: 250 kcal, Protein: 15g, Fat: 15g, Carbohydrates: 15g, Fiber: 5g

15. Tuna steak with papaya sauce

Ingredients: Tuna steak (2 fillets of approximately 150g each), papaya (1, ripe and peeled), red onion (1/2, finely chopped), red chili pepper (1/2, finely chopped), lime (the juice of 2 limes), fresh coriander (a handful, chopped), salt, black pepper, extra virgin olive oil.

Preparation:

- Start by making the papaya sauce. Cut the papaya into cubes and place it in a large bowl.
- Add the chopped red onion and red chili to the papaya.
- Squeeze the juice of the two limes onto the fruit and vegetables and mix everything well. Add chopped coriander and a pinch of salt and black pepper. Mix again and leave aside.
- Preheat a grill or a nonstick skillet to medium-high heat.
- Lightly brush the tuna fillets with a little olive oil and season with salt and black pepper to taste.
- Cook the tuna on the grill or in the pan for about 2-3 minutes per side. The tuna should remain pink inside.
- Serve the grilled tuna fillets with the papaya sauce on top and garnish with a few fresh coriander leaves.

Nutritional Values (per serving): Calories: 300 kcal, Protein: 30g, Fat: 8g, Carbohydrates: 30g, Fiber: 5g

16. Baked salmon with chili lime sauce

Ingredients: Salmon (4 fillets of approximately 150g each), fresh red chili pepper (1, finely chopped), garlic (2 cloves, chopped), lime (the juice of 2 limes), honey (2 tablespoons), soy sauce (2 tablespoons), fresh ginger (1 teaspoon, grated), extra virgin olive oil, salt, black pepper, fresh parsley (for garnish).

Preparation:

- Preheat the oven to 180°C and prepare a baking sheet with parchment paper on it.
- In a bowl, mix the crushed red chili pepper, minced garlic, lime juice, honey, soy sauce and grated ginger to make the marinade.

- Place the salmon fillets in the prepared baking dish and season with salt and black pepper to taste.
- Pour the marinade over the salmon, making sure each fillet is well coated.
- Wrap the baking dish in aluminum foil and bake for 15-20 minutes, or until the salmon has been cooked and it flakes easily with a fork.
- Meanwhile, prepare the chili lime sauce. In a small saucepan, heat some olive oil and add the chili pepper
- remaining chopped red. Cook over low heat for a few minutes until fragrant.
- Add the remaining lime juice and cook for another minute.
- Serve the salmon fillets with the chili lime sauce on top and garnish with some chopped fresh parsley.

Nutritional Values (per serving): Calories: 350 kcal, Protein: 30g, Fat: 20g, Carbohydrates: 15g, Fiber: 1g

17. Chicken curry with coconut and pineapple

Ingredients: Chicken breast (2 breasts, diced), onion (1, chopped), garlic (2 cloves, chopped), fresh ginger (1 teaspoon, grated), red chili pepper (1, finely chopped), curry powder (2 tablespoons), coconut milk (400 ml), pineapple (200g, cut into cubes), extra virgin olive oil, salt, black pepper, fresh parsley (for garnish).

Preparation:

- In a large nonstick skillet, heat some olive oil over medium heat. Cook the onion for 5 minutes or until it becomes transparent.
- Add minced garlic, grated ginger and crushed red chili to the pan. Cook for about 2 minutes or until they release their aroma.
- Add the curry powder and mix well for about a minute.
- Cook until the chicken breast cubes become golden on all sides in the skillet. Pour the coconut milk into the pan and mix well with the chicken and spices. Let cook for about 10-15 minutes over medium-low heat or until the chicken is cooked and the sauce has thickened.
- Add the pineapple cubes to the pan and stir gently. Let cook for another 2-3 minutes to heat the pineapple.
- For tasting, season with salt and pepper to your liking. Serve the chicken curry with coconut and pineapple on a bed of brown rice or quinoa, garnished with chopped fresh parsley.

Nutritional Values (per serving): Calories: 380 kcal, Protein: 30g, Fat: 20g, Carbohydrates: 20g, Fiber: 3g

18. Beef steak with truffle sauce

Ingredients: Beef steak (2 pieces, approx. 2.5 cm thick), sea salt, black pepper, extra virgin olive oil, fresh porcini mushrooms (200g, sliced), shallots (1, finely chopped), non-salted butter salted (2 tablespoons), fresh cream (120 ml), white truffle sauce (2 tablespoons), fresh parsley (for garnish).

Preparation:

- Preheat the oven to 200°C.
- Before cooking steaks, make sure they are at room temperature. You can leave them out of the refrigerator for about 30 minutes before cooking.
- Heat an ovenproof skillet over medium-high heat. Incorporate a little extra virgin olive oil.
- Season the steaks on each side with sea salt and freshly ground black pepper.

- Once the pan is hot, add the steaks and cook for about 2-3 minutes per side to achieve even browning.
- Transfer the pan with steaks to the preheated oven and cook for an additional 5 to 7 minutes for medium-rare, or longer depending on your desired doneness. (Cooking time will vary based on thickness of steaks and personal preference.)
- While the steaks rest, prepare the truffle sauce. In the same pan, add the butter and chopped shallots. Brown everything for about 2 minutes.
- Add the sliced porcini mushrooms and cook until soft and golden.
- Pour the fresh cream and white truffle sauce into the pan with the mushrooms. Mix well and cook for a further 2-3 minutes until the sauce has thickened slightly.
- Try the sauce and season with salt and pepper as needed. Pour the truffle sauce over the steaks.
- Sprinkle with fresh parsley and serve quickly.

Nutritional Values (per serving): Calories: 450 kcal, Protein: 36g, Fat: 30g, Carbohydrates: 7g, Fiber: 1g

19. Turkey meatballs with avocado sauce

Ingredients: Ground turkey (500g), breadcrumbs (1/2 cup), egg (1), red onion (1, finely chopped), garlic (2 cloves, finely chopped), fresh parsley (2 tablespoons, chopped), salt marine (1/2 teaspoon), black pepper (1/2 teaspoon), extra virgin olive oil (2 tablespoons), avocado (2, peeled and pitted), lime juice (1), Greek yogurt (120 ml), garlic powder (1/2 teaspoon), cumin powder (1/2 teaspoon), smoked paprika (1/2 teaspoon), salt (1/2 teaspoon), black pepper (1/4 teaspoon), fresh parsley (for garnish).

Preparation:

- In a large bowl, combine the ground turkey, breadcrumbs, egg, red onion, garlic, parsley, sea salt and black pepper. Check that all of the ingredients are properly incorporated.
- Take a small amount of the turkey mixture and shape it into round patties with your hands. Repeat the process until you run out of dough.
- In a nonstick skillet over a medium-high flame, warmth the olive oil. Add the turkey meatballs to the skillet and cook for about 4-5 minutes per side or until cooked through and golden brown.
- While the meatballs are cooking, prepare the avocado sauce. In a blender, combine the avocado, lime juice, Greek yogurt, and garlic
- powder, cumin powder, smoked paprika, salt and black pepper. Mix until a creamy sauce forms.
- Serve the turkey meatballs hot, accompanied by the avocado sauce. Garnish with chopped fresh parsley.

Nutritional Values (per serving, excluding sauce): Calories: 250 kcal, Protein: 25g, Fat: 10g, Carbohydrates: 16g, Fiber: 2g

20. Fish tacos with orange and cilantro salsa

Ingredients: White fish fillets (600g, e.g. cod or sea bass), corn tortillas (8), lettuce leaves (1 cup, chopped), red onion (1/2, thinly sliced), fresh coriander (1/2 cup, chopped), orange (2, juice and grated peel), lemon (1, juice), extra virgin olive oil (2 tablespoons), black pepper (1/2 teaspoon), sea salt (1/2 teaspoon), green chili (1, finely chopped), garlic (2 cloves, finely chopped).

Preparation:

- In a bowl, mix the orange juice, lemon juice, grated orange peel, olive oil, black pepper, sea salt, green chile and minced garlic to create the marinade.

- Dip the fish fillets into the marinade, making sure they are well covered. Cool for at least 30 minutes to give the flavors to combine.
- While the marinated fish rests, prepare the orange and coriander sauce. In a bowl, mix the chopped fresh coriander, orange juice, grated orange peel, black pepper and salt. Set aside.
- Temperature a non-stick skillet or grill pan over a medium-high flame. Cook the marinated fish fillets for about 3-4 minutes per side or until the fish is cooked through and has a golden crust.
- Heat the corn tortillas in a hot skillet for about 20-30 seconds per side.
- To assemble the tacos, place a portion of grilled fish on each tortilla, then add chopped lettuce, thin red onion and a generous dollop of orange-cilantro salsa.
- Roll the tortillas around the filling and serve the tacos hot.

Nutritional Values (per portion, considering 2 tacos): Calories: 320 kcal, Protein: 25g, Fat: 10g, Carbohydrates: 35g, Fiber: 4g

21. Duck breast with honey and ginger sauce

Ingredients: 2 duck breasts, 2 tablespoons of honey, 1 teaspoon of grated fresh ginger, 2 tablespoons of soy sauce, 2 finely chopped garlic cloves, Salt and black pepper (to taste), chopped fresh parsley for garnish.

Preparation:
- Start by making the sauce. In a small bowl, mix honey, grated ginger, soy sauce, and minced garlic. Mix the ingredients well until you obtain a smooth sauce.
- Preheat the oven to 180°C (350°F).
- Score the skin of the duck breasts with a sharp knife to create a diagonal grid. Make sure you don't cut the meat, just the skin.
- Heat a nonstick skillet over medium-high heat. There is no need to add oil as the fat from the duck will be released during cooking. In the pan, place the duck's breasts skin side down.
- Cook the duck breasts for 4-5 minutes or until the skin is crisp and golden.
- Cook the duck breasts for an additional 2-3 minutes on the other opposite side.
- Place the duck breasts, skin side up, on a baking sheet.
- Brush the duck breasts generously with the honey-ginger sauce.
- Place the duck breasts in the preheated oven and cook for about 10-12 minutes for medium-rare, or longer if you prefer your meat rarer.
- Once cooked, remove the duck breasts from the oven and let them rest for a few minutes before cutting them into thin slices.
- Serve the duck breast cut into slices, sprinkled with fresh chopped parsley as a garnish. You can accompany the dish with side dishes such as basmati rice or grilled vegetables.

Nutritional Values (per serving): Calories: 350 kcal, Protein: 25g, Fat: 20g, Carbohydrates: 18g, Fiber: 0.5g

22. Grilled salmon with basil and garlic sauce

Ingredients: 4 salmon fillets, 2 cups fresh basil leaves, 4 cloves of garlic, 1/2 cup extra virgin olive oil, 2 tablespoons lemon juice, salt and freshly ground black pepper (to taste)

Preparation:
- Start by making the basil and garlic sauce. In a blender, add the basil leaves, garlic cloves, lemon juice, and a pinch of salt and pepper.
- Start the blender and start mixing the ingredients. While the blender is running, slowly pour in the olive oil to emulsify the sauce. Continue blending until you obtain a smooth, creamy sauce. Test and modify the salt and pepper as needed.
- Preheat grill to medium-high heat and brush lightly with oil to prevent salmon from sticking.
- Brush both sides of the salmon fillets with a little olive oil and season with salt and pepper to taste.
- Place the salmon fillets on the pre-heated grill, skin side down.
- Cook the salmon for about 4-5 minutes per side or until the meat flakes easily with a fork and is golden brown and slightly crispy on the outside.
- During the last minutes of cooking, generously brush the basil-garlic sauce over the salmon fillets.
- Remove the salmon from the grill and serve hot with additional basil and garlic sauce on top, if desired.

Nutritional Values (per serving): Calories: 350 kcal, Protein: 25g, Fat: 25g, Carbohydrates: 3g, Fiber: 1g.

23. Lemon chicken with asparagus and almonds

Ingredients: 4 chicken breasts (about 170g each), 1 bunch of fresh asparagus (about 450g) with ends split, 2 lemons (juice and zest), 1/4 cup (25g) sliced almonds, 2 tablespoons extra virgin olive oil, 2 cloves of garlic, chopped, Salt and freshly ground black pepper (to taste), fresh parsley, chopped (for garnish, to taste).

Preparation:
- Start by preparing the chicken breast. Split each chicken breast in half lengthwise, resulting in two thin slices of chicken breast from each breast. This will make the chicken more tender and quicker to cook.
- In a bowl, mix the juice and zest of a lemon with a tablespoon of olive oil, chopped garlic, a pinch of salt and pepper. This will be the marinade for the chicken.
- Dip the chicken breast slices into the marinade, making sure they are well coated. Allow for at least 15-30 minutes of marinating time.
- In the meantime, preheat a large nonstick skillet over a medium-high flame.
- Add the sliced almonds and toast lightly, stirring constantly, until golden and fragrant. Place aside the almonds in a mixing bowl.
- Pour the remaining olive oil into the same pan. Drain and add the chicken breast slices from the marinade.
- Cook the chicken for about 3-4 minutes per side or until browned and cooked through. To maintain the chicken warm, put it on a plate and protect with foil.
- In the same pan, add the split asparagus and cook for about 5-7 minutes or until tender but still crunchy. You can add a little water to create steam and cover with a lid to cook them faster.
- Once the asparagus is cooked, remove it from the pan.
- Add the chicken back to the pan, pour the juice of the second lemon over it and cook for another minute.
- You are now ready to serve. Place the chicken on top of the asparagus, sprinkle the toasted almonds over the top, and garnish with fresh parsley, if desired.

Nutritional Values (per serving): Calories per serving: 320-350 kcal, Protein: 30-35g, Fat: 15-18g, Carbohydrates: 20-25g, Sodium: Approximately 450-500mg

24. Grilled Tofu with Chili Peanut Sauce

Ingredients:
Extra-Strength Tofu (250g), Low Sodium Soy Sauce (2 tablespoons), Sesame Oil (2 tablespoons), Chili Powder (1 teaspoon), Roasted Peanuts (2 tablespoons), Green Onion (2 tablespoons), grated fresh ginger (1 teaspoon), garlic (1 clove), lemon juice (juice of half a lemon), salt and black pepper (to taste), fresh parsley (1 tablespoon, for garnish).

Preparation:
- In a bowl, mix the soy sauce, sesame oil, chili powder, garlic, grated ginger and lemon juice to create the marinade.
- Add the tofu cubes to the marinade and make sure they are well coated. Leave to marinate for at least 15-20 minutes, stirring occasionally.
- While the tofu is marinating, preheat a grill or nonstick skillet over medium-high heat.
- Once the tofu has marinated enough, place the cubes on the grill or in the pan and cook for about 3-4 minutes per side or until golden and crispy.
- While the tofu cooks, prepare the chili peanut sauce. In a small bowl, mix the finely chopped peanuts with the green onion. Add some ground black pepper and mix well.
- When tofu is done, remove from grill or pan and place on a serving platter.
- Sprinkle the tofu with the previously prepared chili and peanut sauce.
- Garnish with chopped fresh parsley.
- Serve the grilled tofu with chili and peanut sauce hot, perhaps accompanied by brown rice or grilled vegetables.

Nutritional values: Calories: 280-300 kcal; Protein: 15-18g; Fat: 20-23g (Saturated Fat: 2-3g, Monounsaturated Fat: 10-12g, Polyunsaturated Fat: 4-5g); Carbohydrates: 10-12g (Fibre: 2-3g, Sugars: 2-3g); Sodium: 350-400mg

25. Duck breast with raspberry sauce

Ingredients: Duck breast (2 breasts), raspberries (200g), sugar (3 tablespoons), balsamic vinegar (2 tablespoons), chicken broth (250 ml), butter (2 tablespoons), salt and black pepper (to taste), olive oil (1 tablespoon).

Preparation:
- Preheat the oven to 180°C.
- Score the skin of the duck breasts with a sharp knife, forming a diagonal grid. Make sure not to cut into the meat.
- Heat a nonstick skillet over medium-high heat. There is no need to add oil as the duck breast will release enough fat.
- Set the skin-side into duck breasts in the pan. Cook for 5-6 minutes, so that the skin is crispy and brown. Turn the breasts and cook for another 2-3 minutes.
- Transfer the duck breasts to the oven rack and cook for about 10-12 minutes for rare or longer for well done.
- Meanwhile, prepare the raspberry sauce. In a small saucepan, melt the sugar over medium heat until golden caramel.
- Add the balsamic vinegar and raspberries. Let cook over medium-low heat for about 5 minutes or until the sauce thickens. Cook for an additional 5 minutes after adding the chicken broth.
- Strain the sauce through a fine sieve to remove the raspberry seeds. Add the butter and mix until the sauce is smooth.
- Season with salt and pepper.
- When the duck breasts are ready, remove from the oven and let rest for a few minutes before cutting them into slices.
- Serve sliced duck breast with raspberry sauce on top.
- Sprinkle with fresh parsley and an addition of olive oil.

Nutritional values (per approximate serving): Calories: 400-450 kcal, Protein: 25-30g, Fat: 25-30g, Carbohydrates: 15-20g

26. Mustard Pork with Asparagus and Mushrooms

Ingredients: Pork (4 thin slices), Dijon mustard (2 tablespoons), Salt, Black pepper, Asparagus (200g), Mushrooms (200g), Olive oil (2 tablespoons), Shallot (1, chopped), Chicken broth (250ml), Heavy cream (120ml)

Preparation:
- Spread the Dijon mustard on the pork slices and season with salt and black pepper.
- In a pan, heat the olive oil and cook the pork until golden brown on both sides. Transfer the pork to a plate.
- In the same pan, add the asparagus, mushrooms, and shallot. Cook until the asparagus become tender.
- Pour in the chicken a broth and heavy cream. Bring the sauce to a boil and continue to cook until it thickens.
- Return the pork to the pan to heat it through.
- Serve the pork with asparagus, mushrooms, and the sauce.

Nutritional Values: Calories: 350-400 kcal, Protein: 30-35g, Fat: 20-25g, Carbohydrates: 10-15g

27. Tuna Steak with Rosemary and Lemon Sauce

Ingredients: Tuna steak (2 thick slices), Fresh rosemary (2 tablespoons, chopped), Lemon (juice and grated zest), Olive oil (2 tablespoons), Salt, Black pepper

Preparation:
- In a bowl, mix the chopped rosemary, lemon juice, lemon zest, olive oil, salt, and black pepper.
- Spread this mixture on the tuna slices and let them marinate for about 15-30 minutes.
- Preheat a grill or a nonstick skillet in a medium-high flame.
- Cook the tuna for 2-3 minutes on each side or until it's pink in the middle but still slightly pink at the center.
- Serve with an extra drizzle of lemon juice if desired.

Nutritional Values: Calories: 250-300 kcal, Protein: 40-45g, Fat: 10-15g, Carbohydrates: 5-10g

28. Quinoa Meatballs with Tomato and Parsley Sauce

Ingredients: Cooked quinoa (2 cups), Eggs (2), Breadcrumbs (1/2 cup), Onion (1, chopped), Garlic (2 cloves, minced), Parsley (2 tablespoons, chopped), Salt, Black pepper, Olive oil, Tomato passata (400g)

Preparation:
- In a bowl, mix the cooked quinoa, eggs, breadcrumbs, chopped onion, minced garlic, parsley, salt, and black pepper.
- Form the mixture into meatballs.
- Heat olive oil in a pan and cook the meatballs until they are golden brown on both sides.

- Meanwhile, prepare the tomato sauce by heating the tomato passata with garlic, parsley, salt, and pepper.
- Spoon the tomato sauce over the meatballs and serve.

Nutritional Values: Calories: 300-350 kcal, Protein: 12-15g, Fat: 8-10g, Carbohydrates: 45-50g

29. Baked Salmon with Pink Peppercorn and Dill Sauce

Ingredients:4 salmon fillets (approximately 150g each),1 tablespoon whole pink peppercorns, 1 tablespoon fresh dill, chopped,2 tablespoons olive oil,2 tablespoons lemon juice, Salt and freshly ground black pepper

Preparation:

- Preheat the oven to 180°C (350°F). Line a baking tray with parchment paper or lightly grease it with olive oil.
- In a bowl, mix the pink peppercorns, fresh dill, olive oil, and lemon juice.
- Place the salmon fillets on the prepared tray and evenly brush the pink peppercorn and dill mixture over the fillets.
- Season the salmon fillets with a pinch of salt and freshly ground black pepper.
- Bake in the preheated oven for about 15-20 minutes or until the salmon flakes easily with a fork and is lightly golden on the surface.
- Serve the baked salmon hot, garnished with additional fresh dill if desired.

Nutritional Values: Calories: 300-350 kcal, Protein: 30-35g, Fat: 18-20g, Carbohydrates: 2-3g

30. Chicken curry with pumpkin and spinach

Ingredients: 4 boneless, skinless chicken breasts, 1 teaspoon olive oil, 1 chopped onion, 3 chopped garlic cloves, 1 teaspoon grated fresh ginger, 2 tablespoons red curry paste, 400g chopped pumpkin diced, 200 g of fresh spinach, 400 ml of coconut milk, 1 teaspoon of lime juice, Salt and pepper, to taste.

Preparation:

- In a big skillet over a medium-high flame, warm the olive oil. Cook approximately 5 minutes, or until the onion is translucent.
- Add the chopped garlic and grated ginger to the onion and cook for a minute until they release their aroma.
- Add the red curry paste and mix well with the other vegetables.
- Add the pumpkin cubes and stir so they are coated with the curry mixture.
- Add the chicken breasts and cook until golden on both sides.
- Pour the coconut milk over the meat and vegetables, bring everything to the boil, then reduce the heat and simmer covered for about 15-20 minutes or until the chicken is cooked and the squash is soft.
- Add the fresh spinach at the end and let it sweat in the curry mixture.
- Add lime juice, salt, and pepper according to preference.
- Serve your pumpkin and spinach chicken curry hot and garnish with fresh coriander leaves if desired.

Nutritional Values (per serving): Calories: 350 kcal, Protein: 30 g, Fat: 22 g, Carbohydrates: 10 g, Fibre: 3 g

31. Beef steak with white wine sauce and parsley

Ingredients: 4 beef steaks (approximately 200 g each), 2 tablespoons olive oil, 1 chopped onion, 2 chopped garlic cloves, 120 ml dry white wine, 1 teaspoon Dijon mustard, 2 tablespoons sliced fresh parsley, pepper and salt according to preference

Preparation:

- In a nonstick skillet in a medium-high flame, heat the olive oil. Add the beef steaks and cook them for the desired time depending on the desired doneness (for thick steaks about 3-4 minutes per side for rare).
- Remove the steaks from the pan and transfer them to a plate. Cover them with aluminum foil and let them rest while you prepare the sauce.
- In the same pan, add the chopped onion and chopped garlic. Cook for 2-3 minutes or until tender.
- Bring to a boil with the dry white wine. Reduce the heat to low and continue to simmer until the wine has been reduced by half.
- Add the Dijon mustard and chopped parsley to the sauce and mix well. Cook for another minute or two.
- Season with salt and pepper as desired. Pour the sauce over the beef steaks and serve hot.

Nutritional Values (per serving): Calories: 400 kcal, Protein: 40 g, Fat: 22 g, Carbohydrates: 4 g, Fibre: 1 g

32. Turkey meatballs with tzatziki sauce and tomato

Ingredients:500 g of minced turkey meat, 1/2 chopped red onion, 2 chopped garlic cloves, 1 teaspoon of dried oregano 1 teaspoon of cumin powder, 1 egg, 50 g of breadcrumbs, Salt and pepper, to taste, Olive oil for cooking

For the tzatziki sauce: 200 g of Greek yogurt, 1 cucumber, peeled and grated, 2 cloves of garlic, chopped, 1 tablespoon of chopped fresh mint, Juice of 1/2 lemon, Salt and pepper, to taste, For the tomato sauce: 2 ripe tomatoes, diced, 1/2 chopped red onion, 1 tablespoon chopped fresh parsley, Juice of 1/2 lemon, Salt and pepper, to taste.

Preparation:

- In a bowl, mix the ground turkey, chopped red onion, chopped garlic cloves, oregano, cumin, egg, and breadcrumbs. Season with salt and pepper as desired.
- With wet hands, form small meatballs from the mixture and place them on a tray.
- Heat a nonstick skillet over a medium-high flame with a small amount of olive oil. Cook the meatballs until evenly browned and cooked through, about 4-5 minutes per side.
- Meanwhile, prepare the tzatziki sauce by mixing the Greek yogurt, grated cucumber, chopped garlic cloves, mint, lemon juice, salt and pepper in a bowl.
- Also, prepare the tomato sauce by mixing the diced tomatoes, chopped red onion, parsley, lemon juice, salt and pepper in another bowl.
- Serve the turkey meatballs with the tzatziki sauce and tomato dressing. You can add a generous amount of leafy green vegetables for a complete meal.

Nutritional Values (per serving): Calories: 350 kcal, Protein: 30 g, Fat: 15 g, Carbohydrates: 22 g, Fiber: 4 g.

33. Chicken tacos with avocado and cucumber salad

Ingredients:2 chicken breasts, cut into strips,2 tablespoons of olive oil,2 teaspoons smoked paprika,1 teaspoon cumin powder 1/2 teaspoon chili powder (optional), Salt and black pepper, to taste,8 corn or flour tortillas,

For the avocado and cucumber salad:2 ripe avocados, peeled, pitted and diced,1 cucumber, diced,1/2 red onion, chopped

1 red chili, finely chopped (optional), Juice of 2 limes,2 tablespoons chopped fresh coriander (or parsley), Salt and black pepper, to taste
To serve: Chili sauce (optional), Greek yogurt or sour cream (optional)
Preparation:
- In a bowl, toss the chicken breast strips with the olive oil, smoked paprika, cumin powder, chili powder (if desired), salt and black pepper. Check that the chicken is thoroughly coated in the spices.
- Heat a nonstick pan over medium-high heat. Cook the marinated chicken for about 5-7 minutes per side or until it is fully cooked and has developed a golden crustPlace the chicken on a plate and protect with aluminum foil to maintain it warm.
- Prepare the avocado and cucumber salad in a large bowl. Mix together the diced avocados, diced cucumber, chopped red onion, red chili (if desired), lime juice and chopped coriander.
- Season your liking with salt and black pepper. Heat the tortillas in a hot skillet or in the microwave until hot and soft.
- To serve, fill each tortilla with the grilled chicken and avocado-cucumber salad. Add chili sauce, Greek yogurt or sour cream if desired.

Nutritional Values (per serving, includes 2 tortillas): Calories: 480 kcal, Protein: 35 g, Fat: 24 g, Carbohydrates: 35 g, Fiber: 9 g.

34. Grilled salmon with tarragon and lemon sauce
Ingredients: 4 salmon fillets, 2 tablespoons olive oil, 1 clove of garlic, chopped, 2 tablespoons chopped fresh tarragon
Grated zest of 1 lemon, Juice of 1 lemon, Salt and black pepper, to taste.
For the sauce: 1/2 cup sour cream, 2 tablespoons Dijon mustard, 2 tablespoons honey, 1 teaspoon chopped fresh tarragon, Salt and black pepper, to taste.
Preparation:
- Preheat grill to medium-high heat.
- In a bowl, combine the olive oil, minced garlic, chopped fresh tarragon, grated lemon zest, lemon juice, salt and black pepper. Spread this marinade on the salmon fillets.
- In a separate bowl, mix the sour cream, Dijon mustard, honey, chopped tarragon, salt and black pepper to make the sauce.
- Grill the salmon for about 4-5 minutes per side or until the fish is cooked through and has developed a golden crust.
- Serve the salmon with the tarragon and lemon sauce.

Nutritional Values (per serving): Calories: 420 kcal, Protein: 32 g, Fat: 26 g, Carbohydrates: 14 g, Fiber: 1 g.

35. Duck Breast with Black Cherry and Port Sauce
Ingredients:4 duck breasts, Salt and black pepper, to taste,1 cup black cherries, pitted and halved,1/2 cup port,2 tablespoons of sugar,1 tablespoon balsamic vinegar,1 tablespoon butter,1 teaspoon chopped fresh rosemary
Preparation:
- Preheat the oven to 180°C.
- Make shallow incisions in the skin of the duck breasts, then season with salt and black pepper.
- In a nonstick pan, heat the duck breasts over medium-high heat, skin side down. Cook for five minutes at a time or until the skin becomes crispy.
- Turn the breasts and cook for another 3-4 minutes.

- Transfer the duck breasts to a baking tray and cook in the oven for 10-12 minutes until medium rare (or to your taste). Take away from the oven and set aside for a few minutes before slicing.
- Meanwhile, prepare the sauce. In a small saucepan, combine the black cherries, port, sugar, balsamic vinegar, butter and rosemary. Cook over medium heat until the sauce has thickened slightly and the cherries are soft.
- Serve the sliced duck breasts with the black cherry and port sauce on top.

Nutritional Values (per serving): Calories: 350 kcal, Protein: 28 g, Fat: 12 g, Carbohydrates: 30 g, Fiber: 2 g.

36. Mustard Pork with Carrots and Sweet Potatoes
Ingredients:4 pork steaks, Salt and black pepper, to taste,2 tablespoons of mustard,2 tablespoons of olive oil,4 carrots, peeled and cut into thin slices,2 sweet potatoes, peeled and diced,2 cloves garlic, minced,1 teaspoon dried rosemary,1/2 cup chicken broth
Preparation:
- Preheat the oven to 200°C.
- Season the pork steaks with salt, pepper, and mustard.
- Heating the olive oil in an ovenproof skillet over a medium-high flame. Brown the pork steaks for about 2-3 minutes per side or until browned.
- Take the steaks out of the pan and set them aside.In the same pan, add the carrots, sweet potatoes, garlic, rosemary, chicken broth, salt and pepper. After completely combining, bring to a boil.
- Place the steaks back on top of the vegetables and transfer the pan to the oven. Cook for about 20-25 minutes or until the vegetables are tender and the pork is fully cooked.
- Serve the pork with the carrots and sweet potatoes, adding broth as a sauce, if desired.

Nutritional Values (per serving): Calories: 420 kcal, Protein: 34 g, Fat: 16 g, Carbohydrates: 32 g, Fibre: 5 g.

37. Tuna Steak with Basil and Cherry Tomato Sauce
Ingredients:4 tuna steaks, Salt and black pepper, to taste,2 tablespoons of olive oil,2 cups cherry tomatoes, cut in half
1/2 cup fresh basil leaves,2 cloves garlic, minced,2 tablespoons lemon juice, Grated zest of 1 lemon
Preparation:
- In a pan over a medium-high flame, heat the olive oil. Season both sides of the tuna steaks with pepper and salt.
- Cook the tuna for about 2-3 minutes per side or until cooked to your liking. Transfer it to a plate.
- In the same pan, add the cherry tomatoes, basil, garlic, lemon juice and grated lemon zest. Cook for about 2-3 minutes or until the tomatoes soften.
- Serve the tuna with the basil and cherry tomato sauce.

Nutritional Values (per serving): Calories: 310 kcal, Protein: 39 g, Fat: 14 g, Carbohydrates: 8 g, Fiber: 2 g.

38. Quinoa Meatballs with Tzatziki Sauce and Olives
Ingredients:1 cup cooked quinoa,1/2 cup crumbled feta cheese
1/4 cup chopped fresh parsley,1 egg,2 cloves garlic, minced, Salt and black pepper, to taste,1/2 cup breadcrumbs
For the tzatziki sauce: 1 cup Greek yogurt, grated cucumber, minced garlic, fresh mint, lemon juice, salt and pepper.

Black olives for garnish.
Preparation:
- In a bowl, mix the cooked quinoa, feta cheese, parsley, egg, garlic, salt and pepper.
- Gradually add the breadcrumbs until you get a consistency that can be shaped into meatballs.
- Form meatballs with the mixture and cook them in a pan with olive oil until golden.
- For the tzatziki sauce, mix the Greek yogurt, grated cucumber, garlic, mint, lemon juice, salt and pepper.
- Serve the meatballs with the tzatziki sauce and garnish with black olives.

Nutritional Values (per serving): Calories: 310 kcal, Protein: 12 g, Fat: 11 g, Carbohydrates: 41 g, Fibre: 5 g.

39. Turmeric Tofu with Peppers and Zucchini

Ingredients:14 ounces extra firm tofu, cut into cubes 1 teaspoon of turmeric, Salt and black pepper, to taste,2 tablespoons of olive oil,1 red pepper, cut into strips,2 courgettes, cut into slices,2 cloves garlic, minced,1 teaspoon grated fresh ginger,2 tablespoons low-sodium soy sauce,2 tablespoons sesame seeds,1 tablespoon chopped chives
Preparation:
- In a bowl, mix the tofu with the turmeric, salt and pepper.
- In a pan over a medium-high flame, heat the olive oil. Cook the tofu until golden brown. Removed it from the pan and put it aside.
- In the same pan, add the bell pepper, zucchini, garlic and ginger. Cook until the vegetables become tender.
- Add the previously cooked tofu and season with soy sauce. Cook for a few more minutes.
- Serve the tofu with the vegetables and sprinkle with sesame seeds and chives.

Nutritional Values (per serving): Calories: 240 kcal, Protein: 14 g, Fat: 16 g, Carbohydrates: 14 g, Fiber: 4 g.

40. Baked Salmon with Cilantro Lime Sauce

Ingredients:4 salmon fillets, Salt and black pepper, to taste,1 teaspoon coriander powder,2 cloves garlic, minced, Juice and grated zest of 2 limes,1/4 cup chopped fresh cilantro,2 tablespoons of olive oil
Preparation:
- Preheat the oven to 180°C.
- Season the salmon fillets with salt, pepper, coriander powder and garlic.
- Place the fillets on a lightly greased baking tray.
- Mix the lime juice, lime zest, fresh cilantro and olive oil in a bowl. Pour the sauce over the salmon.
- Cover the pan with foil and bake in the oven for about 15-20 minutes or until the salmon flakes easily with a fork.
- Serve the salmon with plenty of coriander and lime sauce.

Nutritional Values (per serving): Calories: 280 kcal, Protein: 28 g, Fat: 16 g, Carbohydrates: 6 g, Fiber: 2 g.

41. Tuna Steak with Sesame and Soy Sauce

Ingredients:4 tuna steaks,2 tablespoons low-sodium soy sauce 2 tablespoons sesame oil,2 tablespoons sesame seeds, 1 minced garlic clove Depending on your preference, season with salt and black pepper. sliced spring onions for garnish
Preparation:
- In a bowl, mix the soy sauce, sesame oil, sesame seeds, garlic, salt and pepper.
- Marinate the tuna steaks in the mixture for at least 30 minutes.
- Preheat your grill or nonstick skillet over medium-high heat.
- Cook the tuna steaks for about 2-3 minutes per side to keep them pink inside.
- Serve the steaks with the remaining sauce and garnish with chopped spring onions.

Nutritional Values (per serving): Calories: 310 kcal, Protein: 42 g, Fat: 13 g, Carbohydrates: 3 g, Fiber: 1 g.

42. Quinoa Meatballs with Chilli Ginger Sauce

Ingredients:1 cup cooked quinoa,1 egg,1/4 cup chopped onion 2 tablespoons chopped fresh parsley,2 teaspoons grated fresh ginger,2 cloves garlic, minced, Salt and black pepper, to taste 2 tablespoons sweet chili sauce,1 tablespoon olive oil
For the sauce: 1/4 cup Greek yogurt, grated ginger, lemon, salt and pepper.
Preparation:
- In a bowl, mix the cooked quinoa, egg, onion, parsley, ginger, garlic, salt and pepper.
- Form meatballs with the mixture and cook them in a pan with olive oil until golden.
- For the sauce, mix the Greek yogurt, grated ginger, lemon juice, salt and pepper.
- Serve the meatballs with the sauce.

Nutritional Values (per serving): Calories: 260 kcal, Protein: 9 g, Fat: 12 g, Carbohydrates: 29 g, Fiber: 3 g.

43. Baked Salmon with Dijon Mustard Dressing

Ingredients:4 salmon fillets,2 tablespoons Dijon mustard,2 tablespoons honey,1 clove garlic, minced,2 tablespoons lemon juice, Salt and black pepper, to taste,1 tablespoon chopped fresh parsley
Preparation:
- Preheat the oven to 180°C.
- In a bowl, mix the mustard, honey, garlic, lemon juice, salt and pepper.
- Place the salmon fillets on a lightly greased baking tray.
- Spread the mustard and honey sauce over the salmon fillets.
- Bake for about 12-15 minutes or until salmon flakes easily with a fork.
- Serve the salmon with a sprinkling of chopped parsley.

Nutritional Values (per serving): Calories: 290 kcal, Protein: 24 g, Fat: 12 g, Carbohydrates: 22 g, Fibre: 1 g.

44. Duck Breast with Pomegranate Sauce

Ingredients:2 duck breasts, Salt and black pepper, to taste 1 cup pomegranate juice,1/4 cup brown sugar,1/4 cup balsamic vinegar,1 tablespoon corn starch (cornflour), Pomegranate seeds for garnish (optional)
Preparation:
- Before starting, make sure the duck breasts are at room temperature.
- Preheat the oven to 200°C.
- Make diamond-shaped cuts on the skin of the duck breasts, being careful not to cut the meat underneath.
- Generously salt and pepper the duck breasts on both sides.
- In a cold non-stick pan, place the duck breasts skin side down.
- Turn the heat on to medium and cook the duck breasts for about 10-12 minutes, turning them once or twice during cooking to obtain a crispy skin.

- In the meantime, prepare the pomegranate sauce. In a small saucepan, combine the pomegranate juice, brown sugar and balsamic vinegar.
- Bring to the boil, then reduce the heat and simmer for about 15-20 minutes or until the sauce thickens.
- Mix the cornstarch with a little water to form a thick mixture, then add it to the pomegranate sauce.
- Continue cooking for another 2-3 minutes until the sauce thickens further.
- When the duck breasts are cooked, remove them from the pan and let them rest for a few minutes.
- Trim the duck breasts into small slices.
- Serve the duck breast slices with the pomegranate sauce and garnish with pomegranate seeds if desired.

Nutritional Values (per serving): Calories: 350 kcal, Protein: 25 g, Fat: 18 g, Carbohydrates: 26 g, Fibre: 1 g.

45. Beef Steak with Black Pepper and Rosemary

Ingredients:2 beef steaks (about 200-250 g each), Kosher salt, to taste, Ground black pepper, to taste, Fresh rosemary, finely chopped, to taste, Olive oil, to taste

Preparation:
- Preheat the grill or a nonstick skillet over medium-high heat.
- While the grill or pan heats, prepare the steaks. Make sure they are at room temperature for even cooking. Using paper towels, let the steaks dry.
- Brush both sides of the steaks with a drizzle of olive oil.
- Sprinkle plenty of ground black pepper on both sides of the steaks, then add a generous amount of chopped rosemary. Lightly press the black pepper and rosemary so that they adhere to the meat.
- When the grill or pan is hot, gently place the steaks on the hot surface.
- Cook the steaks for about 3-4 minutes per side for rare. If you prefer different cooking, adjust the cooking time to your liking. The entire time needed for cooking will vary according to the thickness of the steaks.
- During cooking, avoid continually turning the steaks; turn them only once to obtain a nice golden crust.
- Once you reach the desired doneness, transfer the steaks to a cutting board and let them rest for a few minutes.
- This step is important to allow the juices to redistribute into the meat, keeping it juicy.
- Thinly cut the steaks against the grain. Serve the beef steaks with a sprinkle of kosher salt and garnish with fresh rosemary if desired.

Nutritional Values (per serving): Calories: 300 kcal, Protein: 25 g, Fat: 20 g, Carbohydrates: 1 g, Fibre: 0 g.

46. Quinoa Meatballs with Peppers and Onions

Ingredients:1 cup cooked and cooled quinoa,1 red pepper, finely chopped,1 red onion, finely chopped,2 cloves garlic, finely chopped,1 egg,1/2 cup low-fat shredded cheese (of your choice) 1/4 cup fresh parsley, chopped,1 teaspoon cumin powder,1 teaspoon smoked paprika, Salt and black pepper, to taste, Olive oil for cooking

Preparation:
- In a large bowl, combine the cooked quinoa, red bell pepper, red onion, garlic, egg, shredded cheese, parsley, cumin, smoked paprika, salt and black pepper.
- Mix the ingredients well until a uniform mixture is obtained.

- Cover the bowl with cling film and place it in the refrigerator for at least 30 minutes to let the mixture rest. This will help compact the meatballs and make them easier to handle.
- After the resting time, form the mixture into round and flattened meatballs of the desired size.
- Heat a nonstick skillet over a medium-high flame with a small amount of olive oil. Place the meatballs in the hot pan and cook them for about 3-4 minutes per side or until they are golden brown and cooked inside.
- Once cooked, transfer the meatballs to a plate lined with kitchen paper to absorb excess oil.
- Serve the quinoa meatballs with a sauce of your choice or on a bed of fresh salad.

Nutritional Values (per serving): Calories: 220 kcal, Protein: 10 g, Fat: 7 g, Carbohydrates: 30 g, Fiber: 5 g.

47. Tuna Steak with Mango Chili Sauce

Ingredients:2 fresh tuna steaks (about 200 g each),1 ripe mango, peeled, pitted and cut into cubes,1 red chili pepper, finely chopped (remove seeds for less spicy flavor, if desired) Juice of 1 lime,2 tablespoons chopped fresh coriander,1 clove garlic, finely chopped, Salt and black pepper, to taste, Olive oil for cooking

Preparation:
- In a bowl, mix the mango cubes with the chopped chili pepper, lime juice, coriander, garlic, salt and pepper. This will be the mango and chili sauce.
- Make sure all the ingredients are well combined and let sit in the refrigerator while you prepare the tuna.
- Heating a nonstick skillet over a medium-high flame with a drizzle of olive oil. Season the tuna steaks on each side with salt and pepper.
- Cook the tuna steaks in the hot pan for about 2-3 minutes per side, depending on the thickness of the steaks. The tuna should be pink inside.
- After the desired cooking time, remove the steaks from the pan and set aside.
- Pour the mango and chili sauce over the tuna steaks.
- Serve the tuna steaks with the mango and chili sauce, garnished with lime slices and fresh coriander leaves.

Nutritional Values (per serving): Calories: 350 kcal, Protein: 40 g, Fat: 6 g, Carbohydrates: 30 g, Fiber: 4 g.

48. Baked Salmon with Lemon Dill Sauce

Ingredients:4 salmon fillets (about 150 g each),2 tablespoons of olive oil, Juice of 1 lemon,2 cloves garlic, finely chopped,2 tablespoons chopped fresh dill, Salt and black pepper, to taste

Preparation:
- Preheat the oven to 180 degrees Celsius and line the surface of the oven with parchment paper.
- In a bowl, mix the olive oil, lemon juice, minced garlic, fresh dill, salt and black pepper.
- Arrange the salmon fillets in the baking dish that has been prepared.
- Pour the prepared marinade over the salmon fillets, making sure to cover them evenly.
- Bake the salmon in the preheated oven for about 15 to 20 minutes or until the fish flakes easily with a fork and turns pale pink.
- Serve the salmon hot, garnished with lemon slices and sprigs of fresh dill.

Nutritional Values (per serving): Calories: 250 kcal, Protein: 30 g, Fat: 12 g, Carbohydrates: 2 g, Fiber: 1 g.

49. Turkey Meatballs with Curry Sauce and Almonds

Ingredients:

For the meatballs:500 g of minced turkey meat,1/2 onion, finely chopped,2 cloves garlic, finely chopped,1 egg,1/4 cup almond flour,2 tablespoons chopped fresh parsley,1 teaspoon curry powder, Salt and black pepper, to taste, Olive oil for cooking Ingredients for the sauce:1/2 cup heavy cream,1 tablespoon red curry paste,1/4 cup toasted almonds, chopped, Salt and black pepper, to taste, Chopped fresh parsley for garnish

Preparation: For the meatballs:

- In a bowl, mix the ground turkey, chopped onion, minced garlic, egg, almond flour, chopped parsley, curry powder, salt and black pepper.
- With wet hands, form evenly sized meatballs.
- In a skillet with a nonstick coating over medium-high heat, heat some olive oil.
- Cook the meatballs in the pan, turning occasionally, until golden brown and fully cooked (about 12-15 minutes). Make sure they are cooked evenly.
- For the sauce:
- Heat the cream in a small saucepan over a medium-low flame.
- Add the red curry paste and mix until well incorporated.
- Add the chopped almonds and continue to cook for a few minutes until the sauce thickens slightly.
- The season your liking with salt and black pepper.
- To serve:
- Arrange the turkey meatballs on a serving platter.
- Pour the curry and almond sauce over the meatballs.
- Garnish with chopped fresh parsley.
- Serve hot and accompany with rice or steamed vegetables.

Nutritional Values (per portion, with sauce included): Calories: 380 kcal, Protein: 30 g, Fat: 24 g, Carbohydrates: 15 g, Fiber: 4 g.

50. Chicken curry with chickpeas and spinach

Ingredients:

1 pound (450g) boneless, skinless chicken breasts or thighs, cut into bite-sized pieces, 1 can (15 oz) chickpeas, drained and rinsed, 2 cups fresh spinach or frozen spinach, thawed and drained, 1 onion, finely chopped, 3 cloves garlic, minced, 1-inch piece of fresh ginger, grated, 1 can (14 oz) diced tomatoes, 1 cup coconut milk, 2 tablespoons olive oil, 2 teaspoons curry powder, 1 teaspoon ground turmeric,1 teaspoon ground cumin,1/2 teaspoon ground coriander,1/2 teaspoon ground cinnamon, Salt and pepper to taste, Fresh cilantro leaves for garnish (optional)

Preparation:

- Heating the olive oil in a big skillet over a medium-high flame.
- Cook the chicken cubes until golden. Use them out of the pan and place them aside.
- Add the minced garlic and onion to the same pan. Cook, stirring occasionally, for just a few minutes, until all of the onions are transparent.
- Add the curry paste to the pan and mix well with the onion and garlic. Continue cooking for another minute to let the curry flavors develop.
- Return the browned chicken to the pan with the curry and stir to coat with the curry.
- Add the drained and rinsed chickpeas and mix well.

- Pour the coconut milk into the pan and bring everything to the boil. Then reduce the heat and simmer for about 15 minutes or until the chicken is cooked and the sauce has thickened.
- Add the fresh spinach and cook until it softens and reduces in volume. Season with salt and pepper to taste. If desired, add a little lemon juice for a touch of freshness.

Nutritional values per serving: Calories: 400-500 kcal, Protein: 25-30 g, Fat: 20-25 g, Carbohydrates: 20-25 g, Fiber: 5-8 g

51. Turmeric Chicken with Roasted Carrots

Ingredients:4 chicken breasts,2 tablespoons of olive oil,1 teaspoon of turmeric powder,4 carrots, peeled and cut into sticks,2 cloves of garlic, minced, Salt and black pepper, to taste. Chopped fresh parsley (optional)

Preparation:

- Preheat the oven to 200°C.
- In a bowl, mix the olive oil, turmeric powder, minced garlic, salt and pepper.
- Grease a baking tray with olive oil or line it with baking paper. Place the chicken breasts on the baking tray and brush them with half the oil and turmeric mixture.
- Arrange the carrot sticks around the chicken in the baking dish and toss with the rest of the oil and turmeric mixture.
- Place the pan in the preheated oven and bake for about 25-30 minutes or until the chicken is cooked through and the carrots are tender, turning the chicken halfway through cooking.
- When the chicken and carrots are done, remove them from the oven.
- Sprinkle with chopped parsley (if desired) and serve hot.

Nutritional values per portion: Calories: 350-400 kcal, Protein: 25-30 g, Fat: 10-15 g, Carbohydrates: 25-30 g, Fibers: 5-7 g

52. Grilled salmon with ginger-lime sauce

Ingredients: 4 salmon fillets, 2 tablespoons of olive oil, Salt and black pepper, to taste, For the sauce: 2 tablespoons of grated fresh ginger, Juice of 2 limes, 2 tablespoons of soy sauce, 1 tablespoon honey, 2 cloves garlic, minced, 1 teaspoon dried red chili (optional), chopped fresh chives or parsley for garnish (optional).

Preparation:

- Preheat grill to medium-high heat.
- In a bowl, mix the olive oil with the juice of one lime, salt and pepper. Brush this mixture over the salmon fillets on both sides.
- Place the salmon fillets on the preheated grill and cook for about 4-5 minutes per side or until the salmon is cooked through and has nice grilled streaks.
- Meanwhile, prepare the sauce. In a small bowl, mix the juice of the second lime, grated ginger, soy sauce, honey, minced garlic, and, if desired, dried red chili pepper.
- Pour the ginger-lime sauce over the grilled salmon fillets just before serving.
- Garnish with chives or chopped fresh parsley, if desired.

Nutritional values per serving: Calories: 300-350 kcal, Protein: 25-30 g, Fat: 15-20 g, Carbohydrates: 10-15 g, Fibers: 1-2 g

53. Beef steak with chimichurri and sautéed spinach

Ingredients:4 beef steaks, Salt and black pepper, to taste, For the chimichurri:1 cup fresh parsley, chopped,4 cloves of garlic, minced,1 teaspoon dried red chili pepper (optional),2 tablespoons of red wine vinegar,1/2 cup olive oil, Salt and black pepper, to taste.

For the sautéed spinach:500 g of fresh spinach,2 tablespoons of olive oil,2 cloves of garlic, minced, Juice of 1 lemon, Salt and black pepper, to taste.

Preparation:

- Start by making the chimichurri. In a bowl, mix the chopped parsley, minced garlic, dried red chili pepper (if you want a spicy kick), red wine vinegar and olive oil. Add salt and black pepper to taste. Combine all of the ingredients and set away.
- Preheat a grill or a skillet with a nonstick coating to medium-high temperature.
- Preheat the oven to 180°C if you prefer to finish cooking in the oven.
- Before cooking the steaks, make sure they are at room temperature. Brush them lightly with olive oil and season with salt and black pepper on both sides.
- Cook the steaks on the grill or in the hot pan for the desired time depending on how you prefer doneness. For rare cooking, about 3-4 minutes per side; for medium-rare, 4-5 minutes per side. If you prefer more thorough cooking, cook for a longer time. If you want a golden crust, you can finish cooking the steaks in a preheated oven at 180°C for a few minutes.
- While the steaks rest after cooking, prepare the sautéed spinach. Warm the olive oil in a skillet over a medium-high flame.
- Add the minced garlic and cook for about a minute or until aromatic. Add the fresh spinach and sauté until it softens and reduces in volume, which will only take a few minutes. Squeeze the lemon juice over the spinach and season with salt and black pepper to taste.
- Serve the steaks hot, garnish with the fresh chimichurri sauce and accompany them with the sautéed spinach.

Nutritional values per serving: Calories: 350-450 kcal, Protein: 30-40 g, Fat: 20-25 g, Carbohydrates: 5-10 g, Fibers: 3-5 g

54. Mustard pork with asparagus and sweet potatoes

Ingredients:4 pork fillets, 600 g of asparagus,600 g of sweet potatoes,4 tablespoons of mustard,4 tablespoons of olive oil, Salt and pepper to taste, Fresh rosemary sprigs (optional)

Preparation:

- Preheat the oven to 200°C.
- Dice the sweet potatoes and the asparagus into pieces. Arrange them on a baking tray and season them with olive oil, salt, pepper and rosemary.
- Bake the potatoes and asparagus in the preheated oven for about 25-30 minutes or until soft and lightly browned.
- Meanwhile, prepare the marinade for the pork by mixing the mustard with olive oil, salt, pepper and rosemary.
- Brush the pork with the marinade and cook in a hot skillet or on a hot grill until cooked to your desired doneness. Cooking time will vary based on the thickness of the piece of pork, but should usually be about 4-5 minutes per side for medium-rare.

- Once cooked, let the pork rest for a few minutes before slicing.
- Serve the sliced pork with the asparagus and roasted sweet potatoes.

Nutritional values for portion: Calories: 350-400 kcal, Protein: 25-30 g, Fat: 15-20 g, Carbohydrates: 30-35 g, Fibers: 5-8 g

55. Baked salmon with ginger and citrus sauce

Ingredients:4 salmon fillets,2 oranges (both juice and zest),1 lemon (both juice and zest),2 tablespoons grated fresh ginger,2 tablespoons of olive oil, Salt and black pepper, to taste, Fresh parsley for garnish (optional)

Preparation:

- Preheat the oven to 180 degrees Celsius and accordance a baking sheet with the parchment paper.
- In a bowl, mix the juice and zest of the oranges and lemon. Add the grated ginger and olive oil. Mix the sauce well and adjust the salt and pepper to taste.
- Place the salmon fillets in the prepared baking dish and pour the ginger-citrus sauce evenly over the fish.
- Cover the baking tray with foil and cook in the preheated oven for approximately 15-20 minutes or until the salmon is cooked to the desired point. You can uncover the salmon for the last 5 minutes to brown it slightly.
- While the salmon cooks, prepare the side of your choice, such as steamed vegetables or brown rice.
- Once cooked, remove the salmon from the oven and garnish with chopped fresh parsley (if desired).
- Serve the baked salmon with the hot ginger-citrus sauce and the prepared side dish.

Nutritional values per serving: Calories: 250-300 kcal, Protein: 25-30g, Fat: 12-15 g, Carbohydrates: 10-12g, Fiber: About 2-3 g

56. Quinoa salad with avocado and black beans

Ingredients:1 cup quinoa,2 cups of water,2 ripe avocados, cut into cubes,1 can of black beans (about 400 g), drained and rinsed,1 medium tomato, cut into cubes,1/2 red onion, finely chopped, Juice of 2 limes,3 tablespoons of olive oil, Salt and black pepper, to taste, Fresh coriander (optional) for garnish

Preparation:

- Start by rinsing the quinoa well under cold running water. This will help remove excess starch which can impart a bitter taste.
- Put the two cups of water to a boil in a saucepan. Add the rinsed quinoa and boil over medium heat for about 15 minutes or until the grains open and become tender. Drain it and let it cool.
- In a large bowl, combine the cooled quinoa, avocado cubes, drained black beans, tomato cubes, and chopped red onion.
- In a small bowl, make a vinaigrette by mixing the lime juice, olive oil, salt, and black pepper. Pour the vinaigrette over the ingredients in the large bowl and mix well to coat everything evenly.
- Garnish the salad with fresh cilantro (if desired) and serve.

Nutritional values: Calories: 300-350 kcal, Protein: 8-10 g, Fat: 15-18 g, Carbohydrates: 35-40 g, Fiber: 10-12 g

57. Grilled tofu with roasted vegetables

Ingredients:1 block extra-firm tofu (about 400 g), drained and pressed to remove excess water,4 cups mixed vegetables of your choice (e.g., peppers, zucchini, tomatoes, eggplant),2 tablespoons of olive oil,2 tablespoons soy sauce (or tamari sauce for a gluten-free version),2 cloves of garlic, minced, Juice of 1 lemon, Salt and black pepper, to taste., Fresh herbs (for example, thyme or rosemary, to taste)

Preparation:

- Preheat the oven to 200°C and prepare a baking tray lined with baking paper.
- According to your preference, cut the tofu into cubes or slices.
- In a bowl, mix the olive oil, soy sauce (or tamari), minced garlic, lemon juice, salt and pepper. This will be the seasoning for the tofu.
- Place the tofu on one side of the prepared baking sheet. Brush generously with the dressing.
- Cut the vegetables into pieces and arrange them on the other side of the baking tray. Season the vegetables with a little olive oil, salt and pepper, and add fresh herbs if desired.
- Cook the tofu and vegetables in the preheated oven for about 20-25 minutes or until the tofu is golden brown and the vegetables are cooked al dente.
- While the tofu and vegetables are cooking, you can prepare a salad or side of your choice.
- Once cooked, serve the grilled tofu with the roasted vegetables and garnish with fresh herbs, if desired.

Nutritional values: Calories: 250-300 kcal, Protein: 15-18 g, Fat: 15-18 g, Carbohydrates: 15-20 g, Fiber: 5-8 g

58. Kale salad with pumpkin seeds and feta

Ingredients:1 bunch of black cabbage (about 200 g), washed and stripped of the stems, 1/4 cup toasted pumpkin seeds,100g feta or goat's cheese, crumbled,2 tablespoons of extra virgin olive oil, the juice of 1 lemon, Salt and black pepper, to taste., Honey or maple syrup (optional, to sweeten the vinaigrette)

Preparation:

- Cut the kale into thin strips and place it in a large bowl.
- In a dry skillet, toast the pumpkin seeds over medium heat until they begin to turn golden brown and release an aromatic scent. Fill the pan with pumpkin seeds without overlapping them, so that they toast evenly. Transfer the toasted seeds to a plate and let them cool.
- In a small bowl, prepare the vinaigrette by mixing the olive oil, lemon juice, salt, pepper, and, if desired, a little honey or maple syrup to sweeten the vinaigrette. Mix well.
- Pour the vinaigrette over the kale and gently massage the leaves with your hands to soften them slightly. This will help tenderize the cabbage.
- Add the toasted pumpkin seeds and crumbled feta cheese to the salad. Mix well so that the ingredients are distributed evenly.
- Allow at least 30 minutes for the salad to settle in the fridge before serving. This allows the tastes to blend.
- Before serving, you can garnish with additional toasted pumpkin seeds and crumbled feta, if desired.

Nutritional values: Calories: 200-250 kcal, Protein: 7-10 g, Fat: 12-15 g, Carbohydrates: 15-20 g, Fiber: 4-6 g

59. Vegetarian Taco Bowl

Ingredients:2 cups cooked brown rice,2 cups canned black beans, drained and rinsed, 2 cups canned corn, drained,2 cups diced tomatoes (you can use fresh or canned tomatoes),1 cup diced avocado,1 cup thinly striped lettuce,1/2 cup shredded cheddar cheese (optional), Tomato sauce (taco sauce) to taste, Sour cream (optional), Salt and black pepper, to taste, Chilli powder, cumin and paprika for seasoning

Preparation:

- In a large bowl, prepare cooked brown rice according to package instructions.
- Heating the black beans in a pan over medium heat. Season with chili powder, cumin, and paprika.
- Stir well and cook for a few minutes until the beans are hot.
- Prepare diced tomatoes if using fresh tomatoes. If using canned tomatoes, drain them.
- Cut the avocado into cubes.
- To assemble the taco bowls, spread the cooked brown rice in the bottom of each bowl. Then add the black beans, corn, tomatoes, avocado and lettuce on top of the rice.
- You can add grated cheese if you like.
- Top each taco bowl with tomato salsa and sour cream, if desired. Season with salt and pepper to taste.
- Serve vegetarian taco bowls with spoons or forks and enjoy this delicious creation.

Nutritional values: Calories: 350-400 kcal, Protein: 10-15 g, Fat: 8-10 g, Carbohydrates: 60-70 g, Fiber: 10-15 g

60. Paprika chicken with steamed broccoli

Ingredients:4 boneless, skinless chicken breasts,2 teaspoons of sweet paprika,1 teaspoon smoked paprika (optional, for an extra twist), Salt and black pepper, to taste.,2 tablespoons of olive oil,1 lemon, cut into thin slices,4 cups broccoli, washed and cut into small pieces, Juice of 1 lemon, Fresh herbs (for example, parsley or thyme, for garnish)

Preparation:

- In a bowl, combine sweet paprika, smoked paprika (if using), salt, pepper, and 1 tablespoon olive oil. This will be the marinade for the chicken.
- Spread the marinade evenly on both sides over the chicken breast slices. Let the chicken marinate for at least 15-30 minutes.
- While the chicken marinates, prepare the steamer to cook the broccoli. You can steam broccoli in a basket or with a steamer until tender but still crunchy.
- In a skillet, heat the other tablespoon of olive oil over medium-high heat.
- Add the marinated chicken and cook on both sides until fully cooked and golden, about 5-6 minutes per side, depending on the thickness of the chicken breasts.
- Meanwhile, you can cook the lemon slices in a separate pan until they are lightly caramelized and golden.
- When the chicken is done, serve each breast with a slice of caramelized lemon on top.
- Serve the paprika chicken with steamed broccoli alongside.
- Garnish with fresh herbs and drizzle with fresh lemon juice before serving.

Nutritional values: Calories: 300-350 kcal, Protein: 30-35 g, Fat: 12-15 g, Carbohydrates: 15-20 g, Fiber: 5-7 g

61. Aubergine flan

Ingredients:2 medium aubergines, cut into thin slices,2 ripe tomatoes, cut into thin slices,1/2 cup fresh basil, chopped,200 g of low-fat cheese (for example, low-fat ricotta or low-fat fresh cheese),2 eggs,2 tablespoons of olive oil, Salt and black pepper, to taste., Low-fat grated cheese for garnish (optional)

Preparation:

- Preheat the oven to 180°C and grease a baking tray.
- In a non-stick pan, grill the aubergine slices on both sides until well-marked and soft. You can lightly

brush the eggplant slices with olive oil before grilling. This will require approximately 2-3 minutes per side. Once ready, set them aside.

- In a bowl, beat the eggs and then mix in the low-fat cheese. Add chopped basil, salt and pepper. Mix well.
- Start assembling the flan: arrange a layer of grilled aubergines on the bottom of the baking tray. Add a layer of tomato slices on top of the eggplant.
- Pour half of the egg and cheese mixture over the first layer of eggplant and tomatoes.
- Repeat the process with another layer of eggplant, tomatoes, and egg-cheese mixture. Proceed until the ingredients run out.
- If desired, you can garnish the top with a little shredded low-fat cheese.
- Bake the flan in the preheated oven for about 30-35 minutes or until golden brown on top and the egg mixture has set.
- Remove the flan from the oven and let it rest for a few minutes before cutting it into slices and serving it.

Nutritional values: Calories: 150-200 kcal, Protein: 10-12 g, Fat: 8-10 g, Carbohydrates: 10-12 g, Fibers: 3-5 g

62. Tuna steak with mango sauce and cucumber

Ingredients:4 fresh tuna steaks (about 150 g each),2 ripe mangoes, peeled, pitted and cut into cubes,1 cucumber, peeled, seeded and cut into cubes,1/4 red onion, finely chopped, Juice of 2 limes, 2 tablespoons chopped fresh coriander,2 tablespoons soy sauce (or tamari sauce for a gluten-free version), Salt and black pepper, to taste., Olive oil

Preparation:
- In a bowl, combine the diced mango, cucumber, red onion, lime juice and cilantro. Mix well to create the mango and cucumber salsa. Modify the flavor with pepper and salt according to liking.
- Refrigerate the bowl after it has been covered.
- Preheat a grill or nonstick skillet over medium-high heat. Brush the tuna steaks lightly with a little olive oil and season with salt and black pepper.
- Cook the tuna steaks on the grill or in the hot skillet for about 2-3 minutes per side or until golden brown on the outside but still pink on the inside. The cooking time will vary according to the size of the steaks.
- While the tuna cooks, you can reheat the mango and cucumber salsa over medium-low heat in a small pot, if you prefer to serve it slightly warmed.
- Once cooked, serve the tuna steaks with the mango-cucumber salsa on or next to them.
- Garnish with some chopped fresh coriander and offer immediately.

Nutritional values: Calories: 250-300 kcal, Protein: 30-35 g, Fat: 5-7 g, Carbohydrates: 20-25 g, Fibers: 3-4 g

63. Mushroom risotto with spinach

Ingredients:2 cups risotto rice (such as Arborio or Carnaroli rice),200 g of fresh mushrooms, cleaned and sliced,2 handfuls of fresh spinach, washed and chopped,1 onion, finely chopped,2 cloves of garlic, minced,1/2 cup dry white wine,4 cups vegetable broth (you can make your own or use canned broth),2 tablespoons of olive oil,2 tablespoons butter,1/2 cup grated Parmigiano-Reggiano cheese, Salt and black pepper, to taste, Chopped fresh parsley for garnish (optional)

Preparation:
- Warm the veggie broth in a large pot over medium heat. Keep it heated but not boiling.

- In a large skillet, heat the olive oil and 1 tablespoon butter over medium heat. Add the chopped onion and garlic and sauté until translucent.
- Cook until the sliced mushrooms begin to exude their liquid and become golden.
- Add the risotto rice to the pan and toast for a few minutes, stirring constantly, until the grains become slightly translucent.
- Pour the dry white wine into the pan and stir until the wine has been absorbed by the rice.
- Begin adding the hot vegetable broth one ladle at a time, stirring constantly and waiting for the broth to be absorbed before adding more broth. Continue this process until the rice is cooked al dente and the risotto is creamy, which will take about 18-20 minutes.
- Add the chopped spinach to the risotto and stir until softened and wilted.
- Remove the pan from the heat and add the remaining tablespoon of butter and the grated Parmigiano-Reggiano cheese. Mix well.
- Taste the risotto and adjust the flavor with salt and pepper to taste.
- If preferred, garnish with minced fresh parsley and dish hot.

Nutritional values: Calories: 350-400 kcal, Protein: 8-10 g, Fat: 10-12 g, Carbohydrates: 60-70 g, Fibers: 5-7 g

64. Curry turkey meatballs with yogurt sauce

Ingredients:

For the turkey meatballs:500 g of minced turkey meat,1 small onion, finely chopped,2 cloves of garlic, finely chopped,1 teaspoon curry powder,1/2 teaspoon cumin powder,1/2 teaspoon coriander powder,1/4 teaspoon chili powder (optional, for a spicy kick), Salt and black pepper, to taste.,2 tablespoons of olive oil

For the yogurt sauce:1 cup Greek yogurt,1 cucumber, peeled, seeded and grated,2 tablespoons chopped fresh mint, Juice of 1/2 lemon, Salt and black pepper, to taste.

Preparation:
- For the turkey meatballs:
- In a large bowl, mix the ground turkey with the chopped onion, minced garlic, curry powder, cumin powder, coriander powder, chili powder (if desired), salt, and pepper black. Stir everything together thoroughly.
- Shape the meat mixture into small, around patties. You can moisten your hands with a little water to make it easier to form the meatballs.
- Heating the olive oil in a nonstick skillet over a medium-high flame. Cook turkey meatballs until golden brown and fully cooked, about 4 to 5 minutes per side. Make sure they are cooked completely.
- For the yogurt sauce:
- In a bowl, mix the Greek yogurt with the grated cucumber, chopped mint, lemon juice, salt and black pepper. Mix well.
- Serve the turkey meatballs warm with the yogurt sauce as a side dish or dip.

Nutritional values : Calories : 250-300 kcal, Protein : 25-30 g Fat: 10-12 g, Carbohydrates: 15-20 g, Fibers: About 2-3 g

65. Pumpkin soup with coconut and ginger

Ingredients:1 kg of pumpkin, peeled and cut into cubes,1 onion, chopped,2 cloves of garlic, finely chopped,2cm fresh ginger root, peeled and grated,1 can (400 ml) coconut milk,4 cups of vegetable broth,2 tablespoons of olive oil, Salt and black pepper, to taste, Toasted pumpkin seeds and coriander leaves for garnish (optional)

Preparation:

- Warm the olive oil in a big pot over medium heat. Sauté the chopped onion and garlic mince until transparent.
- Add the pumpkin cubes and grated ginger root to the pot. Mix well and cook for a few minutes until the ingredients begin to soften.
- Pour the vegetable broth into the pan and bring everything to the boil. Then reduce the heat and simmer until the squash is tender, which will take about 20-25 minutes.
- Mix the soup with an immersion blender or food processor until creamy and smooth.
- Add coconut milk to the soup and mix well. Heat it over medium-low heat for another 5-7 minutes, stirring occasionally.
- Taste the soup and season with pepper and salt according to your liking.
- Serve the soup hot, garnished with toasted pumpkin seeds and fresh coriander leaves, if desired.

Nutritional values: Calories: 250-300 kcal, Protein: 4-6 g, Fat: 20-25 g, Carbohydrates: 20-25 g, Fiber: 5-7 g

66. Quinoa and vegetable pie

Ingredients:1 cup quinoa,2 cups of water,2 cups chopped leafy greens (such as spinach, kale, or chard),1 onion, finely chopped,2 cloves of garlic, finely chopped,1/2 cup grated low-fat cheese (e.g. low-fat cheese or low-fat cream cheese),2 eggs,2 tablespoons of olive oil, Salt and black pepper, to taste.

Preparation:

- Preheat the oven to 180°C and grease a cake pan or baking dish.
- In a sieve, rinse the quinoa well under cold running water.
- Put a pair of cups of water to a boil in a saucepan. Add the rinsed quinoa and cook over medium-low heat for about 15-20 minutes or until the liquid has been absorbed and the quinoa is cooked. Let the cooked quinoa cool.
- Heating the olive oil in a pan over a medium-high flame. Sauté the onion that has been chopped and minced garlic until transparent.
- Add the chopped leafy greens to the pan and cook until wilted and reduced in volume.
- In a bowl, whisk the eggs and then mix the cooked quinoa with the browned vegetables, grated low-fat cheese and beaten eggs. Modify the seasoning according to your liking with salt and pepper.
- Put the contents into the oiled baking dish.
- Bake the pie in the preheated oven for about 30-35 minutes or until golden on top and the egg mixture is set.
- Remove the cake from the oven, let it rest for a few minutes, then cut it into slices and serve.

Nutritional values: Calories: 250-300 kcal, Protein: 10-12 g, Fat: 10-12 g, Carbohydrates: 30-35 g, Fibers: 5-7 g

67. Grilled salmon with avocado and lime sauce

Ingredients:4 salmon fillets (about 150 g each),2 ripe avocados, cut into thin slices,2 limes, one for the juice and one for the thin slices,2 tablespoons of olive oil, Salt and black pepper, to taste., Chopped fresh coriander for garnish (optional)

For the lime sauce: Juice of 2 limes,2 tablespoons of olive oil,1 clove of garlic, finely chopped,1 teaspoon honey or maple syrup (to make the sauce slightly sweet), Salt and black pepper, to taste.

Preparation:

- For the grilled salmon:
- Preheat the grill to medium-high heat and lightly brush the salmon fillets with olive oil. Sprinkle with salt and black pepper according to your liking.
- Place the salmon fillets on the heated grill and cook for about 3-4 minutes per side or until the salmon is cooked through and has nice grill marks.
- While the salmon is cooking, you can also grill the avocado slices for a couple of minutes on each side, until they are lightly charred and hot.
- For the lime sauce:
- In a bowl, mix lime juice, olive oil, minced garlic, honey or maple syrup, salt and black pepper. Mix well.
- When the salmon is done, serve each fillet with avocado slices and a generous dollop of lime sauce on top.
- Garnish with chopped fresh cilantro, if desired, and serve immediately.

Nutritional values: Calories: 350-400 kcal, Protein: 30-35 g, Fat: 20-25 g, Carbohydrates: 10-15 g, Fibers: 5-7 g

68. Herb omelet with dried tomatoes and olives

Ingredients:8 eggs,2 tablespoons of milk (or vegetable milk),2 tablespoons chopped fresh herbs (such as parsley, basil or chives),1/4 cup dried tomatoes in oil, drained and chopped,1/4 cup pitted and chopped black olives,1/4 cup crumbled feta cheese (optional), Sprinkle with salt and black pepper according to your liking, 2 tablespoons of olive oil, Fresh herbs for garnish (optional)

Preparation:

- In a bowl, beat the eggs with the milk and add the chopped fresh herbs. Season with salt and black pepper to taste.
- In a 10- to 12-inch nonstick skillet, heat the olive oil over medium heat.
- Pour the egg mixture into the pan and cook over medium-low heat for about 3-4 minutes or until the edges start to set.
- While the omelette is still a little runny on top, spread the chopped sun-dried tomatoes, chopped black olives, and feta cheese (if using) over the surface of the omelette.
- Transfer the pan to the preheated broiler (oven broiler) and cook for a further 2-3 minutes or until the omelet is golden brown and the feta cheese has melted slightly.
- Remove the pan from the grill carefully (use a protected handle) and let cool slightly.
- Cut the herb omelet into wedges and serve hot, garnished with fresh herbs, if desired.

Nutritional values: Calories: 200-250 kcal, Protein: 12-15 g, Fat: 15-20 g, Carbohydrates: 5-7 g, Fibers: 2-3 g

69. Wholemeal couscous with grilled vegetables

Ingredients:1 cup wholemeal couscous,2 cups of water,2 medium courgettes, cut into long slices,1 aubergine, cut into long slices,1 red pepper, cut into strips,1 red onion, sliced,1 lemon, juice,3 tablespoons of olive oil, Salt and black pepper, to taste, Fresh herbs (such as mint or parsley) for garnish (optional)

Preparation:

- Put a pair of cups of water to a boil in a saucepan.

- When the water is boiling, pour in the wholemeal couscous, cover with a lid and remove from the heat source.
- Let rest for 5 minutes, then uncover and use a fork to separate the couscous grains. Put to a large mixing bowl once cool.
- While the couscous is cooking, you can prepare the grilled vegetables. Brush the courgettes, aubergine, pepper and onion with a little olive oil and season with salt and black pepper.
- Heat a grill or nonstick skillet over medium-high heat. Grill the prepared vegetables until well-marked and cooked through, turning occasionally. This will take approximately 8-10 minutes.
- In a small bowl, mix the lemon juice with 3 tablespoons of olive oil. This will be your simple vinaigrette.
- Once cooked, cut the grilled vegetables into small pieces.
- Add the grilled vegetables to the couscous and season everything with the lemon and olive oil vinaigrette. Mix thoroughly to disperse the flavors evenly.
- Garnish with fresh herbs, if desired, and serve at room temperature or cold.

Nutritional values: Calories: 300-350 kcal, Protein: 7-9 g, Fat: 10-12 g, Carbohydrates: 50-55 g, Fibers: 7-9 g

70. Turmeric chicken with brown rice

Ingredients:
For the turmeric chicken:4 boneless, skinless chicken breasts,1 teaspoon of turmeric powder,1/2 teaspoon sweet paprika, Salt and black pepper, to taste,2 tablespoons of olive oil
For the brown rice:1 cup brown rice, 2 cups of water, Salt to taste.
For the vegetables (you can choose your favorites):2 courgettes, cut into cubes,1 red pepper, cut into strips,1 red onion, cut into thin slices,1 clove of garlic, minced,2 tablespoons of olive oil, Salt and black pepper, to taste.

Preparation:
- For the turmeric chicken:
- In a bowl, mix the turmeric powder, sweet paprika, salt and black pepper. Sprinkle this spice mixture on both sides of the chicken breasts.
- Heat 2 tablespoons of olive oil in a nonstick skillet over a medium-high flame.
- Add the seasoned chicken breasts and cook for about 5-7 minutes per side or until browned and cooked through. Put the chicken breasts away after removing them from the pan.
- For the brown rice:
- Put 2 cups of water to a boil in a saucepan. Brown rice with a sprinkle of salt.
- Reduce the heat, cover the pot and cook the rice for about 40-45 minutes or until cooked and the water has been absorbed.
- Allow it to cool for just a few minutes before dishing.
- For the vegetables:
- Heating the two tablespoons of olive oil in a pan over medium heat. Add the minced garlic and sauté until it starts to smell.
- Combine the zucchini, red bell pepper, and red onion in a mixing bowl. Sauté the vegetables until they are cooked but still crisp. Season with salt and black pepper.
- Assembly:

- Serve the turmeric chicken over brown rice and with grilled vegetables on the side.

Nutritional values: Calories: 400-450 kcal, Protein: 30-35 g, Fat: 10-12 g, Carbohydrates: 40-45 g, Fibers: 5-7

71. Courgette spaghetti with Basil pesto

Ingredients:
For the courgette spaghetti:4 medium courgettes, Salt to taste.
For the basil pesto:2 cups fresh basil leaves,1/2 cup pine nuts,1/2 cup grated Parmigiano-Reggiano cheese,2 cloves of garlic, minced,1/2 cup olive oil, Salt and black pepper, to taste.

Preparation:
- For the courgette spaghetti:
- Use a paring knife to cut the zucchini into thin, long, spaghetti-like strips. Or you can do it manually with a sharp knife.
- Place the zucchini strips in a colander and sprinkle them lightly with salt. Let them rest for about 10-15 minutes to lose excess moisture.
- Rinse the courgettes under cold running water and dry them with a clean cloth.
- For the basil pesto:
- In a blender or food processor, combine the basil leaves, pine nuts, grated Parmigiano-Reggiano cheese, and minced garlic.
- Blend the ingredients on low speed while slowly pouring in the olive oil. Continue blending until you get a creamy consistency. If necessary, adjust the flavor with salt and pepper.
- Assembly:
- In a large bowl, combine the zucchini spaghetti with the prepared basil pesto. Mix well so that the courgettes are evenly coated with the pesto.
- Serve right away as a main course or side dish.

Nutritional values: Calories: 200-250 kcal, Protein: 5-7 g, Fat: 18-20 g, Carbohydrates: 5-7 g, Fiber: 2-3 g

72. Baked salmon with mixed vegetables

Ingredients:4 salmon fillets (about 150 g each),2 courgettes, cut into thin slices,1 red pepper, cut into strips,1 yellow pepper, cut into strips,1 red onion, sliced,4 sprigs of fresh rosemary,4 sprigs of fresh thyme,4 slices of lemon, Salt and black pepper, to taste,2 tablespoons of olive oil, Baking paper or foil for parcels

Preparation:
- Preheat the oven to 180°C.
- Prepare four sheets of baking paper or foil, one for each salmon fillet.
- Place the zucchini slices in the center of each sheet of baking paper or foil.
- Place the salmon fillet on each bed of courgettes.
- Spread pepper strips and onion slices over each salmon fillet.
- Place a sprig of rosemary, a sprig of thyme and a slice of lemon on each fillet.
- Season each parcel with salt, black pepper and a drizzle of olive oil.
- Close each parcel by wrapping baking paper or foil to seal the salmon and vegetables inside well.
- Transfer the parcels to a baking tray and bake for about 15-20 minutes or until the salmon is cooked and the vegetables are tender.
- Remove the parcels from the oven, open them carefully and serve the salmon fillets with the mixed vegetables inside the parcels.

Nutritional values: Calories: 250-300 kcal, Protein: 25-30 g, Fat: 12-15 g, Carbohydrates: 10-12 g, Fiber: 3-5 g

73. Avocado and black pepper salsa with grilled chicken

Ingredients:

For the grilled chicken:4 boneless, skinless chicken breasts, Salt and black pepper, to taste.

For the avocado and black pepper sauce:2 ripe avocados, peeled and pitted,2 cloves of garlic, finely chopped, Juice of 2 lemons,1/4 cup olive oil,1 teaspoon ground black pepper (add more or less depending on your taste), Salt to taste.

Preparation:

- For the grilled chicken:
- Preheat grill to medium-high heat.
- Brush the chicken breasts lightly with olive oil and season with salt and black pepper.
- Place the chicken breasts on the heated grill and cook for about 6-8 minutes per side or until cooked through and have nice grill marks.
- Take the chicken from the grill and set it aside for a few minutes to rest before cutting.
- For the avocado and black pepper sauce:
- In a blender or food processor, add peeled avocados, minced garlic, lemon juice, olive oil, ground black pepper and a generous amount of salt.
- Blend all the ingredients until you obtain a creamy and smooth sauce. Taste and adjust the flavor by adding more salt or black pepper, if necessary.
- Assembly:
- Serve grilled chicken breasts with a generous portion of avocado and black pepper sauce on top.

Nutritional values: Calories: 300-350 kcal, Protein: 25-30 g, Fat: 20-25 g, Carbohydrates: 10-12 g, Fibers: 7-9 g

74. Curried chickpea salad with cucumbers and tomatoes

Ingredients:2 cans of chickpeas (about 400 g each), drained and rinsed,2 cucumbers, cut into cubes,4 fresh tomatoes, cut into cubes,1 red onion, finely chopped,1/4 cup chopped fresh cilantro (optional), Salt and black pepper, to taste.

For the curry vinaigrette:1/4 cup olive oil, Juice of 1 lemon,2 teaspoons curry powder,1 teaspoon honey or maple syrup (for light sweetness), Salt and black pepper, to taste.

Preparation:

- For the curry vinaigrette:
- In a small bowl, combine the olive oil, lemon juice, curry powder, honey or maple syrup, salt and pepper. Mix well until you get a creamy vinaigrette.
- Taste the vinaigrette and adjust the flavor with salt, pepper or curry powder, if necessary.
- For the chickpea salad:
- In a large bowl, combine the drained chickpeas, diced cucumbers, diced tomatoes and chopped red onion. Mix well.
- Pour the curry vinaigrette over the salad and toss so that all the ingredients are evenly seasoned.
- Cover the salad and let it rest in the refrigerator for at least 30 minutes so that the flavors blend.
- Before serving, garnish the salad with chopped fresh cilantro, if desired.

Nutritional values: Calories: 300-350 kcal, Protein: 10-12 g, Fat: 12-15 g, Carbohydrates: 40-45 g, Fiber: 10-12 g

75. Steamed salmon with broccoli and quinoa

Ingredients:

For the steamed salmon:4 salmon fillets (about 150 g each), Juice of 1 lemon, Salt and black pepper, to taste.

For the steamed broccoli:2 cups broccoli florets, Salt to taste.

For the quinoa:1 cup quinoa,2 cups of water, Salt to taste.

Preparation:

- For the steamed salmon:
- Preheat a steamer. You can use a steamer or a pot with a steamer basket.
- Place the salmon fillets in the steamer or steamer basket. Squeeze the lemon juice over the fillets and season them with salt and black pepper.
- Cover the pot and steam for about 8-10 minutes or until the salmon is cooked through and flakes easily with a fork.
- For the steamed broccoli:
- While the salmon is steaming, you can prepare the broccoli. Bring a pot of water to a boil, add a pinch of salt and steam the broccoli florets for about 3-4 minutes or until tender but still crunchy.
- For the quinoa:
- Put a pair of cups of water to a boil in a saucepan. Mix in the quinoa and season with salt.
- Reduce the heat, cover the pot and cook the quinoa for about 15 minutes or until cooked and the water has been absorbed.
- Using a fork, fluff the quinoa and remove any extra water.
- Assembly:
- Serve steamed salmon fillets with steamed broccoli and cooked quinoa on the side.

Nutritional values: Calories: 350-400 kcal, Protein: 30-35 g, Fat: 12-15 g, Carbohydrates: 30-35 g, Fiber: 6-8 g

76. Lemon chicken with steamed spinach

Ingredients:

For the lemon chicken:4 boneless, skinless chicken breasts, Juice of 2 lemons, Grated zest of 1 lemon,2 cloves of garlic, finely chopped,2 tablespoons of olive oil, Salt and black pepper, to taste.

For the steamed spinach:400 g of fresh spinach,1 clove of garlic, finely chopped,1 tablespoon of olive oil, Salt and black pepper, to taste.

Preparation:

- For the lemon chicken:
- In a bowl, mix the lemon juice, grated lemon zest, minced garlic, olive oil, salt and black pepper. This will be the marinade for the chicken.
- Place the chicken breasts on a baking tray or bowl and pour the marinade over the top. Cover and set in the freezer for at least 30 minutes to marinate.
- Preheat a nonstick skillet over medium-high heat. Cook the marinated chicken breasts for about 6-8 minutes per side or until browned and fully cooked.
- For the steamed spinach:
- While the chicken is cooking, you can prepare the steamed spinach. In a steamer pan or pot with a steamer basket, steam the spinach for about 2-3 minutes or until wilted.
- Heating one teaspoon of olive oil in a skillet over a medium-high flame. Add the chopped garlic and sauté briefly. Add the steamed spinach and cook for another minute. Season with salt and pepper.
- Assembly:
- Serve lemon chicken breasts with steamed spinach on the side.

Nutritional values: Calories: 250-300 kcal, Protein: 30-35 g, Fat: 12-15 g, Carbohydrates: 10-12 g, Fiber: 3-5 g

77. Red lentil pasta with courgettes and cherry tomatoes

Ingredients:2 cups red lentil pasta,2 medium courgettes, cut into cubes,2 cups cherry tomatoes, cut in half,2 cloves of garlic, finely chopped,1/4 cup olive oil,1/4 cup grated Parmigiano-Reggiano cheese (optional), Salt and black pepper, to taste.

Preparation:

- Put enough of water to a boil in a large pot. Add a pinch of salt and cook the red lentil pasta following the instructions on the package. Drain al dente and set aside.
- As the pasta cooks, heat the olive oil in a big skillet over a medium-high flame. Add the minced garlic and sauté until it starts to smell.
- Add the courgette cubes and cook for about 4-5 minutes or until tender but still crunchy.
- Add the halved cherry tomatoes and cook for a further 2-3 minutes, until starting to soften but holding their shape.
- Add the cooked red lentil pasta to the pan with the courgettes and cherry tomatoes. Mix well so that the ingredients are combined evenly.
- Modify the flavor with salt and black pepper according to your liking.
- If desired, sprinkle with grated Parmigiano-Reggiano cheese before serving.

Nutritional values: Calories: 350-400 kcal, Protein: 15-18 g, Fat: 15-18 g, Carbohydrates: 40-45 g, Fiber: 8-10 g

78. Avocado and orange salad with nuts

Ingredients:2 ripe avocados, peeled and cut into slices,2 oranges, peeled and cut into slices or wedges,1/2 cup walnuts, toasted and roughly chopped,1/4 cup fresh basil leaves,1/4 cup extra virgin olive oil, Two tablespoons of balsamic vinegar with salt and black pepper, according to liking.

Preparation:

- In a large bowl, combine avocado slices, orange slices or wedges, toasted walnuts, and fresh basil.
- In a small bowl, mix the olive oil, balsamic vinegar, salt and black pepper to create the vinaigrette.
- Pour the vinaigrette over the avocado and orange salad and toss gently to coat all the ingredients.
- Taste and adjust the seasoning with pepper and salt as needed.
- Serve the salad immediately as a side dish or light dish.

Nutritional values: Calories: 250-300 kcal, Protein: 4-6 g, Fat: 22-25 g, Carbohydrates: 15-18 g, Fiber: 6-8 g

79. Grilled sea bass fillet with peperonata

Ingredients:

For the grilled sea bass fillet:4 sea bass fillets (about 150 g each), Juice of 1 lemon,2 tablespoons of olive oil, Salt and black pepper, to taste.

For the peperonata:2 red peppers, cut into thin strips, 2 yellow peppers, cut into thin strips,1 onion, cut into slices,2 cloves of garlic, finely chopped,1/4 cup olive oil, Two teaspoons of balsamic vinegar, salt and black pepper, according to your liking.

Preparation:

- For the grilled sea bass fillet:
- Preheat grill to medium-high heat.
- Brush the sea bass fillets with olive oil and lemon juice. Sprinkle with salt and black pepper according to your liking.
- Place the sea bass fillets on the hot grill and cook for about 3-4 minutes per side or until cooked through and have nice grill marks.
- For the peperonata:
- Heating the olive oil in a big skillet over a medium-high flame.
- Add the pepper strips, onion slices and minced garlic. Cook for about 10-15 minutes or until the vegetables are tender and lightly caramelized.
- Add the balsamic vinegar to the vegetables and mix well. Continue cooking for another 2-3 minutes.
- Assembly:
- Serve the grilled sea bass fillets with a generous portion of peperonata on top or as a side dish.

Nutritional values: Calories: 250-300 kcal, Protein: 25-30 g, Fat: 12-15 g, Carbohydrates: 10-12 g, Fibers: 2-4 g

80. Mushroom risotto with asparagus

Ingredients:2 cups risotto rice (such as Carnaroli or Arborio),200 g of fresh mushrooms (such as champignons or porcini mushrooms), cut into slices,200 g of fresh asparagus, cut into pieces,1 onion, finely chopped,2 cloves of garlic, finely chopped,4 cups of hot vegetable broth,1/2 cup dry white wine,2 tablespoons of olive oil,1/4 cup grated Parmigiano-Reggiano cheese (optional), Salt and black pepper, to taste.

Preparation:

- Warm the olive oil in a big pot over a moderate flame. Add the chopped onion and minced garlic and fry until translucent.
- Add the risotto rice and toast it lightly for a couple of minutes, stirring constantly.
- Add the white wine and stir until it has been absorbed by the rice.
- One ladle at a time, add the heated vegetable broth, stirring continuously. Continue cooking and adding broth as it is absorbed, until the rice is cooked al dente (about 18-20 minutes).
- Meanwhile, in a separate pan, cook the mushrooms and asparagus until tender. Add the mushrooms and asparagus to the risotto when it is almost ready.
- Adjust the flavor of the risotto with salt and black pepper to your liking.
- If desired, sprinkle with grated Parmigiano-Reggiano cheese before serving.

Nutritional values: Calories: 350-400 kcal, Protein: 8-10 g, Fat: 5-7 g, Carbohydrates: 70-75 g, Fiber: 5-7 g

81. Tomato and basil sauce with turkey meatballs

Ingredients:

For the turkey meatballs:500 g of minced turkey meat,1 egg,1/4 cup breadcrumbs,1/4 cup grated Parmigiano-Reggiano cheese,2 cloves of garlic, finely chopped,2 tablespoons chopped fresh basil, Salt and black pepper, to taste.

For the tomato and basil sauce:2 cups tomato puree,1/4 cup chopped fresh basil,2 cloves of garlic, finely chopped, Two teaspoons of olive oil, Salt and black pepper according to your liking.

Preparation:

- For the turkey meatballs:
- In a bowl, combine the ground turkey, egg, breadcrumbs, grated Parmigiano-Reggiano cheese, minced garlic and fresh basil. Mix well until you obtain a homogeneous mixture.

- Shape the mixture into small round meatballs and place them on a tray.
- Heat a non-stick pan with a little olive oil and cook the meatballs over medium-high heat for about 8-10 minutes or until cooked through and golden brown.
- For the tomato and basil sauce:
- Heating the olive oil in a saucepan over a medium-high flame.
- Add the minced garlic and fry until it starts to smell.
- Add the tomato puree and fresh basil. Cook for about 10-15 minutes, stirring occasionally, until the sauce thickens and the basil is well incorporated.
- Adjust the flavor of the sauce with salt and black pepper to your liking.
- Assembly:
- Serve turkey meatballs with a generous portion of tomato basil sauce on top or as a main course.

Nutritional values: Calories: 350-400 kcal, Protein: 25-30 g, Fat: 12-15 g, Carbohydrates: 20-25 g, Fiber: 3-5 g

82. Quinoa with grilled aubergines and feta

Ingredients:1 cup quinoa,2 cups of water,2 medium aubergines, cut into thin slices,1/2 cup feta cheese, crumbled,1/4 cup fresh herbs (such as parsley, basil, mint), chopped, Juice of 1 lemon, 2 tbsp of olive oil, Salt and black pepper according to your liking.

Preparation:

- Put the a pair of cups of water to a boil in a saucepan. Mix in the quinoa and season with salt. Reduce the heat, cover the pot and cook the quinoa for about 15 minutes or until cooked and the water has been absorbed. Remove any extra water from the quinoa and fluff with a fork.
- While the quinoa cooks, heat a grill or nonstick skillet over medium-high heat.
- Brush the aubergine slices with a little olive oil, salt and pepper. Cook the eggplant slices on the grill or in the pan for about 2-3 minutes per side or until tender and have grill marks.
- In a large bowl, combine the cooked quinoa, grilled eggplant slices, crumbled feta cheese, and chopped herbs. Mix well.
- Make a vinaigrette by mixing lemon juice, olive oil, salt and black pepper in a small bowl.
- Pour the vinaigrette over the quinoa and mix well so that all the ingredients are evenly seasoned.
- Serve quinoa with grilled eggplant and feta as a side or main course.

Nutritional values: Calories: 300-350 kcal, Protein: Abut 8-10 g, Fat: 12-15 g, Carbohydrates: 40-45 g, Fibers: 7-9 g

83. Chicken curry with roasted cauliflower

Ingredients:

For the chicken curry:4 boneless, skinless chicken breasts,2 tablespoons curry powder,1/2 cup coconut milk,1 onion, finely chopped,2 cloves of garlic, finely chopped,2 tablespoons of olive oil, Salt and black pepper, to taste.

For the roasted cauliflower:1 medium cauliflower, cut into florets,2 tablespoons of olive oil,1 teaspoon cumin powder,1 teaspoon sweet paprika, Salt and black pepper, to taste.

Preparation:

- For the chicken curry:
- In a bowl, mix the curry powder with the coconut milk. This will be the marinade for the chicken.
- Place the chicken breasts on a baking tray or bowl and pour the marinade over the top. Cover and leave to marinate in the refrigerator for at least 30 minutes.
- Preheat a nonstick skillet over medium-high heat. Cook the marinated chicken breasts for about 6-8 minutes per side or until browned and fully cooked.
- For the roasted cauliflower:
- Preheat the oven to 200°C.
- In a bowl, toss the cauliflower florets with olive oil, cumin powder, sweet paprika, salt and black pepper.
- Spread the cauliflower onto a baking tray lined with baking paper and roast in the oven for about 25-30 minutes or until golden and tender, stirring halfway through.
- Assembly:
- Serve the chicken curry with the roasted cauliflower as a side dish.

Nutritional values: Calories:350-400 kcal, Protein: 30-35 g, Fat: 20-25 g, Carbohydrates: 10-12 g, Fiber: 5-7 g

84. Chickpea soup with spinach and lemon

Ingredients: 2 cups cooked chickpeas (you can use previously cooked canned or dried chickpeas),4 cups of vegetable broth,200 g of fresh spinach, washed and cut, Juice and zest of 1 lemon,1 onion, finely chopped,2 cloves of garlic, finely chopped,2 tablespoons of olive oil,1 teaspoon cumin powder, Salt and black pepper, to taste.

Preparation:

- Heating the olive oil in a big pot over a medium-high flame. Add the chopped onion and minced garlic and fry until translucent.
- Add the cumin powder and stir for about a minute or until fragrant.
- Add the cooked chickpeas and vegetable broth. Bring everything to the boil, then reduce the heat and leave to simmer for about 10-15 minutes.
- Add the chopped spinach to the soup and cook for another 3-4 minutes or until wilted.
- Add the lemon juice and grated lemon zest. Mix well and adjust the flavor with salt and black pepper to your liking.
- Serve the chickpea soup with spinach and lemon hot, perhaps with a slice of crusty bread.

Nutritional values: Calories:250-300 kcal, Protein: 10-12 g, Fat: 7-9 g, Carbohydrates: 35-40 g, Fibers: 7-9 g

85. Turkey Meatloaf with Roasted Pepper Sauce

Ingredients:

For the turkey meatloaf: 500 g of minced turkey meat,1 egg,1/2 cup breadcrumbs,1 onion, finely chopped,2 cloves of garlic, finely chopped,2 tablespoons chopped fresh basil, Salt and black pepper, to taste.

For the roasted pepper sauce:2 red peppers, roasted and peeled,2 tablespoons of olive oil,1 clove of garlic, finely chopped,2 tablespoons of balsamic vinegar, Salt and black pepper, to taste.

Preparation:

- For the turkey meatloaf:
- In a bowl, combine the ground turkey, egg, breadcrumbs, chopped onion, minced garlic and fresh basil. Mix well until you obtain a homogeneous mixture.
- Form the mixture into a large meatloaf, place it on a lightly greased baking sheet, and season with salt and black pepper.

- Cook in a preheated oven at 180°C for approximately 30-35 minutes or until the meatloaf is cooked and golden.
- For the roasted pepper sauce:
- Heating the olive oil in a skillet over a medium-high flame. Add the minced garlic and fry until it starts to smell.
- Add the peeled roasted peppers, balsamic vinegar, and a pinch of salt and pepper.
- While it is cooking, for about 5-7 minutes, stir occasionally, until the sauce has thickened slightly.
- Assembly:
- Cut the turkey meatloaf into slices and serve with the roasted pepper sauce on top or on the side.

Nutritional values: Calories:300-350 kcal, Protein: 25-30 g, Fat: 10-12 g, Carbohydrates: 15-18 g, Fibers: 2-4 g

86. Wholemeal couscous with mint aubergines

Ingredients:

For the wholemeal couscous:1 cup wholemeal couscous,2 cups of water, Salt to taste.

For the aubergines with mint:2 medium aubergines, diced,2 tablespoons of olive oil,2 tablespoons fresh mint, chopped, Juice of 1 lemon, Salt and black pepper, to taste.

For the light vinaigrette:2 tablespoons of olive oil, Juice of 1 lemon,1 clove of garlic, finely chopped, Salt and black pepper, to taste.

Preparation:

- For the wholemeal couscous:
- Put a pair of cups of water to a boil in a saucepan. Add the wholemeal couscous and a pinch of salt.
- Cover the pot, turn off the heat and let sit for about 5 minutes or until the couscous is cooked.
- Drain off any excess water and fluff the couscous with a fork.
- For the minted aubergines:
- Preheat the oven to 200°C.
- In a bowl, toss the diced eggplant with olive oil, chopped fresh mint, lemon juice, salt and black pepper.
- Spread the aubergines onto a baking tray lined with baking paper and roast in the oven for about 20-25 minutes or until tender and lightly browned.
- For the light vinaigrette:
- In a small bowl, mix the olive oil, lemon juice, minced garlic, salt and black pepper.
- Assembly:
- In a large bowl, combine the cooked whole-wheat couscous with the roasted mint eggplant. Mix well.
- Pour the light vinaigrette over the couscous and eggplant mixture and toss until all ingredients are evenly seasoned.
- Serve wholemeal couscous with minted aubergines as a side dish or main course.

Nutritional values: Calories: 300-350 kcal, Protein: 6-8 g, Fat: 10-12 g, Carbohydrates: 50-55 g, Fibers: 7-9 g

87. Grilled chicken salad with fruit

Ingredients:

For the chicken salad:2 grilled chicken breasts, cut into thin strips,8 cups of mixed salad (lettuce, spinach, arugula, etc.),2 cups fresh fruit of your choice (strawberries, blueberries, mango, etc.),1/2 cup walnuts, toasted and roughly chopped,1/4 cup feta cheese, crumbled (optional)

For the vinaigrette:3 tablespoons of olive oil,2 tablespoons of balsamic vinegar,1 teaspoon honey, Salt and black pepper, to taste.

Preparation:

- For the chicken salad:
- Grill the chicken breasts until they are cooked through and have grill marks. Cut the chicken into thin strips.
- In a large bowl, combine the salad greens, fresh fruit, toasted nuts, and feta cheese (if desired).
- For the vinaigrette:
- In a small bowl, mix the olive oil, balsamic vinegar, honey, salt and black pepper. Mix until you get a smooth vinaigrette.
- Assembly:
- Pour the vinaigrette over the salad mixture and toss well to dress evenly.
- Toss the salad with the grilled chicken strips.
- Serve grilled chicken salad with fruit as a main course.

Nutritional values: Calories: 350-400 kcal, Protein: 25-30 g, Fat: 20-25 g, Carbohydrates: 20-25 g, Fiber: 5-7 g

88. Baked salmon with dill and lemon

Ingredients: 4 salmon fillets,2 tablespoons of olive oil, Juice and zest of 1 lemon,2 tablespoons fresh dill, chopped, Salt and black pepper, to taste.

Preparation:

- Preheat the oven to 200°C and line a baking tray with baking paper or lightly greased with oil.
- Whisk together the olive oil, lemon juice, lemon zest, sliced fresh dill, salt, and black pepper in a mixing bowl.
- Arrange the salmon fillets on the baking sheet that has been prepared. Generously brush the lemon-dill marinade over each salmon fillet.
- Bake in the preheated oven for about 12-15 minutes or until the salmon is cooked through and flakes easily with a fork.
- The duration of cooking will depend on the size of the salmon fillets.
- Serve the lemon-dill-baked salmon hot, garnishing with lemon slices or fresh dill, if desired.

Nutritional values: Calories: 300-350 kcal, Protein: 30-35 g, Fat: 18-20 g, Carbohydrates: 2-3 g, Fiber: 1-2 g

89. Brown rice with tofu and wok vegetables

Ingredients: 2 cups cooked brown rice,250g tofu, diced,2 cups mixed vegetables of your choice (peppers, carrots, zucchini, broccoli, etc.), cut into strips or cubes,2 tablespoons of soy sauce,2 tablespoons of sesame oil,2 cloves of garlic, finely chopped,1 teaspoon grated fresh ginger, Salt and black pepper, to taste., Toasted almond flakes (optional, for garnish)

Preparation:

- Heating the sesame oil in a big skillet or wok over a medium-high flame.
- Add the diced tofu and sauté until golden on all sides. This will take approximately 5-7 minutes. Set away the tofu from the pan.
- Place the mixed vegetables in the same pan. Stir-fry them for about 5-7 minutes or until tender but still crunchy.
- Add the minced garlic and grated ginger to the vegetables and cook for a minute until fragrant.
- Add the cooked brown rice to the vegetables and mix well. Pour the soy sauce over the rice and continue stirring until all the ingredients are well combined.

- Add the previously sautéed tofu to the wok and heat for about 2-3 minutes, stirring regularly.
- Taste and season with salt and black pepper according to your liking.
- Serve the brown rice with tofu and hot wok vegetables, garnishing with toasted almond flakes if desired.

Nutritional values: Calories: 350-400 kcal, Protein: 15-18 g, Fat: 10-12 g, Carbohydrates: 50-55 g, Fiber: 6-8 g

90. Baked tortilla with sweet potatoes and peppers

Ingredients: 2 medium sweet potatoes, peeled and thinly sliced,1 red pepper, cut into strips,1 green pepper, cut into strips,1 red onion, cut into thin slices,8 eggs,1/4 cup milk, Salt and black pepper, to taste.,2 tablespoons of olive oil, Shredded cheese (cheddar, Swiss, or your choice, optional)

Preparation:

- Preheat the oven to 180°C.
- Heating the olive oil in a nonstick skillet over a medium-high flame. Add the sweet potato slices and cook until tender and lightly browned. This will take approximately 8-10 minutes. Remove the sweet potatoes from the pan and set aside.
- In the same pan, add the pepper strips and onion slices. Cook until the vegetables are tender and lightly browned, about 5 to 7 minutes.
- In a bowl, beat the eggs with the milk. Season with salt and black pepper according to your liking.
- Arrange the sweet potatoes, peppers, and onions in the pan in an even layer.
- Pour the egg mix into the pan with the vegetables. Sprinkle grated cheese (if desired) over the surface of the egg.
- Transfer the pan to the preheated oven and bake for about 15 to 20 minutes or until the tortilla is puffed and golden.
- Remove from the oven and let rest for a few minutes before cutting into slices.
- Serve the baked tortilla with sweet potatoes and peppers hot.

Nutritional values: Calories: 250-300 kcal, Protein: 10-12 g, Fat: 10-12 g, Carbohydrates: 30-35 g, Fiber: 5-7 g

91. Avocado and cilantro salsa with grilled shrimp

Ingredients:

For the grilled prawns:500 g of prawns, peeled and cleaned,2 tablespoons of olive oil, Salt and black pepper, to taste.
For the avocado and coriander salsa:2 ripe avocados, peeled and stoned,1/4 cup fresh cilantro, chopped, Juice of 1 lime,1 clove of garlic, finely chopped, Salt and black pepper, to taste.

Preparation:

- For the grilled prawns:
- Preheat grill to medium-high heat.
- In a bowl, toss the shrimp with olive oil, salt and black pepper.
- Thread the shrimp onto grilling skewers or use a rack with baskets to prevent the shrimp from falling through the grates.
- Grill the shrimp for about 2-3 minutes per side or until pink and cooked through.
- For the avocado and coriander salsa:
- In a blender or with an immersion blender, blend the avocados, fresh cilantro, lime juice, minced garlic, salt and black pepper until smooth.
- If the sauce is too thick, you can add a little water or more lime juice to get the desired consistency.
- Assembly:

- Serve the grilled prawns hot, accompanied by the avocado and coriander sauce.

Nutritional values: Calories: 250-300 kcal, Protein: 20-25 g, Fat: 15-18 g, Carbohydrates: 12-15 g, Fibers: 7-9 g

92. Sautéed Chinese cabbage with tofu and ginger

Ingredients: 400 g Chinese cabbage, cut into strips,250g tofu, diced,2 tablespoons of sesame oil,2 cloves of garlic, finely chopped,1 teaspoon grated fresh ginger,2 tablespoons of soy sauce, Salt and black pepper, to taste., Toasted sesame seeds (optional, for garnish)

Preparation:

- Heating the sesame oil in a big skillet or wok over a medium-high flame.
- Cook the tofu cubes until golden brown on all sides. This will take approximately 5-7 minutes.
- Take away the tofu from the pan and set it aside.
- Combine the minced garlic and grated ginger in the same pan. Cook for 1 minute, or until fragrant.
- Add the shredded bok choy and soy sauce to the pan. Sauté cabbage until tender but still crunchy, about 5 to 7 minutes.
- Add the previously sautéed tofu to the pan and heat for about 2-3 minutes, stirring regularly.
- Taste and season with salt and black pepper according to your liking. If wanted, garnish with toasted seeds of sesame.
- Serve the sautéed bok choy with tofu and hot ginger.

Nutritional values: Calories: 250-300 kcal, Protein: 15-18 g, Fat: 15-18 g, Carbohydrates: 15-20 g, Fiber: 6-8 g

93. Grilled aubergine salad with tomatoes and mint

Ingredients: 2 medium aubergines, cut into thin slices,4 ripe tomatoes, cut into cubes,1/2 cup fresh mint, chopped,2 cloves of garlic, finely chopped, Juice of 1 lemon,3 tablespoons of olive oil, Salt and black pepper, to taste.

Preparation:

- Preheat a grill or nonstick skillet over medium-high heat.
- Brush the aubergine slices with a little olive oil and grill for about 2-3 minutes per side, or until grill-marked and tender. You can cook them in batches if necessary.
- In a large bowl, combine the grilled eggplant slices, tomato cubes, chopped fresh mint, and minced garlic.
- In a small bowl, prepare the vinaigrette by mixing the lemon juice, olive oil, salt and black pepper.
- Pour the vinaigrette over the eggplant, tomato and mint mixture. Stir gently to season evenly.
- Let the salad sit in the refrigerator for at least 30 minutes before serving to allow the flavors to blend.

Nutritional values: Calories: 150-200 kcal, Protein: 2-3 g, Fat: 10-12 g, Carbohydrates: 15-20 g, Fibers: 6-8 g

94. Salmon baked in foil with thyme vegetables

Ingredients: 4 salmon fillets (about 150 g each),2 medium courgettes, cut into thin slices,2 ripe tomatoes, cut into slices,1 red onion, thinly sliced,4 sprigs of fresh thyme, Juice of 1 lemon,2 tablespoons of olive oil, Salt and black pepper, to taste.

Preparation:

- Preheat the oven to 200°C.
- Prepare four sheets of baking paper or foil, one for each salmon fillet.
- On each of these sheets, place a portion of sliced zucchini, tomato slices and sliced onion.
- Place the salmon fillet on each bed of vegetables.

- Season the salmon with lemon juice, olive oil, fresh thyme leaves, salt and black pepper to taste.
- Close the sheets of baking paper or foil around the fish and vegetables to form well-sealed packages.
- Transfer the packets to a baking sheet and bake for about 20-25 minutes or until the salmon is cooked and the vegetables are tender.
- Remove the packets carefully from the oven (the steam will be very hot) and serve the salmon in foil directly in the packets.

Nutritional values: Calories: 300-350 kcal, Protein: 25-30 g, Fat: 15-20 g, Carbohydrates: 10-15 g, Fibers: 3-4 g

95. Lemon risotto with courgettes and parsley

Ingredients: 2 cups risotto rice (such as Arborio),2 medium courgettes, diced,1 onion, finely chopped,2 cloves of garlic, finely chopped, Grated zest of 1 lemon, Juice of 1 lemon,1/2 cup dry white wine,4-5 cups of hot vegetable broth,1/2 cup grated Parmigiano-Reggiano cheese,2 tablespoons butter,2 tablespoons of olive oil,1/4 cup fresh parsley, chopped, Salt and black pepper, to taste.

Preparation:

- Heating the olive oil in a big pot over a medium-high flame. Cook the chopped onion and garlic until transparent.
- Add the rice and toast it for 1-2 minutes, stirring constantly.
- Add the white wine and cook until the wine is almost completely absorbed.
- Add the diced courgettes and continue to cook, stirring regularly.
- Start adding the hot vegetable broth one ladle at a time, cooking the rice and stirring constantly. Add the next broth only when the previous one has been absorbed.
- Continue this process until the rice is al dente and has reached your desired creamy consistency, usually about 18-20 minutes.
- Remove from the heat and add the lemon juice, grated lemon zest, chopped parsley, grated Parmigiano-Reggiano cheese and butter. Mix well.
- Taste and season with salt and black pepper according to your liking. Serve the lemon risotto with courgettes and hot parsley.

Nutritional values: Calories: 350-400 kcal, Protein: 8-10 g, Fat: 12-15 g, Carbohydrates: 50-55 g, Fiber: 3-4 g

96. Quinoa and black bean meatballs with avocado salsa

Ingredients:

For the meatballs:1 cup cooked quinoa,1 cup cooked black beans, drained and rinsed,1 red onion, finely chopped,2 cloves of garlic, finely chopped,1 teaspoon cumin powder,1 teaspoon paprika, Salt and black pepper, to taste.,1/2 cup breadcrumbs (or cornmeal) for the dough and breading, Olive oil for cooking
For the avocado salsa:2 ripe avocados, peeled and stoned, Juice of 1 lime,1/4 cup fresh cilantro, chopped, Salt and black pepper, to taste.

Preparation:

- For the meatballs:
- In a large bowl, combine cooked quinoa, black beans, chopped red onion, minced garlic, cumin, paprika, salt, black pepper, and breadcrumbs. Make sure the ingredients are well combined.
- Form the mixture into small meatballs and roll them in breadcrumbs or corn flour.
- Heating the olive oil in a nonstick skillet over a medium-high flame. Cook meatballs until golden brown on both sides, about 3 to 4 minutes per side.
- For the avocado salsa:
- In a blender or with an immersion blender, blend the avocados, lime juice, fresh cilantro, salt and black pepper until smooth.
- Assembly:
- Serve the quinoa and black bean meatballs with the avocado salsa as a topping.

Nutritional values: Calories: 300-350 kcal, Protein: 8-10 g, Fat: 15-18 g, Carbohydrates: 30-35 g Fiber: 8-10 g

97. Chickpea pasta with kale and cherry tomatoes

Ingredients: 250 g chickpea pasta (or pasta of your choice),1 head of kale, washed and cut into strips,200 g of cherry tomatoes, cut in half,2 cloves of garlic, finely chopped,1/4 cup olive oil, Red chili pepper (optional, for a touch of spiciness), Salt and black pepper, to taste., Grated Pecorino or Parmesan cheese (optional, for garnish)

Preparation:

- Bring a pot of salted water to a boil and cook the chickpea pasta according to package instructions until al dente. Drain it and keep it aside.
- Heating the olive oil in a big skillet over a medium-high flame. Add the minced garlic and, if you want a spicy touch, the red chili pepper.
- Add the shredded kale and cook for about 5-7 minutes or until tender.
- Add the halved cherry tomatoes and cook for a further 2-3 minutes until starting to soften.
- Add the chickpea paste to the pan with the cabbage and cherry tomatoes. Mix well to blend the flavors.
- Taste and season with salt and black pepper according to your liking.
- Serve the chickpea pasta with kale and cherry tomatoes hot, garnished with grated Pecorino or Parmesan cheese if desired.

Nutritional values: Calories: 350-400 kcal, Protein: 10-12 g, Fat: 15-18 g, Carbohydrates: 45-50 g, Fiber: 8-10 g

98. Grilled steak with black pepper sauce and spinach

Ingredients: 4 beef steaks (about 200 g each),1 cup fresh spinach,1/4 cup heavy cream,2 tablespoons of olive oil,2 tablespoons whole black pepper, Salt and ground black pepper, to taste.

Preparation:

- Start by making the black pepper sauce. In a pan over medium heat, toast the whole black peppercorns until they begin to release their aroma, then add the heavy cream. Let it cook for about 5 minutes until the sauce thickens. Add salt to taste.
- While the sauce is preparing, grill the steaks on a hot grill or in a nonstick skillet. Cook the steaks for the desired time to achieve your preferred doneness (rare, medium rare, medium, etc.), usually 3 to 5 minutes per side depending on the thickness of the steaks.
- While the steaks rest after cooking, in a separate pan, heat the olive oil and add the fresh spinach. Cook the spinach until slightly wilted, stirring occasionally.
- Serve the steaks hot, with the black pepper sauce on top and the sautéed spinach alongside.

Nutritional values: Calories: 350-400 kcal, Protein: 30-35 g, Fat: 20-25 g, Carbohydrates: 2-4 g, Fiber: 1-2 g

99. Coconut Curry Sweet Potato Soup

Ingredients: 2 medium sweet potatoes, peeled and cut into cubes,1 onion, chopped,2 cloves of garlic, finely chopped,1 tablespoon of olive oil,1 tablespoon curry powder,1/2 teaspoon of turmeric,1 can (about 400 ml) of coconut milk,4 cups of vegetable broth, Salt and black pepper, to taste., Fresh coriander or parsley for garnish (optional)

Preparation:

- Heating the olive oil in a big pot over a medium-high flame. Add the chopped onion and garlic and fry until golden.
- Add curry powder and turmeric. Combine well to evenly distribute the spices.
- Add the sweet potato cubes and stir to coat with the spices for about 2-3 minutes.
- Pour the coconut milk and vegetable broth into the pot. Bring to a boil, then minimize to a medium-low flame.
- Cover and let simmer for about 20-25 minutes or until sweet potatoes are tender.
- Use an immersion blender to blend the soup until smooth and lump-free.
- Taste and season with salt and black pepper according to your liking.
- Serve the coconut curry sweet potato soup hot, garnished with fresh cilantro or parsley if desired.

Nutritional values: Calories: 250-300 kcal, Protein: 3-4 g, Fat: 10-12 g, Carbohydrates: 35-40 g, Fiber: 5-6 g

100. Curry Salmon with Steamed Vegetables

Ingredients: 150g salmon fillet, 1 teaspoon curry powder, 1/2 teaspoon turmeric,1/2 teaspoon freshly grated ginger, 1 clove garlic, minced,1 tablespoon olive oil, Salt and pepper to taste 1 cup broccoli, cut into florets, 1 cup carrots, cut into sticks 1 cup cooked quinoa

Instructions:

- Preheat the oven to 200°C (392°F).
- In a small bowl, mix curry powder, turmeric, grated ginger, minced garlic, olive oil, salt, and pepper.
- Place the salmon fillet on a lined baking sheet. Evenly spread the spice mixture over the surface of the salmon.
- Cook the salmon in the heated oven for 15-20 minutes, or until it is cooked. Meanwhile, steam broccoli florets and carrots until tender but still crisp.
- Prepare quinoa according to package instructions.
- Serve the salmon on a bed of quinoa, accompanied by steamed broccoli and carrots.

Nutritional Values (per serving): Calories: approximately 400 kcal, Protein: 25g, Fat: 20g, Carbohydrates: 30g, Fiber: 5g

Chapter 11: Soups and Broths

50 Anti-Inflammatory Soups and Broth Recipes

Nothing beats the feeling of comfort you get while enjoying a hot soup or steaming broth. But what if these dishes were not only delicious, but also beneficial for our body? Welcome to the section of anti-inflammatory soups and broths, where health and the pleasure of the palate meet in perfect harmony. Chronic inflammation is often the underlying cause of a variety of health conditions, from arthritis to heart disease. But the secret to fighting this inflammation and promoting optimal health may be right in our kitchen. Soups and broths are powerful tools for achieving this goal. With carefully selected ingredients and expertly prepared combinations, the recipes you will find in this section will not only pamper your taste buds, but will also help reduce inflammation in your body. Our recipes are based on ingredients rich in anti-inflammatory properties, such as herbs, spices, dark green leafy vegetables and lean proteins. These ingredients not only give soups and broths amazing flavor, but they also provide your body with essential nutrients and antioxidants that will help it fight inflammation.

Regardless of what you are looking for, whether it is a creamy soup, a light broth or a traditional dish reinterpreted with an anti-inflammatory twist, you will find something that will satisfy your gastronomic desires and help you take care of your well-being. So, get ready to discover a wide range of delicious and nutritious recipes that will make your journey to inflammation-free living not only healthy, but also incredibly tasty. Bon appetit and good health!

1. Coconut Turmeric Soup with Vegetables

Ingredients: 1 can (15 oz) coconut milk, 2 cups (about 480ml) vegetable broth, 1 onion, chopped, 2 cloves garlic, minced, 1-inch piece of fresh ginger, peeled and minced, 2 carrots, peeled and chopped, 2 zucchinis, chopped, 1 red bell pepper, chopped, 1 tablespoon ground turmeric (adjust to taste), 1 tablespoon olive oil, Salt and black pepper to taste, Fresh cilantro leaves for garnish (optional).

Preparation:
- In a saucepan, heat some extra virgin olive oil and fry the onion until translucent.
- Add the diced carrots and courgettes and cook for a few minutes.
- Add turmeric powder and mix well.
- Combine the coconut milk and vegetable broth in a mixing bowl.
- Bring everything to a boil, then decrease to a low heat and continue to cook until the vegetables are tender.
- Change your seasoning with pepper and salt according to your liking. Serve the soup hot, garnished with fresh coriander leaves if desired.

Nutritional Values (per serving): Calories, 250-300 kcal. Protein, 5-7g. Fat, 15-18g. Carbohydrates, 20-25g. Fiber, 5-7g.

2. Quinoa and Vegetable Minestrone

Ingredients: 1 cup (185g) quinoa, rinsed, 2 carrots, peeled and chopped, 2 celery stalks, chopped, 1 onion, chopped, 2 cloves garlic, minced, 4 cups (1 liter) vegetable broth, 1 can (15 oz) diced tomatoes, 2 zucchinis, chopped, 1 cup (150g) green beans, chopped, 1 teaspoon dried basil, Salt and black pepper to taste, Olive oil for sautéing, Grated Parmesan cheese for garnish (optional).

Preparation:
- In a large pot, heat some extra virgin olive oil and fry the onion until
- translucent. Add diced celery, carrots and courgettes and cook until the vegetables begin to soften.
- Add the quinoa and mix well. Pour the vegetable broth and the diced tomatoes.
- Bring everything to a boil, then decrease to a low heat and continue to cook until the quinoa is tender and the vegetables are soft.
- Add the chopped green beans and cook for a few minutes.
- Season with pepper, salt and freshly chopped parsley. Serve the soup hot.

Nutritional Values (per serving): Calories, 300-350 kcal., Protein, 10-15g. Fat, 5-8g. Carbohydrates, 50-60g. Fiber, 10-15g.

3. Chicken broth with ginger and parsley

Ingredients: 1 whole chicken (about 3-4 pounds), cut into pieces, 2-3 inches of fresh ginger, sliced, 1 bunch of fresh parsley, 2 onions, peeled and halved, 4 cloves garlic, minced, 2 bay leaves, 10-12 whole black peppercorns, Salt to taste, Water to cover the ingredients.

Preparation:
- In a large pot, place the chicken carcass and cover it with water.
- Add a few slices of fresh ginger and a handful of fresh parsley.
- Bring everything to the boil, then reduce the heat and leave to simmer for at least an hour.
- Take out any foam that has accumulated on the surface.
- Once ready, drain the broth into another pot or container, removing the carcass and herbs.
- Change your seasoning with pepper and salt according to your liking. This homemade chicken stock can be used as a base for many other soups and stews.

Nutritional Values (per serving): Calories, 50-70 kcal. Protein, 3-4g. Fat, 0g. Carbohydrates, 0-2g. Fiber, 0g.

4. Courgette and Avocado Cream

Ingredients: 2 large courgettes (zucchini), chopped, 2 ripe avocados, peeled and pitted, 1 onion, chopped, 2 cloves garlic, minced, 4 cups (1 liter) vegetable broth, 1/2 cup (120ml) heavy cream (or a dairy-free alternative), Juice of 1 lime, Salt and black pepper to taste, Olive oil for sautéing, Fresh basil leaves for garnish (optional).

Preparation:
- In a saucepan, fry the onion until translucent.
- Add the sliced courgettes and cook until tender.
- Add the ripe avocado, vegetable broth and lemon juice.
- Blend everything with an immersion blender until you obtain a smooth cream.
- If necessary, add more vegetable broth to achieve the desired consistency.
- Change your seasoning with pepper and salt according to your liking. Serve the cream hot or cold, depending on your preferences.

Nutritional Values (per serving): Calories, 150-200 kcal. Protein, 2-3g. Fat, 12-15g. Carbohydrates, 10-12g. Fiber, 4-5g.

5. Curry Red Lentil Soup

Ingredients: 1 cup (200g) red lentils, rinsed and drained, 1 onion, chopped, 2 cloves garlic, minced, 1 tablespoon curry powder (adjust to taste), 4 cups (1 liter) vegetable broth, 1 can (15 oz) diced tomatoes, 1 can (15 oz) coconut milk, 2 tablespoons olive oil, Salt and black pepper to taste, Fresh cilantro leaves for garnish (optional).

Preparation:

- In a saucepan, sauté the onion, garlic and ginger until aromatic.
- Add curry powder and mix well.
- Combine the red lentils, vegetable broth, and coconut milk in a mixing bowl.
- Bring everything to the boil, then reduce the heat and simmer until the lentils are soft and the soup has reached the desired consistency.
- Season your liking with pepper, salt, and lemon juice.
- This soup is packed with flavor thanks to the curry and coconut milk.

Nutritional Values (per serving): Calories, 200-250 kcal. Protein, 8-10g. Fat, 8-10g. Carbohydrates, 25-30g. Fiber, 4-5g.

6. Fish Broth with Tomatoes and Basil

Ingredients: 1 pound (450g) fish heads and bones (such as snapper, cod, or any white fish), 2 tomatoes, chopped, 1 onion, chopped, 2 cloves garlic, minced, 1/2 cup (120ml) white wine (optional), 4 cups (1 liter) water, Fresh basil leaves, to taste, Salt and black pepper to taste, Olive oil for sautéing.

Preparation:

- In a large pot, heat some extra virgin olive oil and fry the onion until translucent.
- Add the chopped ripe tomatoes and cook until soft.
- Pour fish stock or water with a fish stock cube and bring to the boil.
- Lower the heat to low and add the fish fillets.
- Simmer until the fish is cooked and tender.
- Season with salt, pepper and fresh basil before serving.

Nutritional Values (per serving): Calories, 150-200 kcal. Protein, 20-25g. Fat, 5-7g. Carbohydrates, 10-15g. Fiber, 2-3g.

7. Roasted Cauliflower Soup

Ingredients: 1 large head of cauliflower, cut into florets, 1 onion, chopped, 2 cloves garlic, minced, 4 cups (1 liter) vegetable broth, 1/2 cup (120ml) heavy cream (or a dairy-free alternative), 2 tablespoons olive oil, 1 teaspoon ground cumin, Salt and black pepper to taste, Fresh parsley leaves for garnish (optional).

Preparation:

- Separate the cauliflower into florets and place them on a baking sheet..
- Drizzle with olive oil, salt and pepper, then roast in the oven at 200°C until the cauliflower is golden and soft.
- In a saucepan, fry the onion until translucent.
- Add the roasted cauliflower and vegetable broth. Bring it all
- to the boil and then reduce the heat and leave to simmer for about 15-20 minutes.
- Combine the soup until it has a creamy texture.
- Serve garnished with toasted walnuts.

Nutritional Values (per serving): Calories, 150-200 kcal. Protein, 4-6g. Fat, 8-10g. Carbohydrates, 15-20g. Fiber, 4-6g.

8. Black Bean and Spinach Minestrone

Ingredients: 2 cans (15 oz each) cleaned and drained black beans, 2 cups (about 180g) fresh spinach, chopped, 1 onion, chopped, 2 cloves garlic, minced, 1 can (15 oz) diced tomatoes, 4 cups (1 liter) vegetable broth, 1 cup (200g) small pasta (e.g., ditalini or small shells), 1 teaspoon dried basil, Salt and black pepper to taste, Olive oil for sautéing, Grated Parmesan cheese for garnish (optional).

Preparation:

- In a saucepan, fry the onion, carrots and celery until soft.
- Add the diced tomatoes and vegetable broth.
- Then bring it to a boil, then remove from the heat.
- Pour in the drained and cleaned black beans.
- Cook for about 10 minutes. Add fresh spinach and cook until wilted.
- Season with salt, pepper and chopped fresh parsley before serving.

Nutritional Values (per serving): Calories, 200-250 kcal. Protein, 8-10g. Fat, 5-7g. Carbohydrates, 30-35g. Fiber, 7-9g.

9. Sweet Potato and Carrot Soup with Cinnamon

Ingredients: 2 large sweet potatoes, peeled and chopped, 4 large carrots, peeled and chopped, 1 onion, chopped, 2 cloves garlic, minced, 4 cups (1 liter) vegetable broth, 1 teaspoon ground cinnamon, Salt and black pepper to taste, Olive oil for sautéing, Fresh parsley for garnish (optional).

Preparation:

- In a saucepan, fry the onion until translucent.
- Add the sweet potatoes and chopped carrots.
- Add the vegetable broth, ground cinnamon and nutmeg.
- Then bring it to boiling point, then turn off the heat.
- Cook until vegetables are tender.
- Blend the soup until smooth.
- Season with salt, pepper and a sprinkling of cinnamon before serving.

Nutritional Values (per serving): Calories, 150-200 kcal. Protein, 2-4g. Fat, 1-2g. Carbohydrates, 30-35g. Fiber, 4-6g.

10. Beef Broth with Aromatic Herbs

Ingredients: 1 pound (450g) beef bones (such as marrow or knuckle bones), 2 onions, peeled and halved, 2 carrots, peeled and chopped, 2 celery stalks, chopped, 2 cloves garlic, minced, 2 bay leaves, A few sprigs of fresh thyme, A few sprigs of fresh rosemary, 10-12 whole black peppercorns, Salt to taste, Water to cover the ingredients.

Preparation:

- In a large pot, place the beef bones and cover them with water.
- Add roughly chopped onion, carrots and celery, along with thyme, rosemary and bay leaves.
- Bring everything to a boil, then reduce the heat and simmer for at least 4-6 hours to develop a rich flavor.
- Take out any foam that has accumulated on the surface.
- Once ready, drain the broth into another pot or container, removing the bones and herbs.
- Season according to liking with pepper and salt.
- This homemade beef stock is a versatile base for many soup and sauce recipes.

Nutritional Values (per serving): Calories, 150-200 kcal. Protein, 2-4g. Fat, 1-2g. Carbohydrates, 4-6g. Fiber, 0-1g.

11. Chickpea and Tomato Soup with Cumin

Ingredients: 2 cans (15 oz each) washed and drained chickpeas, 1 onion, chopped, 2 cloves garlic, minced, 1 can (15 oz) diced tomatoes, 4 cups (1 liter) vegetable broth, 1 teaspoon ground cumin, Salt and black pepper to taste, Olive oil for sautéing, Fresh cilantro leaves for garnish (optional).

Preparation:
- In a pan, fry the onion and garlic with a little olive oil until golden.
- Add cumin and red chili powder if you want a spicy kick.
- Cook up until the diced tomatoes are softened. Add the drained and rinsed chickpeas. Bring to a boil with the broth made from vegetables.
- Reduce the heat and let it simmer for about 15-20 minutes.
- Mix the soup in a blender until it has a creamy texture.
- Season with salt and pepper. Garnish with fresh parsley before being served.

Nutritional Values (per serving): Calories, 150-200 kcal. Protein, 5-8g. Fat, 3-5g. Carbohydrates, 25-30g. Fiber, 5-7g.

12. Pea and Mint Cream

Ingredients: 2 cups (about 400g) fresh or frozen peas, 1 onion, chopped, 2 cloves garlic, minced, 4 cups (1 liter) vegetable broth, 1/2 cup (120ml) heavy cream (or a dairy-free alternative), Fresh mint leaves, to taste, Salt and black pepper to taste, Olive oil for sautéing.

Preparation:
- In a saucepan, fry the onion and garlic in a little butter until translucent.
- Cook for just a few minutes after adding the peas. Bring to a boil with the vegetable broth.
- Change the heat to low and continue to cook until the peas are softened.
- Mix in the freshly chopped mint until the soup is smooth.
- If desired, add a little fresh cream for extra creaminess.
- Season with salt and pepper. Serve with parmesan flakes and fresh mint leaves to garnish.

Nutritional Values (per serving): Calories, 100-150 kcal. Protein, 2-4g. Fat, 4-6g. Carbohydrates, 10-15g. Fiber, 2-3g.

13. Chicken and Lemon Broth

Ingredients: 1 whole chicken (about 3-4 pounds), cut into pieces, 2 lemons, sliced, 2 onions, peeled and halved, 4 cloves garlic, minced, 4 cups (1 liter) chicken broth, 2 bay leaves, Fresh thyme sprigs, Salt and black pepper to taste, Water to cover the ingredients.

Preparation:
- In a large pot, place the chicken breast, onion, carrots, celery, a slice of lemon, fresh parsley,
- bay leaves, salt and pepper.
- Cover everything with water.
- Bring to a boil, then minimize to a low heat and cook for at least 45 minutes.
- Cut the chicken breast into small pieces after removing it from the pan.
- Remove flavorings and solid ingredients from the pot.
- Return the cut chicken to the pot. Squeeze the lemon juice into the soup and mix well.
- Season with salt and pepper to taste. Serve hot.

Nutritional Values (per serving): Calories, 150-200 kcal. Protein, 15-20g. Fat, 5-8g. Carbohydrates, 10-15g. Fiber, 2-4g.

14. Pumpkin and Ginger Soup

Ingredients: 2 pounds (about 900g) pumpkin, peeled and diced, 1 onion, chopped, 2 cloves garlic, minced, 1-inch piece of fresh ginger, peeled and minced (adjust to taste), 4 cups (1 liter) vegetable broth, 1/2 cup (120ml) coconut milk (or a dairy-free alternative), 1 teaspoon ground cinnamon, Salt and black pepper to taste, Olive oil for sautéing, Fresh cilantro leaves for garnish (optional).

Preparation:
- Cut the pumpkin into small pieces. In a pan, fry the onion and garlic with a little olive oil until golden.
- Add the pumpkin and grated ginger. Cook for a few minutes.
- Add the vegetable a broth and let it come to a boil.
- Lower the heat and continue to cook until the pumpkin is softened.
- Blend the soup until smooth.
- If desired, add a little fresh cream for extra creaminess.
- Season with salt and pepper. To decoration, sprinkle with toasted pumpkin seeds.

Nutritional Values (per serving): Calories, 150-200 kcal. Protein, 2-4g. Fat, 2-4g. Carbohydrates, 30-40g. Fiber, 4-6g.

15. Quinoa and Black Cabbage Minestrone

Ingredients: 1 cup (185g) quinoa, rinsed, 1 small head of black cabbage (also known as Lacinato or Tuscan kale), chopped, 1 onion, chopped, 2 cloves garlic, minced, 1 can (15 oz) diced tomatoes, 4 cups (1 liter) vegetable broth, 1 teaspoon dried thyme, Salt and black pepper to taste, Olive oil for sautéing, Grated Parmesan cheese for garnish (optional).

Preparation:
- In a saucepan, fry the onion, carrots and celery until soft.
- Add the black cabbage cut into thin strips and cook until wilted.
- Add the diced tomatoes, vegetable broth, quinoa and herbs (rosemary and thyme).
- Then bring it to a boil, then remove from the heat.
- Cook until the quinoa is tender.
- Season with salt and pepper. If wanted, top with grated parmesan.

Nutritional Values (per serving): Calories, 250-300 kcal. Protein, 10-15g. Fat, 4-7g. Carbohydrates, 40-50g. Fiber, 8-10g.

16. Lentil and Spinach Soup

Ingredients: 1 cup (200g) green or brown lentils, rinsed and drained, 1 onion, chopped, 2 cloves garlic, minced, 4 cups (1 liter) vegetable broth, 2 cups (about 180g) fresh spinach, chopped, 2 carrots, peeled and chopped, 2 celery stalks, chopped, 1 teaspoon ground cumin, Salt and black pepper to taste, Olive oil for sautéing.

Preparation:
- In a pan, sauté the onion, carrots, celery and garlic with a little olive oil until soft.
- Add the lentils and fresh rosemary.
- Add the vegetable broth and let it come to a boil.
- Reduce heat and simmer until lentils are tender.
- Cook until the spinach is wilting.
- Season with salt and pepper to taste. Serve hot.

Nutritional Values (per serving): Calories, 200-250 kcal. Protein, 10-15g. Fat, 2-4g. Carbohydrates, 30-40g. Fiber, 8-10g.

17. Fish Broth with Chilli

Ingredients: 1 pound (450g) fish heads and bones (such as snapper, cod, or any white fish), 2 red chilli peppers, chopped (adjust to taste), 1 onion, chopped, 2 cloves garlic, minced, 2 tomatoes, chopped, 2 bay leaves, 4 cups (1 liter) water, Salt and black pepper to taste, Olive oil for sautéing.

Preparation:

- In a large pot, sauté the onion, celery, carrots and chilli with a little olive oil until golden brown.
- Cook the fish heads and bones until they start to turn red. Add the diced tomatoes, fresh parsley and cover everything with water.
- Bring to a boil, then turn off the heat. Let at least 30 minutes for it to simmer.
- Strain the broth to remove solid ingredients. Season with salt and pepper to taste. You can use it as a base for fish or seafood soups.

Nutritional Values (per serving): Calories, 150-200 kcal. Protein, 20-25g. Fat, 4-6g. Carbohydrates, 8-10g. Fiber, 2-4g.

18. Cabbage and Onion Soup with Parsley

Ingredients: 1 small head of cabbage, shredded, 2 onions, chopped, 2 cloves garlic, minced, 4 cups (1 liter) vegetable broth, 2 tablespoons olive oil, 1/2 cup (120ml) heavy cream (or a dairy-free alternative), Salt and black pepper to taste, Fresh parsley leaves for garnish (optional).

Preparation:

- In a pan, fry the onion and garlic with a little olive oil until golden.
- Add the cabbage cut into thin strips and cook until wilted.
- Let the vegetable broth come to a boil.
- Lower the heat to low and continue to cook until cabbage is tender.
- Season your liking with pepper and salt as needed. Serve with fresh parsley on top.

Nutritional Values (per serving): Calories, 80-120 kcal. Protein, 2-4g. Fat, 0-2g. Carbohydrates, 15-20g. Fiber, 4-6g.

19. Carrot and Star Anise Cream

Ingredients: 1 pound (450g) carrots, peeled and chopped, 1 onion, chopped, 2 cloves garlic, minced, 2-3 whole star anise pods, 4 cups (1 liter) vegetable broth, 1/2 cup (120ml) heavy cream (or a dairy-free alternative), Salt and black pepper to taste, Olive oil for sautéing, Fresh cilantro leaves for garnish (optional).

Preparation:

- In a pan, fry the onion and garlic in a little butter until golden brown.
- Add the carrots cut into slices and the star anise.
- Cook for a few minutesSet the vegetable broth to a boil in the meantime.
- Reduce the heat and cook until the carrots are soft.
- Remove the star anise. Blend the soup until it has a silky texture.
- If desired, add a little fresh cream for extra creaminess.
- Season your liking with pepper and salt as needed

Nutritional Values (per serving): Calories, 100-130 kcal. Protein, 2-3g. Fat, 4-6g. Carbohydrates, 15-20g. Fiber, 4-6g.

20. Turkey Broth with Shiitake Mushrooms

Ingredients: Turkey carcass or bones (leftover from a roast turkey), 1 onion, chopped, 2 carrots, peeled and chopped, 2 celery stalks, chopped, 2 cloves garlic, minced, 8-10 shiitake mushrooms, dried or fresh, 2 bay leaves, 4-5 sprigs fresh thyme, 10-12 whole black peppercorns, 8 cups (2 liters) water, Salt to taste.

Preparation:

- In a large pot, place the turkey carcass, shiitake mushrooms, onion, celery, carrots, thyme, rosemary, salt and pepper.
- Cover everything with water. Bring to a boil, then reduce heat and simmer for at least 1-2 hours.
- Strain the broth to remove solid ingredients.
- Season with salt and pepper to taste. You can use it as a base for soups or stews.

Nutritional Values (per serving): Calories, 70-90 kcal. Protein, 7-9g. Fat, 1-2g. Carbohydrates, 6-8g. Fiber, 2-3g.

21. Eggplant and pepper soup

Ingredients: 2 large eggplants, peeled and diced, 2 red bell peppers, chopped, 1 onion, chopped, 2 cloves garlic, minced, 4 cups (1 liter) vegetable broth, 2 tablespoons olive oil, 1 teaspoon dried thyme, Salt and black pepper to taste, Fresh parsley for garnish (optional).

Preparation:

- In a pan, fry the onion and garlic with a little olive oil until golden.
- Add the diced aubergines and peppers and cook until soft.
- Add the peeled tomatoes and the vegetable broth.
- Then bring it to a boil, afterwards remove from the heat.
- Simmer it for a minimum of 30 minutes.
- Season according to liking with salt, pepper, and fresh basil. Serve immediately.

Nutritional Values (per serving): Calories, 80-100 kcal. Protein, 2-4g. Fat, 2-3g. Carbohydrates, 14-18g. Fiber, 4-6g.

22. White Bean and Cauliflower Minestrone

Ingredients: 1 can (15 oz) white beans, drained and rinsed, 1 small head of cauliflower, cut into florets, 1 onion, chopped, 2 cloves garlic, minced, 1 can (15 oz) diced tomatoes, 4 cups (1 liter) vegetable broth, 1 cup (200g) small pasta (e.g., ditalini or small shells), 1 teaspoon dried oregano, Salt and black pepper to taste, Olive oil for sautéing, Grated Parmesan cheese for garnish (optional).

Preparation:

- In a pan, fry the onion, carrots and celery with a little olive oil until soft.
- Cook for 5 minutes, or until the cauliflower is softened.
- Add the drained and rinsed white beans, then pour in the vegetable broth.
- Bring it to a boil, afterwards reduce the heat. Allow it to cook for 20 to 30 minutes.
- Season your liking with pepper, salt, and freshly chopped parsley.

Nutritional Values (per serving): Calories, 150-180 kcal. Protein, 7-9g. Fat, 1-2g. Carbohydrates, 25-30g. Fiber, 6-8g.

23. Chickpea Soup with Rosemary

Ingredients: 2 cans (15 oz each) chickpeas, drained and rinsed, 1 onion, chopped, 2 cloves garlic, minced, 2 sprigs fresh rosemary, leaves removed and chopped (or 1 teaspoon dried rosemary), 4 cups (1 liter) vegetable broth, 2 tablespoons olive oil, Salt and black pepper to taste, Fresh rosemary sprigs for garnish (optional).

Preparation:

- In a pan, fry the onion and garlic with a little olive oil until golden.
- Add the fresh rosemary and the drained and rinsed chickpeas.
- Add the vegetable broth and bring to boiling point.
- Reduce the heat and let it simmer for about 15-20 minutes.
- Season with salt and pepper to taste.

Nutritional Values (per serving): Calories, 250-300 kcal. Protein, 10-12g. Fat, 6-8g. Carbohydrates, 40-45g. Fiber, 8-10g.

24. Beef Broth with Leeks and Thyme

Ingredients: 1 pound (450g) beef bones (such as marrow or knuckle bones), 2 leeks, white and light green parts, cleaned and chopped, 1 onion, chopped, 2 cloves garlic, minced, 2 bay leaves, 4 cups (1 liter) water, A few sprigs of fresh thyme (or 1 teaspoon dried thyme), Salt and black pepper to taste.

Preparation:
- Place the beef bones, leeks, carrots, celery and thyme in a large pot.
- Cover everything with water. Bring to the boil, then reduce the heat and simmer for at least 2-3 hours.
- Remove the solid ingredients and filter the broth.
- Season your liking with pepper and salt as needed.
- You can use it as a base for other soups or as a broth to enjoy on its own.

Nutritional Values (per serving): Calories, 150-200 kcal. Protein, 10-12g. Fat, 5-7g. Carbohydrates, 15-20g. Fiber, 3-4g.

25. Tomato and Basil Soup

Ingredients: 4 cups (800g) ripe tomatoes, chopped, 1 onion, chopped, 2 cloves garlic, minced, 1 cup (240ml) vegetable broth, 1/2 cup (120ml) heavy cream (or a dairy-free alternative), 1/4 cup (10g) fresh basil leaves, chopped, 1 tablespoon olive oil, Salt and black pepper to taste.

Preparation:
- In a pan, fry the onion and garlic with a little olive oil until golden.
- Add the diced tomatoes and fresh basil.
- Pour in the vegetable broth and bring to the boil.
- Reduce the heat and let it simmer for about 20-30 minutes.
- Season with salt and pepper to taste. Serve with fresh basil leaves.

Nutritional Values (per serving): Calories, 100-150 kcal. Protein, 2-3g. Fat, 4-6g. Carbohydrates, 15-20g. Fiber, 2-3g.

26. Asparagus and Lemon Cream

Ingredients: 1 bunch of asparagus, tough ends trimmed and chopped, 1 onion, chopped, 2 cloves garlic, minced, Zest and juice of 1 lemon, 4 cups (1 liter) vegetable broth, 1/2 cup (120ml) heavy cream (or a dairy-free alternative), Salt and black pepper to taste, Olive oil for sautéing, Fresh parsley for garnish (optional).

Preparation:
- In a pan, fry the onion and garlic with a little olive oil until golden.
- Add the chopped asparagus and cook until soft.
- Pour in the vegetable broth and bring to the boil.
- Reduce the heat and let it simmer for about 20-30 minutes.
- Use an immersion blender to cream the soup.
- Add lemon juice, salt and pepper to taste.
- Add fresh cream if you want a creamier consistency.

Nutritional Values (per serving): Calories, 150-200 kcal. Protein, 2-3g. Fat, 12-15g. Carbohydrates, 8-10g. Fiber, 3-4g.

27. Chicken Broth with Turmeric and Black Pepper

Ingredients: 1 whole chicken (about 3-4 pounds), cut into pieces, 2 onions, peeled and halved, 2 carrots, peeled and chopped, 2 celery stalks, chopped, 2 bay leaves, 1-inch piece of fresh turmeric, peeled and sliced (or 1 teaspoon ground turmeric), 10-12 whole black peppercorns, Salt to taste, Water to cover the ingredients.

Preparation:
- In a large pot, place the chicken and cover with water.
- Bring to the boil, then reduce the heat and simmer for at least 1-2 hours.
- Add turmeric powder, black peppercorns and salt while cooking.
- Set the chicken aside after removing it from the broth.
- You can use it as a base for other soups or as a broth to enjoy on its own.

Nutritional Values (per serving): Calories, 50-70 kcal. Protein, 8-10g. Fat, 1-2g. Carbohydrates, 1-2g. Fiber, 0g.

28. Pumpkin and Cinnamon Soup

Ingredients: 1 small pumpkin (about 2-3 pounds), peeled, seeded, and diced, 1 onion, chopped, 2 cloves garlic, minced, 4 cups (1 liter) vegetable broth, 1 teaspoon ground cinnamon, 1/2 teaspoon ground nutmeg, Salt and black pepper to taste, Olive oil for sautéing, Cream or coconut milk for garnish (optional), Fresh parsley for garnish (optional).

Preparation:
- In a pan, fry the onion and garlic with a little olive oil until golden.
- Add the diced pumpkin and cook until soft.
- Pour in the vegetable broth and bring to the boil.
- Reduce the heat and let it simmer for about 20-30 minutes.
- Use an immersion blender to cream the soup.
- Add ground cinnamon, nutmeg, salt and pepper to taste.
- Add fresh cream if you want a creamier consistency.

Nutritional Values (per serving): Calories, 100-120 kcal. Protein, 2-3g. Fat, 1-2g. Carbohydrates, 20-25g. Fiber, 5-6g.

29. Quinoa and Broccoli Minestrone

Ingredients: 1 cup (185g) quinoa, rinsed, 1 head of broccoli, cut into florets, 1 onion, chopped, 2 cloves garlic, minced, 1 can (15 oz) diced tomatoes, 4 cups (1 liter) vegetable broth, 1 teaspoon dried basil, 1 teaspoon dried oregano, Salt and black pepper to taste, Olive oil for sautéing, Grated Parmesan cheese for garnish (optional).

Preparation:
- In a pan, fry the onion, carrots and celery with a little olive oil until soft.
- Cook, stirring occasionally, for 5 minutes, or until the broccoli is cooked.
- Add the quinoa and pour in the vegetable broth.
- Stir to a boil, then withdraw from the heat.
- Let it simmer for about 15-20 minutes.
- Season your liking with pepper, salt, and freshly chopped parsley.

Nutritional Values (per serving): Calories, 250-300 kcal. Protein, 10-12g. Fat, 5-7g. Carbohydrates, 40-45g. Fiber, 8-10g.

30. Lentil Soup with Rosemary

Ingredients: 1 cup (200g) green or brown lentils, rinsed and drained, 1 onion, chopped, 2 carrots, peeled and chopped, 2 celery stalks, chopped, 2 cloves garlic, minced, 2 sprigs fresh rosemary, leaves removed and chopped (or 1 teaspoon dried rosemary), 4 cups (1 liter) vegetable broth, 2 tablespoons olive oil, Salt and black pepper to taste, Fresh parsley for garnish (optional).

Preparation:
- In a pan, fry the onion and garlic with a little olive oil until golden.
- Add the dried lentils and fresh rosemary.
- Pour in the vegetable broth and bring to the boil.

- Reduce the heat and let simmer for about 30-40 minutes or until the lentils aresoft.
- Season your liking with pepper and salt as needed.

Nutritional Values (per serving): Calories, 250-300 kcal. Protein,1 2-15g.Fat,3-5g. Carbohydrates,40-45g. Fiber 10-12g.

31. Fish Broth with Saffron

Ingredients: 1 pound (450g) fish heads and bones (such as snapper, cod, or any white fish), 1 onion, chopped, 2 cloves garlic, minced, 2 tomatoes, chopped, 2 bay leaves, A pinch of saffron threads, 4 cups (1 liter) water, Salt and black pepper to taste, Olive oil for sautéing.

Preparation:

- In a large pot, boil the water with the coarsely chopped onions, carrots and celery.
- Add the fish and cook until the fish is fully cooked and the vegetables are tender.
- Add saffron to give color and flavor to the broth.
- Season your liking with pepper and salt as needed.
- Strain the broth to remove the vegetables and fish.
- You can serve the broth on its own or as a base for other fish soups.

Nutritional Values (per serving): Calories, 150-200 kcal. Protein, 15-20g. Fat, 5-7g. Carbohydrates, 10-15g. Fiber, 2-3g.

32. Cauliflower and Curry Soup

Ingredients: 1 head of cauliflower, cut into florets, 1 onion, chopped, 2 cloves garlic, minced, 1 tablespoon curry powder (adjust to taste), 4 cups (1 liter) vegetable broth, 1 can (15 oz) coconut milk, Salt and black pepper to taste, Olive oil for sautéing, Fresh cilantro leaves for garnish (optional).

Preparation:

- In a pan, fry the onion and garlic with a little olive oil until golden.
- Add the chopped cauliflower and curry powder.
- Simmer for just a few minutes in order for the flavors to combine.
- Pour in the vegetable broth and bring to the boil. Reduce heat and let simmer until cauliflower is tender.
- Use an immersion blender to cream the soup.
- Add coconut milk to give it a creamier consistency.
- Season with salt, pepper and fresh coriander to taste.

Nutritional Values (per serving): Calories, 150-200 kcal. Protein, 5-7g. Fat, 8-10g. Carbohydrates, 15-20g. Fiber, 5-7g.

33. Sweet Potato and Cinnamon Cream

Ingredients: 2 large sweet potatoes, peeled and diced, 1 onion, chopped, 2 cloves garlic, minced, 1 teaspoon ground cinnamon, 4 cups (1 liter) vegetable broth, 1/2 cup (120ml) coconut milk (or a dairy-free alternative), Salt and black pepper to taste, Olive oil for sautéing, Fresh cilantro leaves for garnish (optional).

Preparation:

- In a pan, fry the onion and garlic with a little olive oil until golden.
- Add the diced sweet potatoes and ground cinnamon.
- Sauté for just a few minutes to allow the flavors to mix together.
- Pour in the vegetable broth and bring to the boil.
- Lower the temperature to low and simmer until the potatoes are tender.
- Use an immersion blender to cream the soup.
- Add milk to give it a creamier consistency.
- Season your liking with pepper and salt as needed.

Nutritional Values (per serving): Calories, 200-250 kcal. Protein, 2-4g. Fat, 7-9g. Carbohydrates, 35-40g. Fiber, 5-7g.

34. Chicken Broth with Garlic and Parsley

Ingredients: 1 whole chicken (about 3-4 pounds), cut into pieces, 2 onions, peeled and halved, 4 cloves garlic, minced, 1 bunch fresh parsley, stems and leaves included, 10-12 whole black peppercorns, Salt to taste, Water to cover the ingredients.

Preparation:

- In a large pot, place the chicken and cover with water.
- Bring to the boil, then reduce the heat and simmer for at least 1-2 hours.
- Add garlic, fresh parsley, celery and carrots during cooking to flavor the broth.
- Remove the chicken and strain the broth.
- You can use it as a base for other soups or as a broth to enjoy on its own.

Nutritional Values (per serving): Calories, 40-50 kcal. Protein, 3-5g. Fat, 1-2g. Carbohydrates, 4-6g. Fiber, 1-2g.

35. Chickpea and Dried Tomato Soup

Ingredients: 1 can (15 oz) chickpeas, drained and rinsed, 1/2 cup (100g) dried tomatoes, chopped, 1 onion, chopped, 2 cloves garlic, minced, 4 cups (1 liter) vegetable broth, 1 teaspoon dried basil, 1 teaspoon dried oregano, Salt and black pepper to taste, Olive oil for sautéing, Fresh basil leaves for garnish (optional).

Preparation:

- In a pan, fry the onion and garlic with a little olive oil until golden.
- Add the drained chickpeas and the chopped dried tomatoes.
- Cook for a few minutes to let the flavors blend.
- Pour in the vegetable broth and bring to the boil.
- Reduce heat and simmer until chickpeas are soft.
- Add fresh rosemary, pepper and salt to taste.
- You can serve the soup with a drizzle of olive oil and toasted bread.

Nutritional Values (per serving): Calories, 150-200 kcal. Protein, 5-7g. Fat, 2-3g. Carbohydrates, 25-30g. Fiber, 5-7g.

36. Black Bean and Chard Minestrone

Ingredients: 1 cup (200g) dried black beans, soaked and cooked, or 2 cans (15 oz each) of black beans, drained and rinsed, 1 bunch Swiss chard, chopped, 1 onion, chopped, 2 cloves garlic, minced, 1 can (15 oz) diced tomatoes, 6 cups (1.5 liters) vegetable broth, 1 cup (200g) small pasta (e.g., ditalini or small shells), 2 bay leaves, 1 teaspoon dried oregano, Salt and black pepper to taste, Olive oil for sautéing, Grated Parmesan cheese for garnish (optional).

Preparation:

- In a large pot, sauté the onion and garlic with a little olive oil until golden brown.
- Add the diced tomatoes and the chard leaves cut into strips.
- Cook for a few minutes to soften the chard.
- Pour in the vegetable broth and add the drained black beans.
- Add fresh rosemary, salt and pepper.
- Let simmer until the chard is tender.
- You can serve this soup with toasted bread croutons.

Nutritional Values (per serving): Calories, 200-250 kcal. Protein, 8-10g. Fat, 4-5g. Carbohydrates, 30-35g. Fiber, 8-10g.

37. Eggplant Soup with Rosemary

Ingredients: 2 large eggplants, peeled and diced, 1 onion, chopped, 2 cloves garlic, minced, 2 sprigs fresh rosemary, leaves removed and chopped (or 1 teaspoon dried rosemary), 4 cups (1 liter) vegetable broth, 2 tablespoons olive oil, Salt and black pepper to taste, Fresh rosemary sprigs for garnish (optional).

Preparation:
- Cut the aubergines into cubes and set them aside. In a pan, fry the onion and garlic with a little olive oil until golden.
- Add the aubergines and cook until slightly softened.
- Add canned peeled tomatoes, fresh rosemary, salt and pepper.
- Pour in the vegetable broth and bring to the boil.
- Reduce heat and simmer until eggplant is fully cooked and soup has reached desired consistency.

Nutritional Values (per serving): Calories, 150-200 kcal. Protein, 3-4g. Fat, 7-9g. Carbohydrates, 20-25g. Fiber, 6-8g.

38. Turkey broth with rosemary and thyme

Ingredients: Turkey carcass or bones (leftover from a roast turkey), 1 onion, chopped, 2 carrots, peeled and chopped, 2 celery stalks, chopped, 2 cloves garlic, minced, 2 sprigs fresh rosemary, 4-5 sprigs fresh thyme, 10-12 whole black peppercorns, 8 cups (2 liters) water, Salt to taste.

Preparation:
- In a large pot, place the turkey bones, onion, carrots, celery, rosemary and fresh thyme.
- Cover with plenty of water.
- Bring everything to a boil, then reduce the heat and simmer for several hours to make the stock.
- Strain the broth to remove the vegetables and bones.
- You can use this broth as a base for other soups or as a broth to enjoy on its own.

Nutritional Values (per serving): Calories, 50-70 kcal. Protein, 3-5g. Fat, 1-2g. Carbohydrates, 5-7g. Fiber, 1-2g.

39. Tomato and Chilli Soup

Ingredients: 4 cups (800g) ripe tomatoes, chopped, 1 onion, chopped, 2 cloves garlic, minced, 1-2 red chili peppers, seeded and chopped (adjust to taste for spiciness), 4 cups (1 liter) vegetable broth, 1 teaspoon dried basil, 1 teaspoon dried oregano, Salt and black pepper to taste, Olive oil for sautéing, Fresh basil leaves for garnish (optional), Grated Parmesan cheese for garnish (optional).

Preparation:
- In a pan, fry the onion and garlic with a little olive oil until golden.
- Add the canned peeled tomatoes and chili pepper.
- Cook for just a few minutes to allow the flavors to mix together.
- Pour in the vegetable broth and bring to the boil.
- Reduce the heat and let it simmer for about 20-30 minutes.
- Add fresh basil, salt and pepper.
- You can serve the soup with toasted bread croutons.

Nutritional Values (per serving): Calories, 50-70 kcal. Protein, 1-3g. Fat, 1-2g. Carbohydrates, 10-15g. Fiber, 2-4g.

40. Carrot and Ginger Cream

Ingredients: 1 pound (450g) carrots, peeled and chopped, 1 onion, chopped, 2 cloves garlic, minced, 1-inch piece of fresh ginger, peeled and minced, 4 cups (1 liter) vegetable broth, 1/2 teaspoon ground cumin, Salt and black pepper to taste, Olive oil for sautéing, Fresh cilantro or parsley for garnish (optional).

Preparation:
- In a pan, fry the onion, garlic and ginger with a little olive oil until golden brown.

- Add the sliced carrots and cook for a few minutes to blend the flavors.
- Pour in the vegetable broth and bring to the boil.
- Reduce heat and simmer until
- when the carrots are tender.
- Use an immersion blender to cream the soup.
- Add coconut milk to give it a creamier consistency.
- Season your liking with pepper and salt as needed.

Nutritional Values (per serving): Calories, 50-70 kcal. Protein, 1-2g. Fat, 2-3g. Carbohydrates, 5-10g. Fiber, 2-3g.

41. Beef Broth with Celery Roots

Ingredients: 1 pound (450g) beef bones (such as marrow or knuckle bones), 2 celery roots (celeriac), peeled and chopped, 1 onion, chopped, 2 carrots, peeled and chopped, 2 cloves garlic, minced, 2 bay leaves, 4 cups (1 liter) water, Salt and black pepper to taste.

Preparation:
- In a large pot, place the beef chunks, celery roots, onion, carrots and bay leaf.
- Cover with beef broth and water.
- Bring everything to a boil, then reduce the heat and simmer for several hours to make the stock.
- Strain the broth to remove the vegetables and beef bones.
- You can use this broth as a base for other soups or as a broth to enjoy on its own.

Nutritional Values (per serving): Calories, 20-40 kcal. Protein, 1-2g. Fat, 0-1g. Carbohydrates, 3-5g. Fiber, 1-2g.

42. Pumpkin and Nutmeg Soup

Ingredients: 1 small pumpkin (about 2-3 pounds), peeled, seeded, and diced, 1 onion, chopped, 2 cloves garlic, minced, 4 cups (1 liter) vegetable broth, 1/2 teaspoon ground nutmeg, 1/2 teaspoon ground cinnamon, Salt and black pepper to taste, Olive oil for sautéing, Cream or coconut milk for garnish (optional), Fresh parsley for garnish (optional).

Preparation:
- Cut the pumpkin into cubes and set aside. In a pan, fry the onion and garlic with a little butter and olive oil until golden brown.
- Add the pumpkin and cook until slightly softened.
- Add the nutmeg and vegetable broth.
- Bring to the boil and cook until the squash is fully cooked.
- To purée the soup, utilize an immersion blender.
- Add the cream, salt and pepper.
- Mix well and serve.

Nutritional Values (per serving): Calories, 50-80 kcal. Protein, 1-2g. Fat, 1-3g. Carbohydrates, 10-15g. Fiber, 2-4g.

43. Quinoa and Brussels Sprouts Minestrone

Ingredients: 1 cup (185g) quinoa, rinsed, 1 cup (200g) Brussels sprouts, trimmed and halved, 1 onion, chopped, 2 cloves garlic, minced, 1 can (15 oz) diced tomatoes, 4 cups (1 liter) vegetable broth, 1 teaspoon dried oregano, 1 teaspoon dried basil, Salt and black pepper to taste, Grated Parmesan cheese for garnish (optional).

Preparation:
- In a pan, fry the onion, carrots and celery with a little olive oil until golden brown.
- Add the halved Brussels sprouts and cook until lightly browned.
- Add canned diced tomatoes, vegetable broth and quinoa.

- Bring to the boil, then reduce the heat and simmer until the quinoa is cooked and the Brussels sprouts are tender.
- Season with salt and pepper a
- Pleasure.

Nutritional Values (per serving): Calories, 150-200 kcal. Protein, 5-8g. Fat, 3-5g. Carbohydrates, 25-30g. Fiber, 5-7g.

44. Lentil and Cherry Tomato Soup

Ingredients: 1 cup (200g) dried green or brown lentils, rinsed and drained, 1 onion, chopped, 2 cloves garlic, minced, 2 cups (400g) cherry tomatoes, halved, 4 cups (1 liter) vegetable broth, 1 teaspoon ground cumin, 1 teaspoon ground coriander, 1/2 teaspoon smoked paprika, Salt and black pepper to taste, Olive oil for sautéing, Fresh cilantro leaves for garnish (optional).

Preparation:

- In a pan, fry the onion and garlic with a little olive oil until golden.
- Add the halved cherry tomatoes and cook until they start to release their juices.
- Add the lentils, fresh rosemary and vegetable broth.
- Heat to a boil and continue to cook until the lentils completely tender.
- Season your liking with pepper and salt as needed.

Nutritional Values (per serving): Calories, 150-200 kcal. Protein, 7-10g. Fat, 2-3g. Carbohydrates, 25-30g. Fiber, 7-10g.

45. Fish Broth with Mediterranean Herbs

Ingredients: 1 pound (450g) fish heads and bones (such as snapper, cod, or any white fish), 1 onion, chopped, 2 cloves garlic, minced, 2 tomatoes, chopped, 2 bay leaves, 1 sprig of fresh thyme (or 1 teaspoon dried thyme), 1 sprig of fresh rosemary (or 1 teaspoon dried rosemary), 4 cups (1 liter) water, Salt and black pepper to taste, Olive oil for sautéing.

Preparation:

- In a large pot, place the fish bones, onion, celery, carrots, Mediterranean herbs, garlic and black peppercorns.
- Cover with plenty of water.
- Bring everything to a boil, then reduce the heat and simmer for several hours to make the stock.
- Strain the broth to remove the vegetables and fish bones.
- You can use this broth as a base for other fish soups or as a broth to enjoy on its own.

Nutritional Values (per serving): Calories, 150-200 kcal. Protein, 10-15g. Fat, 2-3g. Carbohydrates, 15-20g. Fiber, 5-8g.

46. Cauliflower and Cumin Soup

Ingredients: 1 head of cauliflower, cut into florets, 1 onion, chopped, 2 cloves garlic, minced, 1 teaspoon ground cumin, 4 cups (1 liter) vegetable broth, 2 tablespoons olive oil, Season with salt and black pepper to taste. Garnish with fresh cilantro leaves (optional).

Preparation:

- Cut the cauliflower into pieces and the onion into thin slices. In a pan, fry the onion with a little olive oil until it becomes transparent.
- Add the cauliflower and cumin powder and cook for a few minutes.
- Mix the vegetable broth and coconut milk in a mixing bowl.
- Bring everything to the boil, then reduce the heat and cook until the cauliflower is tender.
- Mix the soup with an immersion blender until homogeneous.

- Season your liking with pepper and salt as needed.
- Serve with fresh parsley if desired.

Nutritional Values (per serving): Calories, 100-150 kcal. Protein, 3-5g. Fat, 4-6g. Carbohydrates, 15-20g. Fiber, 4-6g.

47. Sweet Potato and Rosemary Cream

Ingredients: 2 large sweet potatoes, peeled and diced, 2 tablespoons olive oil, 1 onion, chopped, 2 cloves garlic, minced, 1 sprig of fresh rosemary, leaves removed and chopped (or 1 teaspoon dried rosemary), 4 cups (1 liter) vegetable broth, Salt and black pepper to taste, 1/2 cup (120ml) heavy cream (or a dairy-free alternative), Fresh rosemary sprigs for garnish (optional).

Preparation:

- Peel and cut the sweet potatoes into bite-sized pieces.
- In a pan, fry the onion and garlic with a little olive oil until golden.
- Add the sweet potatoes and fresh rosemary and cook for a few minutes.
- Heat to a boil with the veggie broth.
- Decrease the temperature and continue to simmer until the potatoes are tender.
- To purée the soup, utilize an immersion blender.
- Add cream if you want a richer cream.
- Season your liking with pepper and salt as needed.

Nutritional Values (per serving): Calories, 150-200 kcal. Protein, 2-3g. Fat, 6-8g. Carbohydrates, 20-25g. Fiber, 3-5g.

48. Chicken Broth with Bay Leaf and Black Pepper

Ingredients: 1 whole chicken (about 3-4 pounds), cut into pieces, 2 onions, peeled and halved, 2 carrots, peeled and chopped, 2 celery stalks, chopped, 2 bay leaves, 10-12 whole black peppercorns, Salt to taste, Water to cover the ingredients.

Preparation:

- In a large pot, place the chicken carcasses, onion, carrots, celery, bay leaf, black peppercorns and salt.
- Cover with plenty of water. Bring everything to a boil, then reduce the heat and simmer for several hours to make the broth.
- Strain the broth to remove the vegetables and chicken bones.
- This broth can be used as a base for many soups and cooking recipes.

Nutritional Values (per serving): Calories, 20-30 kcal. Protein, 2-3g. Fat, 1-2g. Carbohydrates, 2-3g. Fiber, 0-1g.

49. Chickpea and Spinach Soup with Lemon

Ingredients: 1 can (15 oz) chickpeas, drained and rinsed, 1 tablespoon olive oil, 1 onion, chopped, 2 cloves garlic, minced, 1 teaspoon ground cumin, 1 teaspoon ground coriander, 4 cups (1 liter) vegetable broth, 4 cups (120g) fresh spinach leaves, Juice of 1 lemon, Salt and black pepper to taste, Lemon wedges and fresh cilantro for garnish (optional).

Preparation:

- In a pan, fry the onion and garlic with a little olive oil until golden.
- Add the drained and rinsed chickpeas, then pour in the vegetable broth.
- Bring to the boil and leave to cook for 10-15 minutes.
- Add fresh spinach and let it sweat in the soup.
- Squeeze the lemon juice into the soup, then season with salt and pepper.

Nutritional Values (per serving): Calories, 100-120 kcal. Protein, 4-5g. Fat, 3-4g. Carbohydrates, 14-16g. Fiber, 4-5g.

50. White Bean and Leek Minestrone

Ingredients: 1 cup (200g) dried white beans, soaked and cooked, or 2 cans (15 oz each) of white beans, drained and rinsed, 2 leeks, washed and sliced, 2 carrots, peeled and diced, 2 celery stalks, diced, 2 cloves garlic, minced, 1 can (15 oz) diced tomatoes, 6 cups (1.5 liters) vegetable broth, 1 cup (200g) small pasta (e.g., ditalini or small shells), 2 bay leaves, 1 teaspoon dried thyme, Salt and black pepper to taste, Fresh parsley, chopped, for garnish, Grated Parmesan cheese for garnish (optional).

Preparation:

- Dice the leeks, carrots and celery. In a pan, fry the leeks, carrots and celery with a little olive oil until golden brown.
- Add canned diced tomatoes, drained and rinsed white beans, fresh rosemary and vegetable broth.
- Heat to a boil and continue to simmer until the vegetables are cooked.
- Season your liking with pepper and salt as needed.

Nutritional Values (per serving): Calories, 180-220 kcal. Protein, 7-8g. Fat, 3-4g. Carbohydrates, 30-35g. Fiber, 6-7g.

Chapter 12: Desserts and sweets

50 anti-inflammatory dessert and sweet recipes

Introduction: Enjoy Dessert Without Inflammation
On the path to a healthier, inflammation-free lifestyle, giving up sweets and desserts doesn't have to mean sacrificing the pleasure of good food. Our collection of over 150 anti-inflammatory dessert and sweets recipes is here to prove that it's possible to satisfy your sweet tooth without compromising your health. In this chapter, we will explore a world of flavors, textures, and ingredients that will not only delight your taste buds but also help reduce inflammation in your body. The recipes presented here have been carefully selected to include ingredients known for their anti-inflammatory properties and health benefits. From fresh, thirst-quenching fruit to creamy spoon delights, from biscuits to chocolate desserts, you will find a wide range of options to satisfy your sweet tooth in a healthy and balanced way. Each recipe has been designed to provide maximum pleasure without the negative effects of inflammation. Get ready to amaze yourself and your guests with desserts that will not only satisfy your sweet tooth but also make you feel energetic and healthy. Whether you are looking for a dessert for a special occasion or simply want to pamper yourself, you will find the perfect solution here.
So, get inspired, put on your apron and start creating delicious desserts that will do your body and spirit good. Welcome to the world of anti-inflammatory desserts!

1. Fresh Fruit Salad with Mint

Ingredients: 1 cup mixed fresh fruit (strawberries, blueberries, pineapple, kiwi, etc.), Some fresh mint leaves, Honey or sweetener, to taste (optional)

Preparation:
- Cut the strawberries, pineapple, kiwi and grapes into small pieces.
- Chop some fresh mint leaves and mix everything in a bowl.
- Add lemon juice and powdered sugar if you want a little sweetness.
- Mix well and serve as a fresh and healthy dessert.

Nutritional Values (per serving): Calories, 70-100 kcal. Protein, 1-2g. Fat, 0-1g. Carbohydrates, 15-20g. Fiber, 2-4g.

2. Coconut Panna Cotta with Berries

Ingredients: 1 can (13.5 oz or 400 ml) of coconut milk, 1/4 cup (60 ml) of whole milk or a milk alternative (such as almond milk or coconut milk), 1/4 cup (60 g) of granulated sugar (adjust to taste), 1 teaspoon of vanilla extract, 2 teaspoons of unflavored gelatin powder, 2 tablespoons of cold water, Mixed berries (e.g., strawberries, blueberries, raspberries) for topping, Mint leaves for garnish (optional).

Preparation:
- Soak the isinglass in cold water. In a saucepan, mix the coconut milk, cream, sugar and vanilla seeds.
- Bring everything to the boil, then add the soaked isinglass and stir until it dissolves completely.
- Pour the mixture into molds and place in the refrigerator for at least 4 hours or until it solidifies.
- Turn it out onto a dessert plate and serve with berries and a sprinkling of icing sugar.

Nutritional Values (per serving): Calories, 150-250 kcal. Protein, 1-3g. Fat, 12-20g. Carbohydrates, 10-20g. Fiber, 1-3g.

3. Gluten Free Lemon Cake

Ingredients: 1 1/2 cups (180g) gluten-free all-purpose flour, 1 1/2 teaspoons gluten-free baking powder, 1/2 teaspoon salt, 1/2 cup (1 stick or 113g) unsalted butter, softened, 1 cup (200g) granulated sugar, 2 large eggs, Zest of 2 lemons, 1/4 cup (60ml) fresh lemon juice, 1/2 cup (120ml) milk or a milk alternative (such as almond milk or coconut milk), 1 teaspoon pure vanilla extract.

Preparation:
- In a bowl, mix the almond flour, icing sugar, eggs, melted butter, grated lemon zest, lemon juice, baking powder and a pinch of salt.
- Place the mixture in a buttered and dusted baking dish.
- Bake in a preheated oven at 180°C for about 25-30 minutes or until the cake is golden and a skewer inserted into the center comes out clean.
- Let cool before serving.

Nutritional Values (per serving): Calories, 250-350 kcal. Protein, 2-4g. Fat, 10-15g. Carbohydrates, 35-45g. Fiber, 1-3g.

4. Banana and Strawberry Ice Cream

Ingredients: 3 ripe bananas, peeled and sliced, 1 cup (150g) strawberries, hulled and halved, 1/2 cup (120ml) plain yogurt or a dairy-free alternative (e.g., coconut yogurt), 2 tablespoons honey or a sweetener of your choice (optional), 1 teaspoon vanilla extract (optional).

Cut ripe bananas into slices and freeze for at least 2 hours.
- Also, freeze strawberries if they aren't already frozen.
- Place the bananas and strawberries in a blender and blend until smooth.
- Add honey or Greek yogurt if you want a little sweetness or a creamier texture.
- Serve immediately as ice cream.

Nutritional Values (per serving): Calories, 100-150 kcal. Protein, 1-2g. Fat, 0-1g. Carbohydrates, 25-30g. Fiber, 2-3g.

5. Almond and Pear Cake

Ingredients: 2 ripe pears, peeled, cored, and sliced, 1 1/2 cups (180g) almond flour or ground almonds, 1/2 cup (60g) all-purpose flour (or a gluten-free flour blend), 1 teaspoon baking powder, 1/2 teaspoon ground cinnamon, 1/4 teaspoon salt, 1/2 cup (1 stick or 113g) unsalted butter, softened, 1/2 cup (100g) granulated sugar, 2 large eggs, 1 teaspoon vanilla extract, Sliced almonds for topping (optional).

Preparation:
- In a bowl, mix the chopped almonds, eggs, sugar, flour, melted butter, baking powder, cinnamon and a pinch of salt.
- Peel and slice the pears and arrange them on the bottom of a baking tray.
- Pour the mixture over the fruit and cook in a preheated oven at 180°C for about 30-40 minutes or until it is golden and a stick inserted into the center comes out clean.

Nutritional Values (per serving): Calories, 200-250 kcal. Protein, 3-4g. Fat, 10-12g. Carbohydrates, 25-30g. Fiber, 2-3g.

6. Blueberry and Oat Tart

Ingredients: 1 1/2 cups (180g) all-purpose flour, 1 cup (90g) rolled oats, 1/2 cup (100g) granulated sugar, 1/2 teaspoon baking powder, 1/4 teaspoon salt, 1/2 cup (1 stick or 113g) unsalted butter, cold and cubed, 1 large egg, 2 cups (300g) fresh blueberries, 1/4 cup (60ml) honey, 1 tablespoon lemon juice, Zest of 1 lemon.

Preparation:
- Prepare the tart dough or use ready-made one. In a bowl, mix the blueberries, sugar, cornstarch and grated lemon zest.
- Roll out the dough into the tart pan and pour the blueberry mixture over the top.
- Cover with oats and bake in a preheated oven at 180°C for about 30-35 minutes or until the crust is golden and the blueberries are soft.

Nutritional Values (per serving): Calories, 150-200 kcal. Protein, 2-3g. Fat, 7-9g. Carbohydrates, 20-25g. Fiber, 2-3g.

7. Whole meal Cinnamon Biscuits

Ingredients: 2 cups (240g) whole wheat flour, 1 tablespoon baking powder, 1/2 teaspoon baking soda, 1/2 teaspoon salt, 1 tablespoon ground cinnamon, 1/4 cup (50g) granulated sugar, 1/2 cup (1 stick or 113g) unsalted butter, cold and cubed, 1 cup (240ml) buttermilk, 1 teaspoon vanilla extract.

Preparation:
- In a bowl, mix the whole-wheat flour, brown sugar, ground cinnamon, melted butter, eggs, baking powder and a pinch of salt.
- Form the dough into a ball and place it in the refrigerator for about 30 minutes.
- Take small portions of dough, shape into balls and flatten them lightly on a baking tray lined with baking paper.
- Bake in a preheated oven at 180°C for about 10-12 minutes or until the biscuits are golden.

Nutritional Values (per serving): Calories, 70-90 kcal. Protein, 1-2g. Fat, 3-4g. Carbohydrates, 10-12g. Fiber, 1-2g.

8. Carrot and Ginger Muffins

Ingredients: 1 1/2 cups (180g) all-purpose flour, 1/2 cup (60g) whole wheat flour, 1/2 cup (100g) granulated sugar, 1 1/2 teaspoons baking powder, 1/2 teaspoon baking soda, 1/2 teaspoon salt, 1 teaspoon ground cinnamon, 1/2 teaspoon ground ginger, 1/4 cup (60ml) vegetable oil, 2 large eggs, 1/2 cup (120ml) plain yogurt, 1/2 cup (120ml) milk, 1 teaspoon vanilla extract, 1 1/2 cups (180g) grated carrots, 1/4 cup (60ml) honey, 1/4 cup (30g) chopped crystallized ginger (optional).

Preparation:
- In a bowl, mix the flour, sugar, grated carrots, grated ginger, eggs, vegetable oil, baking powder, ground cinnamon and a pinch of salt.
- Pour the mixture into muffin molds and bake in a preheated oven at 180°C for about 20-25 minutes or until the muffins are golden and a stick inserted into the center comes out clean.

Nutritional Values (per serving): Calories, 150-200 kcal. Protein, 2-3g. Fat, 6-8g. Carbohydrates, 20-25g. Fiber, 2-3g.

9. Dark Chocolate Mousse with Avocado

Ingredients: 2 ripe avocados, peeled and pitted, 1/2 cup (120g) dark chocolate chips or chopped dark chocolate, 1/4 cup (60ml) unsweetened cocoa powder, 1/4 cup (60ml) honey or a sweetener of your choice, 1 teaspoon vanilla extract, A pinch of salt, Fresh berries for garnish (optional), Whipped cream or coconut whipped cream for garnish (optional).

Preparation:
- In a blender, blend the avocado pulp, melted dark chocolate, cocoa powder, icing sugar (if you want it sweeter), and vanilla extract until creamy.

- Place the mousse in bowls or glasses and leave to cool in the refrigerator for at least an hour before serving.

Nutritional Values (per serving): Calories, 200-250 kcal. Protein, 2-3g. Fat, 15-18g. Carbohydrates, 15-20g. Fiber, 5-7g.

10. Homemade Fruit and Nut Bars

Ingredients: 1 cup (240g) mixed dried fruits (e.g., raisins, apricots, dates, cranberries), 1 cup (120g) mixed nuts (e.g., almonds, walnuts, cashews, pistachios), 1/2 cup (40g) rolled oats, 1/4 cup (60g) nut butter (e.g., almond butter, peanut butter), 1/4 cup (60ml) honey or a sweetener of your choice, 1/2 teaspoon vanilla extract, A pinch of salt (optional), 1/2 cup (90g) chocolate chips (optional).

Preparation:
- Finely chop dried fruit and dehydrated fruit.
- In a bowl, mix the chopped ingredients with honey, cereals and a pinch of vanilla (if desired).
- Roll out the dough on a baking tray lined with baking paper and compact it well.
- Let cool in the refrigerator for a few hours, then cut into bars.

Nutritional Values (per serving): Calories, 150-200 kcal. Protein, 3-4g. Fat, 8-10g. Carbohydrates, 20-25g. Fiber, 4-6g.

11. Vanilla Ice Cream with Maple Syrup

Ingredients: 2 cups (480ml) heavy cream, 1 cup (240ml) whole milk, 3/4 cup (150g) granulated sugar, 2 teaspoons pure vanilla extract, A pinch of salt, Maple syrup, for drizzling (as desired).

Preparation:
- In a saucepan, mix the cream, milk, sugar and vanilla seeds.
- Heat the mixture over medium heat until it begins to boil.
- Whisk the eggs in another basin.
- Slowly pour the hot mixture over the beaten eggs, stirring constantly.
- Return the mixture to the pot and cook over medium-low heat until it thickens slightly.
- Let cool, then add maple syrup.
- Cool completely in the refrigerator before using an ice cream maker or freezing in a container.

Nutritional Values (per serving): Calories, 200-250 kcal. Protein, 2-3g. Fat, 10-12g. Carbohydrates, 25-30g. Fiber, 0-1g.

12. Dark Chocolate Fondue with Fresh Fruit

Ingredients: 8 ounces (226g) dark chocolate, finely chopped, 1/2 cup (120ml) heavy cream, 1 teaspoon vanilla extract, Assorted fresh fruits for dipping (e.g., strawberries, bananas, apple slices, pineapple chunks), Skewers or fondue forks for dipping.

Preparation:
- Put the dark chocolate in a basin and break it up into bits.
- In a saucepan, heat the cream over medium-high heat without letting it boil.
- Pour the hot cream over the chocolate and stir until the chocolate melts completely and you get a smooth consistency.
- Serve the chocolate fondue with fresh fruit for dipping.

Nutritional Values (per serving): Calories, 200-250 kcal. Protein, 2-3g. Fat, 10-12g. Carbohydrates, 25-30g. Fiber, 2-3g.

13. Dairy-Free Tiramisu

Ingredients: 1 cup (240ml) strong brewed coffee, cooled, 1/4 cup (60ml) coffee liqueur (optional), 1 package (14 oz or about 400g) dairy-free ladyfingers, 1 1/2 cups (360g) dairy-free mascarpone-style cheese, 1/2 cup (120ml) unsweetened dairy-free milk (e.g., almond milk, coconut milk), 1/2 cup (100g) granulated sugar, 2 teaspoons vanilla extract, 2 tablespoons unsweetened cocoa powder, Dairy-free chocolate shavings or grated chocolate for garnish (optional).

Preparation:
- In a bowl, mix the coconut cream, powdered sugar and vanilla extract until smooth
- homogeneous cream.
- On a baking tray, alternate layers of ladyfingers soaked in coffee and layers of coconut cream.
- Continue until you run out of ingredients, finishing with a layer of cream.
- Sprinkle cocoa powder on top.
- Leave to cool in the refrigerator for a few hours before serving.

Nutritional Values (per serving): Calories, 250-300 kcal. Protein, 3-4g. Fat, 12-15g. Carbohydrates, 30-35g. Fiber, 1-2g.

14. Coconut and Ginger Cookies

Ingredients: 1 cup (240g) unsalted butter, softened, 1 cup (200g) granulated sugar, 2 cups (240g) all-purpose flour, 1/2 cup (50g) shredded coconut, 2 tablespoons finely grated fresh ginger, 1 teaspoon ground ginger, 1 teaspoon vanilla extract, A pinch of salt, Additional granulated sugar for rolling (optional).

Preparation:
- In a bowl, mix the coconut flour, ground ginger, honey and eggs until smooth.
- Shape small biscuits and place them on a baking tray lined with baking paper.
- Bake in a preheated oven at 180°C for about 10-12 minutes or until golden.

Nutritional Values (per serving): Calories, 150-200 kcal. Protein, 2-3g. Fat, 9-11g. Carbohydrates, 17-20g. Fiber, 1-2g.

15. Gluten-Free Apple and Cherry Pie

Ingredients:

For the Gluten-Free Pie Crust:

2 cups (240g) gluten-free all-purpose flour, 1/2 cup (120g) cold butter, cubed, 1/4 cup (60ml) cold water, 1 teaspoon xanthan gum (if not included in the flour blend), 1/2 teaspoon salt, 1 tablespoon granulated sugar (for sweet pie crust, optional)

For the Pie Filling:

3-4 cups (about 3-4 medium) apples, peeled, cored, and sliced, 1 cup (150g) pitted cherries (fresh or frozen), 1/2 cup (100g) granulated sugar (adjust to taste), 1 teaspoon ground cinnamon, 1/4 teaspoon ground nutmeg, 2 tablespoons gluten-free all-purpose flour (for thickening).

Preparation:
- In a bowl, mix the diced apples, cherries, almond flour, honey, eggs, ground cinnamon and baking powder.
- Pour the mixture into a pan and bake in a preheated oven at 180°C for about 25-30 minutes or until the cake is golden.

Nutritional Values (per serving): Calories, 250-300 kcal. Protein, 3-4g. Fat, 12-15g. Carbohydrates, 35-40g. Fiber, 2-3g.

16. Wholemeal Banana Pancakes

Ingredients: 1 cup (120g) whole wheat flour, 1 tablespoon granulated sugar, 1 teaspoon baking powder, 1/2 teaspoon baking soda, 1/4 teaspoon salt, 1 ripe banana, mashed, 1 cup (240ml) buttermilk or a buttermilk substitute, 1 large egg, 1 teaspoon vanilla extract, 2 tablespoons unsalted butter, melted (plus more for cooking).

Preparation:
- In a bowl, mash the ripe bananas.
- Add whole wheat flour, almond milk, eggs, ground cinnamon, baking powder, and vanilla extract (if desired).
- Blend until the mixture is smooth.
- Cook small quantities of dough in a non-stick pan until bubbles appear on the surface, then turn them over and cook until golden brown.

Nutritional Values (per serving): Calories, 150-200 kcal. Protein, 5-7g. Fat, 2-3g. Carbohydrates, 30-35g. Fiber, 3-4g.

17. Cocoa and Avocado Muffins

Ingredients: 1 1/2 cups (180g) all-purpose flour, 1/2 cup (50g) unsweetened cocoa powder, 1 1/2 teaspoons baking powder, 1/2 teaspoon baking soda, 1/4 teaspoon salt, 2 ripe avocados, peeled and pitted, 3/4 cup (150g) granulated sugar, 2 large eggs, 1 teaspoon vanilla extract, 1 cup (240ml) buttermilk or a buttermilk substitute, 1/2 cup (120ml) vegetable oil, 1/2 cup (90g) chocolate chips (optional).

Preparation:
- In a blender, blend the ripe avocado, cocoa powder, honey, eggs, baking powder and a pinch of salt until smooth.
- Pour the mixture into muffin molds and cook in a preheated oven at 180°C for approximately 15-18 minutes or until the muffins are cooked.

Nutritional Values (per serving): Calories, 150-200 kcal. Protein, 3-4g. Fat, 7-9g. Carbohydrates, 18-22g. Fiber, 3-4g.

18. Chia Pudding with Fresh Fruit

Ingredients: 1/4 cup (48g) chia seeds, 1 cup (240ml) milk of your choice (e.g., almond milk, coconut milk), 1 tablespoon honey or a sweetener of your choice (optional), 1/2 teaspoon vanilla extract, Assorted fresh fruits for topping (e.g., berries, banana slices, kiwi, mango), Nuts or seeds for garnish (optional).

Preparation:
- In a bowl, mix the chia seeds, almond milk, honey and vanilla extract (if desired).
- Mix well and let sit in the refrigerator for at least 3-4 hours or overnight.
- Before serving, add the diced fresh fruit.

Nutritional Values (per serving): Calories, 200-250 kcal. Protein, 5-6g. Fat, 7-9g. Carbohydrates, 25-30g. Fiber, 7-9g.

19. Gluten Free Carrot and Walnut Cake

Ingredients:

For the Cake: 2 cups (240g) gluten-free all-purpose flour, 1 1/2 teaspoons baking powder, 1/2 teaspoon baking soda, 1/2 teaspoon salt, 1 1/2 teaspoons ground cinnamon, 1/2 teaspoon ground nutmeg, 1/2 cup (120ml) vegetable oil, 1 cup (200g) granulated sugar, 2 large eggs, 2 cups (200g) grated carrots, 1/2 cup (60g) chopped walnuts, 1 teaspoon vanilla extract

For the Cream Cheese Frosting:

8 ounces (226g) cream cheese, softened, 1/4 cup (1/2 stick or 56g) unsalted butter, softened, 2 cups (240g) powdered sugar, 1 teaspoon vanilla extract

Preparation:
- In a bowl, mix the grated carrots, chopped walnuts, almond flour, eggs, honey, ground cinnamon and baking powder until smooth.
- Pour the mixture into a pan and bake in a preheated oven at 180°C for about 25-30 minutes or until the cake is golden.

Nutritional Values (per serving): Calories, 250-300 kcal. Protein, 3-4g. Fat, 12-15g. Carbohydrates, 35-40g. Fiber, 3-4g.

20. Watermelon sorbet

Ingredients: 4 cups (about 4 lbs or 1.8 kg) fresh watermelon, seeded and cubed, 1/2 cup (100g) granulated sugar (adjust to taste), 1/4 cup (60ml) fresh lemon juice, 1/4 cup (60ml) water.

Preparation:
- Blend the watermelon until smooth.
- Add lemon juice and, if desired, a little sugar to sweeten.
- Pour the mixture into a container and place it in the freezer.
- Stir every 30 minutes for approximately 2-3 hours or until the sorbet has reached the desired consistency.

Nutritional Values (per serving): Calories, 70-90 kcal. Protein, 1-2g. Fat, 0g. Carbohydrates, 18-20g. Fiber, 0-1g.

21. Chocolate Cream with Banana

Ingredients: 2 ripe bananas, peeled, 1/4 cup (25g) unsweetened cocoa powder, 1/4 cup (60ml) milk of your choice (e.g., almond milk, coconut milk), 2 tablespoons honey or a sweetener of your choice (adjust to taste), 1 teaspoon vanilla extract, A pinch of salt, Whipped cream or a dairy-free alternative for topping (optional), Chocolate shavings for garnish (optional).

Preparation:
- In a blender, blend ripe bananas, cocoa powder, almond milk, honey, and vanilla extract (if desired) until smooth. Pour the cream into bowls and leave to cool in the refrigerator for an hour before serving.

Nutritional Values (per serving): Calories, 200-250 kcal. Protein, 2-4g. Fat, 8-10g. Carbohydrates, 30-35g. Fiber, 3-4g.

22. Oat pancakes with blueberries

Ingredients: 1 cup (90g) rolled oats, 1/2 cup (120ml) milk of your choice (e.g., almond milk, coconut milk), 1 ripe banana, 1 large egg, 1 teaspoon baking powder, 1/2 teaspoon ground cinnamon, 1/4 teaspoon salt, 1/2 cup (75g) fresh blueberries, Maple syrup or honey for drizzling (optional).

Preparation:
- In a bowl, mix the oats, almond milk, fresh blueberries, eggs, honey, ground cinnamon and baking powder until smooth.
- Cook small quantities of dough in a non-stick pan until bubbles appear on the surface, then turn them over and cook until golden brown.

Nutritional Values (per serving): Calories, 250-300 kcal. Protein, 5-7g. Fat, 5-7g. Carbohydrates, 45-55g. Fiber, 5-7g.

23. Cocoa and Cherry Biscuits

Ingredients: 1 1/2 cups (180g) all-purpose flour, 1/3 cup (40g) unsweetened cocoa powder, 1/2 teaspoon baking powder, 1/4 teaspoon salt, 1/2 cup (1 stick or 113g) unsalted butter, softened, 2/3 cup (130g) granulated sugar, 1 large egg, 1 teaspoon vanilla extract, 1/2 cup (75g) dried cherries (or fresh cherries, pitted and chopped), 1/2 cup (90g) chocolate chips or chunks (dark or semisweet).

Preparation:
- In a bowl, mix the oat flour, cocoa powder, dried cherries, honey, eggs, and vanilla extract (if desired) until smooth.
- Shape small biscuits and place them on a baking tray lined with baking paper.
- Bake in a preheated oven at 180°C for about 10-12 minutes or until golden.

Nutritional Values (per serving): Calories, 80-100 kcal. Protein, 1-2g. Fat, 3-5g. Carbohydrates, 12-15g. Fiber, 1-2g.

24. Strawberry Mousse with Greek Yogurt

Ingredients: 2 cups (300g) fresh strawberries, hulled and sliced, 1/4 cup (30g) powdered sugar (adjust to taste), 1 teaspoon lemon juice, 1 cup (240g) Greek yogurt, 1 teaspoon vanilla extract, 1/2 cup (120ml) heavy cream, Fresh strawberries for garnish (optional).

Preparation:
- In a blender, blend fresh strawberries, Greek yogurt, honey, and vanilla extract (if desired) until smooth.
- Pour the mousse into bowls and leave to cool in the refrigerator for at least an hour before serving.

Nutritional Values (per serving): Calories, 120-150 kcal. Protein, 5-7g. Fat, 3-5g. Carbohydrates, 15-20g. Fiber, 1-2g.

25. Gluten Free Pear and Walnut Cake

Ingredients: 2 ripe pears, peeled, cored, and chopped, 1 1/2 cups (180g) gluten-free all-purpose flour, 1 1/2 teaspoons baking powder, 1/2 teaspoon baking soda, 1/4 teaspoon salt, 1 teaspoon ground cinnamon, 1/2 teaspoon ground nutmeg, 1/2 cup (1 stick or 113g) unsalted butter, softened, 1/2 cup (100g) granulated sugar, 2 large eggs, 1 teaspoon vanilla extract, 1/2 cup (60g) chopped walnuts, Powdered sugar for dusting (optional).

Preparation:
- In a bowl, mix the diced pears, chopped walnuts, almond flour, eggs, honey, ground cinnamon and baking powder until smooth.
- Pour the mixture into a pan and bake in a preheated oven at 180°C for approximately 30-35 minutes or until the cake is golden.

Nutritional Values (per serving): Calories, 180-220 kcal. Protein, 3-4g. Fat, 10-12g. Carbohydrates, 20-25g. Fiber, 2-3g.

26. Cocoa and Avocado Smoothie Bowl

Ingredients:

For the Smoothie: 1 ripe avocado, peeled and pitted, 2 tablespoons unsweetened cocoa powder, 1/2 cup (120ml) milk of your choice (e.g., almond milk, coconut milk), 2 tablespoons honey or a sweetener of your choice (adjust to taste), 1/2 teaspoon vanilla extract, A pinch of salt.

For Toppings (Optional):

Sliced bananas, Fresh berries (e.g., strawberries, blueberries), Chia seeds, Shredded coconut, Chopped nuts (e.g., almonds, walnuts).

Preparation:
- In a blender, blend the avocado, banana, almond milk, cocoa powder and honey until you have a creamy smoothie.
- Pour the smoothie into a bowl and garnish with fresh fruit of your choice.

Nutritional Values (per serving): Calories, 250-300 kcal. Protein, 4-5g. Fat, 14-16g. Carbohydrates, 30-35g. Fiber, 8-10g.

27. Chocolate Rice Waffles

Ingredients: 1 cup (200g) uncooked white rice, 2 cups (400ml) milk of your choice (e.g., almond milk, coconut milk), 1/4 cup (25g) unsweetened cocoa powder, 1/4 cup (50g) granulated sugar, 2 teaspoons baking powder, 1/2 teaspoon vanilla extract, 1/4 teaspoon salt, 1/4 cup (60ml) vegetable oil, 2 large eggs.

Preparation:
- Now take and melt the chocolate in the microwave or in a double boiler.
- Mix the melted chocolate with the puffed rice until all the rice grains are well covered.
- Form wafers on a baking tray lined with baking paper and leave to cool in the refrigerator until the chocolate has hardened.

Nutritional Values (per serving): Calories, 150-200 kcal. Protein, 3-4g. Fat, 6-8g. Carbohydrates, 20-25g. Fiber, 1-2g.

28. Gluten-Free Pumpkin and Walnut Cake

Ingredients:

For the Cake:

1 1/2 cups (180g) gluten-free all-purpose flour, 1 1/2 teaspoons baking powder, 1/2 teaspoon baking soda, 1/2 teaspoon salt, 1 teaspoon ground cinnamon, 1/2 teaspoon ground nutmeg, 1/2 teaspoon ground ginger, 1/4 teaspoon ground cloves, 1 cup (240g) canned pumpkin puree, 1/2 cup (120ml) vegetable oil, 1/2 cup (100g) granulated sugar, 1/2 cup (100g) brown sugar, 2 large eggs, 1 teaspoon vanilla extract, 1/2 cup (60g) chopped walnuts

For the Cream Cheese Frosting:

8 ounces (226g) cream cheese, softened, 1/4 cup (1/2 stick or 56g) unsalted butter, softened, 2 cups (240g) powdered sugar, 1 teaspoon vanilla extract

Preparation:

- In a bowl, mix the cooked diced pumpkin, chopped walnuts, almond flour, eggs, honey, ground cinnamon and baking powder until smooth.
- Pour the mixture into a pan and bake in a preheated oven at 180°C for approximately 30-35 minutes or until the cake is golden.

Nutritional Values (per serving): Calories, 200-250 kcal. Protein, 3-4g. Fat, 10-12g. Carbohydrates, 25-30g. Fiber, 2-3g.

29. Mango and Lime Ice Cream

Ingredients: 2 cups (about 2 large) ripe mangoes, peeled and cubed, 1/2 cup (120ml) lime juice (from about 4-6 limes), 1/2 cup (100g) granulated sugar (adjust to taste), 1 cup (240ml) heavy cream, 1/2 cup (120ml) whole milk, Zest of 1 lime, A pinch of salt.

Preparation:

- In a blender, blend the mango, lime juice, Greek yogurt, and honey until smooth.
- Pour the cream into a container and place it in the freezer.
- Stir every 30 minutes for approximately 2-3 hours or until the ice cream has reached the desired consistency.

Nutritional Values (per serving): Calories, 150-200 kcal. Protein, 1-2g. Fat, 1-2g. Carbohydrates, 35-40g. Fiber, 2-3g.

30. Dark Chocolate Panna Cotta

Ingredients: 2 cups (480ml) heavy cream, 1/2 cup (120ml) whole milk, 1/2 cup (100g) granulated sugar, 6 ounces (170g) dark chocolate, finely chopped, 1 1/2 teaspoons unflavored gelatin, 2 tablespoons cold water, 1 teaspoon vanilla extract, A pinch of salt.

Preparation:

- Now take and melt the chocolate in the microwave or in a double boiler.
- Meanwhile, soften the gelatine in cold water.
- In a small saucepan, heat the cream and sugar until the sugar has dissolved.
- Add the melted chocolate and the squeezed gelatine.
- Mix well until all ingredients are well incorporated.
- Pour the panna cotta into molds and leave to cool in the refrigerator for at least 4 hours or until completely solidified.

Nutritional Values (per serving): Calories, 250-300 kcal. Protein, 3-4g. Fat, 15-18g. Carbohydrates, 20-25g. Fiber, 2-3g.

31. Granola with Dried Fruit and Honey

Ingredients: 3 cups (270g) rolled oats, 1 cup (150g) mixed dried fruits (e.g., raisins, apricots, cranberries), 1/2 cup (60g) chopped nuts (e.g., almonds, walnuts), 1/4 cup (30g) seeds (e.g., sunflower seeds, pumpkin seeds), 1/4 cup (60ml) honey or a sweetener of your choice, 1/4 cup (60ml) vegetable oil, 1 teaspoon vanilla extract, A pinch of salt, 1 teaspoon ground cinnamon (optional).

Preparation:

- In a bowl, mix rolled oats, sliced almonds, chopped walnuts, sunflower seeds and pumpkin seeds. In a saucepan, heat the honey and vegetable oil together with the ground cinnamon.
- Pour this liquid mixture over the dry ingredients and mix well.
- Distribute equally on a baking sheet lined with parchment paper.
- Cook in a preheated oven at 160°C for approximately 30-35 minutes, stirring occasionally.
- Once cooled, you can add dried fruit to taste.

Nutritional Values (per serving): Calories, 350-400 kcal. Protein, 7-9g. Fat, 15-18g. Carbohydrates, 50-60g. Fiber, 6-8g.

32. Wholemeal Biscuits with Walnuts and Cinnamon

Ingredients: 1 1/2 cups (180g) whole wheat flour, 1/2 cup (60g) chopped walnuts, 1/2 teaspoon ground cinnamon, 1/2 teaspoon baking powder, 1/4 teaspoon salt, 1/2 cup (1 stick or 113g) unsalted butter, softened, 1/2 cup (100g) granulated sugar, 1 large egg, 1 teaspoon vanilla extract.

Preparation:

- In a bowl, mix the whole-wheat flour, brown sugar, chopped walnuts and ground cinnamon.
- Add the eggs and melted butter and mix until smooth.
- Form small balls of dough and place them on a baking tray lined with baking paper.
- Lightly crush each ball with a fork.
- Bake in a preheated oven at 180°C for about 10-12 minutes or until the biscuits are golden.

Nutritional Values (per serving): Calories, 120-150 kcal. Protein, 2-3g. Fat, 5-7g. Carbohydrates, 15-20g. Fiber, 2-3g.

33. Gluten Free Apricot and Almond Cake

Ingredients:

For the Cake: 1 1/2 cups (150g) almond flour or ground almonds, 1/2 cup (60g) gluten-free all-purpose flour, 1/2 teaspoon baking powder, 1/4 teaspoon salt, 1/2 cup (1 stick or 113g) unsalted butter, softened, 1/2 cup (100g) granulated sugar, 2 large eggs, 1 teaspoon vanilla extract, 1/4 cup (60ml) milk of your choice (e.g., almond milk), 1 cup (150g) dried apricots, chopped

For the Topping:

Sliced almonds, Apricot preserves or jam for glazing (optional)

Preparation:

- In a bowl, mix the ground almonds, sugar, eggs, cornstarch and baking powder until smooth.
- Add the apricots (after draining them if they are canned) and mix gently.
- Pour the mixture into a pan and bake in a preheated oven at 180°C for approximately 30-35 minutes or until the cake is golden.

Nutritional Values (per serving): Calories, 180-220 kcal. Protein, 3-4g. Fat, 8-10g. Carbohydrates, 25-30g. Fiber, 2-3g.

34. Quinoa Pancakes with Berries

Ingredients: 1 cup (185g) cooked quinoa, cooled, 1 cup (240ml) milk of your choice (e.g., almond milk, coconut milk), 2 large eggs, 2 tablespoons honey or a sweetener of your choice, 1 teaspoon vanilla extract, 1 cup (120g) all-purpose flour or a gluten-free flour blend, 2 teaspoons baking powder, 1/4 teaspoon salt, 1 cup (150g) mixed berries (e.g., strawberries, blueberries, raspberries), Butter or oil for cooking.

Preparation:
- In a bowl, mix the cooked quinoa, eggs, milk and honey until a batter forms.
- Heat a non-stick pan and pour a ladle of batter to form the pancakes.
- Be sure to do the baking for each side.
- Serve with fresh or frozen berries as topping.

Nutritional Values (per serving): Calories, 250-300 kcal. Protein, 8-10g. Fat, 5-7g. Carbohydrates, 45-50g. Fiber, 5-6g.

35. Chocolate and Banana Muffins

Ingredients: 2 ripe bananas, mashed, 1/3 cup (80ml) vegetable oil, 1/2 cup (100g) granulated sugar, 1 large egg, 1 teaspoon vanilla extract, 1 1/2 cups (180g) all-purpose flour, 1/4 cup (25g) unsweetened cocoa powder, 1 teaspoon baking powder, 1/2 teaspoon baking soda, 1/4 teaspoon salt, 1/2 cup (90g) chocolate chips, Sliced bananas and additional chocolate chips for topping (optional).

Preparation:
- In a bowl, mash the ripe bananas and mix them with the sugar, eggs and vegetable oil.
- Mix well by adding the baking powder and flour.
- Add the dark chocolate pieces to the mixture.
- Pour the mixture into muffin molds and cook in a preheated oven at 180°C for approximately 20-25 minutes or until the muffins are golden.

Nutritional Values (per serving): Calories, 150-200 kcal. Protein, 3-4g. Fat, 6-8g. Carbohydrates, 25-30g. Fiber, 2-3g.

36. Gluten Free Lemon Coconut Cake

Ingredients:

For the Cake: 1 1/2 cups (180g) gluten-free all-purpose flour, 1/2 cup (60g) almond flour, 1 1/2 teaspoons baking powder, 1/2 teaspoon baking soda, 1/4 teaspoon salt, Zest of 2 lemons, 1/2 cup (1 stick or 113g) unsalted butter, softened, 1 cup (200g) granulated sugar, 3 large eggs, 1/2 cup (120ml) coconut milk, 1/4 cup (60ml) fresh lemon juice, 1 teaspoon vanilla extract, 1/2 cup (40g) shredded coconut

For the Lemon Glaze:

1 cup (120g) powdered sugar, 2-3 tablespoons fresh lemon juice

Preparation:
- In a bowl, mix the coconut flour, sugar, eggs, coconut milk, lemon juice and zest, and baking powder until smooth.
- Pour the mixture into a pan and bake in a preheated oven at 180°C for approximately 30-35 minutes or until the cake is golden.

Nutritional Values (per serving): Calories, 250-300 kcal. Protein, 3-4g. Fat, 12-15g. Carbohydrates, 30-35g. Fiber, 2-3g.

37. Avocado Cocoa Pudding

Ingredients: 2 ripe avocados, peeled and pitted, 1/2 cup (50g) unsweetened cocoa powder, 1/4 cup (60ml) milk of your choice (e.g., almond milk, coconut milk), 1/4 cup (60ml) honey or a sweetener of your choice, 1 teaspoon vanilla extract, A pinch of salt, Fresh berries or sliced bananas for topping (optional).

Preparation:
- In a blender, blend the ripe avocado, cocoa powder, milk, honey, vanilla extract and a pinch of salt until smooth.
- Transfer the pudding to individual bowls and let it rest in the refrigerator for at least an hour before serving.

- You can garnish with fresh fruit, nuts or chocolate chips.

Nutritional Values (per serving): Calories, 150-200 kcal. Protein, 2-3g. Fat, 12-15g. Carbohydrates, 10-15g. Fiber, 5-7g.

38. Cereal Bars with Dried Fruit

Ingredients: 1 cup (240g) dried fruit (e.g., dates, apricots, figs), finely chopped, 1 cup (90g) rolled oats, 1/2 cup (60g) chopped nuts (e.g., almonds, walnuts), 1/4 cup (30g) seeds (e.g., chia seeds, flaxseeds), 1/4 cup (60ml) honey or a sweetener of your choice, 1/4 cup (60ml) nut butter (e.g., almond butter, peanut butter), 1/2 teaspoon vanilla extract, A pinch of salt.

Preparation:
- In a bowl, mix the oat flakes, chopped nuts, dried fruit to taste and, if desired, chia seeds.
- In a small saucepan, heat the honey and peanut butter until liquid.
- Pour this mixture over the cereals and mix well.
- Transfer the mixture to a baking tray lined with baking paper and compact well.
- Leave to cool in the refrigerator for a few hours before cutting the bars.

Nutritional Values (per serving): Calories, 150-200 kcal. Protein, 2-4g. Fat, 5-8g. Carbohydrates, 25-30g. Fiber, 3-5g.

39. Mint and Spinach Ice Cream

Ingredients: 2 cups (about 2.5 oz or 70g) fresh spinach leaves, washed and dried, 1 cup (240ml) heavy cream, 1 cup (240ml) whole milk, 3/4 cup (150g) granulated sugar, 1/2 teaspoon vanilla extract, 1/2 teaspoon peppermint extract, Green food coloring (optional), Chocolate chips or chunks (optional).

Preparation:
- In a blender, blend ripe bananas, fresh spinach, milk and mint extract until creamy.
- Add dark chocolate pieces to the mixture if preferred.
- Pour the ice cream into an airtight container and freeze for a few hours before serving.

Nutritional Values (per serving): Calories, 120-150 kcal. Protein, 2-3g. Fat, 7-9g. Carbohydrates, 15-18g. Fiber, 1-2g.

40. Coconut and Pineapple Cream

Ingredients: 1 can (about 13.5 oz or 400ml) coconut milk, 1 cup (240ml) pineapple juice (fresh or canned), 1/4 cup (60g) granulated sugar (adjust to taste), 1/2 cup (120ml) heavy cream, 1 teaspoon vanilla extract, 1 cup (150g) fresh pineapple chunks, Shredded coconut and additional pineapple chunks for garnish (optional).

Preparation:
- In a blender, blend coconut milk, fresh or canned pineapple (after draining if canned), honey, vanilla extract, and a pinch of salt until smooth.
- Pour the cream into individual bowls and let it cool in the refrigerator for at least an hour before serving.

Nutritional Values (per serving): Calories, 200-250 kcal. Protein, 1-2g. Fat, 15-20g. Carbohydrates, 15-20g. Fiber, 2-3g.

41. Banana and Cocoa Fritters

Ingredients: 2 ripe bananas, mashed, 1/4 cup (25g) unsweetened cocoa powder, 1/2 cup (60g) all-purpose flour, 2 tablespoons granulated sugar, 1/2 teaspoon baking powder, A pinch of salt, 1 large egg, 1/2 cup (120ml) milk of your choice (e.g., almond milk, coconut milk), 1 teaspoon vanilla extract, Oil for frying (e.g., vegetable oil), Powdered sugar for dusting (optional).

Preparation:

- In a bowl, mash the ripe bananas and mix them with the eggs, cocoa powder and baking powder until smooth.
- Heat a non-stick pan and pour a ladle of dough to form the pancakes.
- Cook on both sides until golden brown.

Nutritional Values (per serving): Calories, 100-150 kcal. Protein, 1-2g. Fat, 4-6g. Carbohydrates, 20-25g. Fiber, 2-3g.

42. Almond Flour and Cinnamon Cookies

Ingredients: 2 cups (200g) almond flour, 1/2 teaspoon ground cinnamon, 1/4 teaspoon baking soda, A pinch of salt, 1/4 cup (60ml) melted coconut oil or butter, 1/4 cup (60ml) honey or a sweetener of your choice, 1 large egg, 1 teaspoon vanilla extract.

Preparation:

- In a bowl, mix the almond flour, brown sugar and ground cinnamon.
- Add the eggs and butter (or almond butter) and mix until smooth.
- Form small balls of dough and place them on a baking tray lined with baking paper.
- Lightly crush each ball with a fork.
- Bake in a preheated oven at 180°C for about 10-12 minutes or until the biscuits are golden.

Nutritional Values (per serving): Calories, 60-80 kcal. Protein, 1-2g. Fat, 4-6g. Carbohydrates, 5-8g. Fiber, 1-2g.

43. Gluten Free Blueberry and Almond Cake

Ingredients:

For the Cake: 1 1/2 cups (180g) almond flour, 1/4 cup (30g) coconut flour, 1/2 teaspoon baking powder, 1/4 teaspoon baking soda, 1/4 teaspoon salt, 1/2 cup (1 stick or 113g) unsalted butter, softened, 1/2 cup (100g) granulated sugar, 2 large eggs, 1 teaspoon vanilla extract, 1/4 cup (60ml) milk of your choice (e.g., almond milk), 1 1/2 cups (180g) fresh or frozen blueberries

For the Topping:

Sliced almonds, Powdered sugar for dusting (optional)

Preparation:

- Mix the ground almonds, brown sugar, eggs, melted butter, cornstarch, baking powder and vanilla extract until smooth.
- Add the blueberries and mix gently.
- Pour the batter into a baking tray coated with parchment paper and bake at 180°C for 30-35 minutes, or until the cake is brown and a toothpick placed into the center comes out clear.

Nutritional Values (per serving): Calories, 150-180 kcal. Protein, 3-4g. Fat, 10-12g. Carbohydrates, 15-18g. Fiber, 2-3g.

44. Cocoa and Avocado Smoothie

Ingredients: 1 ripe avocado, peeled and pitted, 2 tablespoons unsweetened cocoa powder, 1/2 cup (120ml) milk of your choice (e.g., almond milk, coconut milk), 2 tablespoons honey or a sweetener of your choice (adjust to taste), 1/2 teaspoon vanilla extract, A pinch of salt.

Preparation:

- In a blender, blend the ripe avocado, milk, cocoa powder, honey, vanilla extract and ice until smooth and creamy.
- Serve immediately.

Nutritional Values (per serving): Calories, 250-300 kcal. Protein, 4-5g. Fat, 15-18g. Carbohydrates, 25-30g. Fiber, 7-8g.

45. Coconut Flour Waffles

Ingredients: 1/2 cup (60g) coconut flour, 1/2 teaspoon baking powder, A pinch of salt, 4 large eggs, 1/4 cup (60ml) coconut oil, melted, 1/4 cup (60ml) milk of your choice (e.g., almond milk, coconut milk), 2 tablespoons honey or a sweetener of your choice (adjust to taste), 1 teaspoon vanilla extract.

Preparation:

- In a bowl, mix the coconut flour, coconut sugar, eggs, melted butter, vanilla extract and a pinch of salt until smooth.
- Heat a waffle iron and cook the dough according to your iron's instructions until you get golden waffles.

Nutritional Values (per serving): Calories, 250-300 kcal. Protein, 6-7g. Fat, 12-15g. Carbohydrates, 25-30g. Fiber, 5-6g.

46. Gluten Free Cherry and Almond Cake

Ingredients:

For the Cake:

1 1/2 cups (180g) almond flour, 1/2 cup (60g) gluten-free all-purpose flour, 1 1/2 teaspoons baking powder, 1/4 teaspoon salt, 1/2 cup (1 stick or 113g) unsalted butter, softened, 1/2 cup (100g) granulated sugar, 2 large eggs, 1 teaspoon almond extract, 1/2 cup (120ml) milk of your choice (e.g., almond milk), 1 1/2 cups (225g) fresh or frozen cherries, pitted

For the Topping:

Sliced almonds, Powdered sugar for dusting (optional)

Preparation:

- Mix the ground almonds, brown sugar, eggs, melted butter, cornstarch, baking powder and vanilla extract until smooth.
- Add the cherries and mix gently.
- Pour the batter into a baking tray coated with parchment paper and bake at 180°C for 30-35 minutes, or until the cake is brown and a toothpick placed into the center comes out clear.

Nutritional Values (per serving): Calories, 200-250 kcal. Protein, 4-5g. Fat, 9-11g. Carbohydrates, 25-30g. Fiber, 3-4g.

47. Banana and Walnut Pancakes

Ingredients: 1 cup (120g) all-purpose flour, 2 tablespoons granulated sugar, 2 teaspoons baking powder, 1/2 teaspoon salt, 2 ripe bananas, mashed, 1/2 cup (120ml) milk of your choice (e.g., almond milk), 1 large egg, 2 tablespoons unsalted butter, melted, 1/2 cup (60g) chopped walnuts, Butter or oil for cooking.

Preparation:

- Mash the ripe bananas in a bowl and mix them with the eggs, oat flour, chopped walnuts, ground cinnamon and a pinch of salt until smooth.
- Heat a non-stick pan and pour a ladle of batter to form the pancakes.
- Cook till golden brown on each side.

Nutritional Values (per serving): Calories, 250-300 kcal. Protein, 5-6g. Fat, 12-15g. Carbohydrates, 30-35g. Fiber, 4-5g.

48. White Chocolate and Raspberry Muffins

Ingredients: 1 3/4 cups (220g) all-purpose flour, 2 teaspoons baking powder, 1/2 teaspoon salt, 1/2 cup (1 stick or 113g) unsalted butter, softened, 3/4 cup (150g) granulated sugar, 2 large eggs, 1 teaspoon vanilla extract, 1/2 cup (120ml) milk of your choice (e.g., whole milk, almond milk), 1 cup (150g) fresh or frozen raspberries, 1/2 cup (90g) white chocolate chips.

Preparation:

- In a bowl, mix the flour, sugar, baking powder and a pinch of salt.
- In another bowl, whisk the eggs, milk and melted butter.

- Combine the liquid ingredients with the dry ones and mix until smooth.
- Add the chopped white chocolate and raspberries and mix gently.
- Pour the mixture into muffin molds and bake in a preheated oven at 180°C for approximately 20-25 minutes or until the muffins are golden and when a toothpick inserted into the center comes out clean.

Nutritional Values (per serving): Calories, 350-400 kcal. Protein, 5-6g. Fat, 15-18g. Carbohydrates, 45-50g. Fiber, 2-3g.

49. Gluten Free Chocolate Avocado Cake

Ingredients:

For the Cake: 2 ripe avocados, peeled and pitted, 1/2 cup (50g) unsweetened cocoa powder, 1/2 cup (120ml) maple syrup or a sweetener of your choice, 2 large eggs, 1 teaspoon vanilla extract, 1/2 cup (60g) almond flour, 1/2 teaspoon baking soda, 1/4 teaspoon salt

For the Chocolate Ganache:

1/2 cup (120ml) coconut milk, 4 ounces (115g) dark chocolate, finely chopped

Preparation:

- In a blender, blend the ripe avocado, melted dark chocolate, sugar, eggs, cocoa powder, vanilla extract and a pinch of salt until smooth.
- Pour the mixture into a baking tray lined with baking paper and bake in a preheated oven at 180°C for approximately 25-30 minutes or until the cake is dry in the centre.

Nutritional Values (per serving): Calories, 250-300 kcal. Protein, 3-4g. Fat, 15-18g. Carbohydrates, 25-30g. Fiber, 4-5g.

50. Kiwi sorbet

Ingredients: 4-5 ripe kiwi fruits, peeled and sliced, 1/2 cup (100g) granulated sugar, 1/2 cup (120ml) water, 2 tablespoons fresh lime juice.

Preparation:

- Peel and cut the kiwis into pieces.
- Blend them together with the sugar and lemon juice until you obtain a creamy mixture.
- Place the mixture in a container and place in the freezer for at least 4 hours.
- Fill your sorbet into cups and serve.

Nutritional Values (per serving): Calories, 100-150 kcal. Protein, 1-2g. Fat, 0-1g. Carbohydrates, 25-30g. Fiber, 2-3g.

8-Week Meal-Plan

Week 1

	Breakfast	Lunch	Dinner
Day 1	Buckwheat Porridge with Apples and Cinnamon	Quinoa Salad with Chickpeas and Olives	Baked salmon with lemon and rosemary sauce
Day 2	Green smoothie with spinach, banana and avocado.	Lentil Salad with Carrots and Spinach	Curry turkey meatballs with yogurt sauce
Day 3	Buckwheat Pancakes with Honey and Fresh Fruit	Lemon Chicken with Broccoli	Baked salmon with mixed vegetables
Day 4	Greek Yogurt Parfait with Blueberries and Walnuts	Tuna Steak with Mango Salsa	Lemon chicken with steamed spinach
Day 5	Scrambled Eggs with Tomatoes and Spinach	Baked Trout Fillet with Aromatic Herbs	Grilled sea bass fillet with peperonata
Day 6	Garnish of Peppers Stuffed with Brown Rice	Beef Steak with Chimichurri	Mushroom risotto with asparagus
Day 7	Herb Omelet with Asparagus and Sun-Dried	Duck Breast with Cranberry Sauce	Grilled Tofu with Chili Peanut Sauce

Week 2

	Breakfast	Lunch	Dinner
Day 1	Sweet potato pancakes with maple syrup.	Turkey Meatballs with Curry Sauce and Almonds	Courgette and Avocado Cream
Day 2	Dark Chocolate Fondue with Fresh Fruit	Avocado and black pepper salsa with grilled chicken	Beef steak with green pepper sauce
Day 3	Millet porridge with apples and cinnamon.	Baked Salmon with Dijon Mustard Dressing	Quinoa and Broccoli Minestrone
Day 4	Mushroom omelet with parsley.	Turmeric Tofu with Peppers and Zucchini	Chicken curry with coconut and pineapple
Day 5	Coconut Parfait with Pineapple and Mango	Beef steak with white wine sauce and parsley	Grilled Salmon with Avocado Sauce
Day 6	Kamut Porridge with Pears and Walnuts	Mustard Pork with Asparagus and Mushrooms	Tuna Steak with Mango Salsa
Day 7	Buckwheat Pancakes with Honey and Fresh Fruit	Duck Breast with Black Cherry and Port Sauce	Chicken broth with ginger and parsley

Week 3

	Breakfast	Lunch	Dinner
Day 1	Buckwheat Porridge with Apples and Cinnamon	Zucchini Spaghetti with Basil Pesto	Grilled Salmon with Citrus Sauce
Day 2	Green smoothie with spinach, banana and avocado.	Grilled Chicken with Peppers and Onions	Tuna Steak with Lime and Coriander Sauce
Day 3	Buckwheat Pancakes with Honey and Fresh Fruit	Sweet Potato and Carrot Soup with Cinnamon	Duck Breast with Blackcurrant Sauce
Day 4	Greek Yogurt Parfait with Blueberries and Walnuts	Curry Chicken Meatballs	Beef Steak with Green Pepper Sauce
Day 5	Scrambled Eggs with Tomatoes and Spinach	Chili Chicken with Peppers and Onions	Pork Curry with Mango
Day 6	Buckwheat Pancakes with Honey and Fresh Fruit	Chicken Broth with Garlic and Parsley	Grilled Salmon with Avocado and Cucumber Sauce
Day 7	Green smoothie with spinach, banana and avocado.	Quinoa Salad with Chickpeas and Olives	Mustard Chicken with Sweet Potatoes

Week 4

	Breakfast	Lunch	Dinner
Day 1	Green smoothie with spinach, banana and avocado.	Duck Breast in Port	Grilled tilapia with basil and tomato sauce.
Day 2	Buckwheat Crepes with Honey and Nuts	Pumpkin and Cinnamon Soup	Quinoa Meatballs with Peppers and Onions
Day 3	Garnish of Peppers Stuffed with Brown Rice.	Cotechino with Lentils and Carrots	Quinoa and vegetable pie
Day 4	Avocado Toast with Sunny-Side-Up Eggs	Mustard Chicken with Asparagus	Turmeric chicken with brown rice
Day 5	Coconut Parfait with Pineapple and Mango	Quinoa Salad with Chickpeas and Olives	Baked salmon with mixed vegetables
Day 6	Whole Wheat Carrot and Walnut Muffins	Grilled Pork with Apple Sauce	Curry Salmon with Steamed Vegetables
Day 7	Buckwheat Pancakes with Maple Syrup	Lentil and Cherry Tomato Soup	Chickpea pasta with kale and cherry tomatoes

Week 5

	Breakfast	Lunch	Dinner
Day 1	Oatmeal with Strawberries and Chia Seeds	Quinoa Meatballs with Tzatziki Sauce	Baked Salmon with Cilantro Lime Sauce
Day 2	Dark Chocolate Fondue with Fresh Fruit	Chicken Tacos with Avocado and Tomato Sauce	Tuna Steak with Basil and Cherry Tomato Sauce
Day 3	Millet porridge with apples and cinnamon.	Lemon Chicken with Olives and Parsley	Mustard pork with asparagus and sweet potatoes
Day 4	Avocado Toast with Sunny-Side-Up Eggs	White Bean and Leek Minestrone	Quinoa and Brussels Sprouts Minestrone
Day 5	Coconut Parfait with Pineapple and Mango	Grilled Salmon with Mango and Chili Sauce	Grilled salmon with ginger-lime sauce
Day 6	Sweet Potato Pancakes with Maple Syrup	Chicken Tacos with Lime and Coriander Sauce	Beef steak with red wine sauce and mushrooms
Day 7	Buckwheat Pancakes with Maple Syrup	Grilled Tofu with Peanut and Ginger Sauce	Cauliflower and Cumin Soup

Week 6

	Breakfast	Lunch	Dinner
Day 1	Buckwheat Porridge with Apples and Cinnamon	Baked Salmon with Pink Pepper Sauce	Kale salad with pumpkin seeds and feta
Day 2	Green smoothie with spinach, banana and avocado.	Grilled Tuna Steak with Basil Sauce	Quinoa salad with avocado and black beans
Day 3	Buckwheat Pancakes with Maple Syrup	Duck Breast with Honey and Lemon Sauce	Beef Broth with Celery Roots
Day 4	Greek Yogurt Parfait with Blueberries and Walnuts	Grilled Pork with Pineapple Sauce	Vegetarian Taco Bowl
Day 5	Scrambled Eggs with Tomatoes and Spinach	Grilled Chicken with Ginger and Lime Sauce	Tuna steak with mango sauce and cucumber
Day 6	Pumpkin Pancakes with Cinnamon	Fish Tacos with Avocado and Tomato Sauce	Aubergine flan
Day 7	Green smoothie with spinach, banana and avocado.	Beef Steak with Porcini Sauce	Eggplant Soup with Rosemary

Week 7

	Breakfast	Lunch	Dinner
Day 1	Whole Wheat Carrot and Walnut Muffins	Duck Breast with Green Pepper	Quinoa and vegetable pie
Day 2	Green smoothie with spinach, banana and avocado.	Turkey Meatballs with Tzatziki Sauce and Cucumbers	Turmeric chicken with brown rice
Day 3	Pumpkin Pancakes with Cinnamon	Chicken Curry with Lentils and Spinach	Black Bean and Chard Minestrone
Day 4	Greek Yogurt Parfait with Blueberries and Walnuts	Tuna steak with lemon and parsley sauce	Herb omelet with dried tomatoes and olives
Day 5	Scrambled Eggs with Tomatoes and Spinach	Baked Trout Fillet with Citrus Sauce	Pumpkin soup with coconut and ginger
Day 6	Oat pancakes with blueberries	Grilled Salmon with Avocado and Cucumber Sauce	Curry turkey meatballs with yogurt sauce
Day 7	Green smoothie with spinach, banana and avocado.	Beef Steak with White Wine Sauce	Fish Broth with Saffron

Week 8

	Breakfast	Lunch	Dinner
Day 1	Buckwheat Porridge with Apples and Cinnamon	Tuna Steak with Mango Sauce	Courgette spaghetti with Basil pesto
Day 2	Green smoothie with spinach, banana and avocado.	Chicken Curry with Mixed Vegetables	Avocado and black pepper salsa with grilled chicken
Day 3	Oat pancakes with blueberries	Grilled Tofu with Garlic Sauce	Red lentil pasta with courgettes and cherry tomatoes
Day 4	Greek Yogurt Parfait with Blueberries and Walnuts	Mustard Pork with Mashed Potatoes	Lemon chicken with steamed spinach
Day 5	Scrambled Eggs with Tomatoes and Spinach	Duck breast with red grape sauce	Beef Broth with Leeks and Thyme
Day 6	Quinoa Pancakes with Berries	Beef Steak with Mushroom Sauce	Avocado and orange salad with nuts
Day 7	Green smoothie with spinach, banana and avocado.	Quinoa Meatballs with Tomato Sauce	Wholemeal couscous with grilled vegetables

15 Day Workouts Plan

Here's a simple 15-day workout plan that can help you burn calories, maintain wellness, and complement your anti-inflammatory diet. This plan includes a combination of cardiovascular and resistance training. Please be sure to consult a fitness professional or doctor before starting any exercise program.

Week 1

Day 1	30 minute brisk walk.
Day 2	Bodyweight exercises (e.g. push-ups, squats) for 20 minutes.
Day 3	Swim or swim freestyle for 30 minutes.
Day 4	20 minute yoga or stretching.
Day 5	Light jog or jog for 20 minutes.
Day 6	Active rest: walks in nature for 30 minutes.
Day 7	Resistance exercises (light weights or elastic bands) for 20 minutes.

Week 2

Day 8	30 minute brisk walk.
Day 9	Bodyweight exercises for 20 minutes.
Day 10	Swim or swim freestyle for 30 minutes.
Day 11	20 minute yoga or stretching.
Day 12	Light jog or jog for 20 minutes.
Day 13	Active rest: walks in nature for 30 minutes.
Day 14	Resistance exercises for 20 minutes.

You can repeat this cycle for a total of 14 days. Be sure to follow the anti-inflammatory diet during this time to maximize the benefits. During training, stay hydrated, listen to your body and be careful not to overdo it.
Remember that it's important to vary your workouts to prevent adaptation and continue burning calories. After these 15 days, you can adapt your training plan according to your personal goals and preferences.

Part III: Tips and Tricks

Chapter 13: Preparation and cooking tips

Tips for cooking healthily and anti-inflammatory - Recommended cooking techniques

Introduction: Flavor and Health in Anti-Inflammatory Cooking

Welcome to the chapter dedicated to "Tips for healthy and anti-inflammatory cooking - Recommended cooking techniques." Here you will discover how to transform anti-inflammatory ingredients into delicious and nutritious dishes through the use of strategically chosen cooking techniques. Anti-inflammatory cooking is much more than just a diet; it is an approach to cooking that aims to maximize the healing power of foods while creating a feast for the palate.

In this chapter, we will guide you through a series of culinary techniques that will help you maintain the maximum nutritional value of ingredients, minimize the use of saturated fats and refined sugars, and make the most of the power of herbs, spices and of natural flavors. You will discover how to cook with creativity and passion, without compromising your health. From using low-fat cooking methods to making delicious dressings and sauces without inflammatory ingredients, this chapter will be your practical guide to creating meals that are both beneficial and tasty.

It will be a culinary journey that will take you through the different nuances of cooking, from grilling and steaming to preparing nutritious soups and baked recipes. You'll learn how to expertly balance flavors and nutrients to create anti-inflammatory dishes that will be a hit at any meal. After exploring these techniques, you'll be ready to put what you've learned into practice with the recipes that follow, each designed to ensure your path to an inflammation-free life is flavorful and fulfilling. Be ready to discover the perfect combination of health and delicious cuisine!

A culinary approach that promotes health and fights inflammation

Cooking for Health

Foods as Medicine: In the context of anti-inflammatory cuisine, the concept of "foods as medicine" represents a key philosophy. It is based on the idea that daily food choices should not only be viewed as a source of nutrition, but also as a means of promoting health and well-being. Here are some key points related to the "food as medicine" concept:

Therapeutic Nutrition: Foods are viewed as therapeutic tools to address specific health conditions, including inflammation. This means that you can choose foods based on their beneficial properties to address or prevent specific health problems.

Fighting Inflammation: In the anti-inflammatory diet, foods are selected so that they have natural anti-inflammatory properties. These foods can help reduce inflammation in the body, alleviating or preventing symptoms related to inflammatory diseases.

Reduce Inflammatory Triggers: The "foods as medicine" approach also involves avoiding or limiting foods that can trigger an inflammatory reaction in the body. These foods include added sugars, saturated fats, highly processed foods and other substances that can contribute to inflammation.

Personalization: An important aspect of the "food as medicine" concept is personalization. There is no universal anti-inflammatory diet, as nutritional needs can vary from person to person. Therefore, it is essential to adapt your food choices to your individual needs and health conditions.

Prevention and Long-Term Wellbeing: This philosophy is not only to address existing diseases, but also to promote long-term well-being and prevent potential health problems. It's about investing in your health through a balanced diet.

Nutritional Balance: Nutritional balance is an essential aspect of anti-inflammatory nutrition and health-focused cooking. It represents the balance between the nutritional intake provided by the foods consumed and the nutritional needs of the body. Here is how the nutritional balance is relevant in this context:

Provide Essential Nutrients: The anti-inflammatory diet aims to provide the body with all the essential nutrients it needs to function properly. These nutrients include proteins, carbohydrates, healthy fats, vitamins, minerals and antioxidants. An adequate nutritional balance ensures that the body receives everything it needs.

Calorie Control: Nutritional balance also involves calorie control. Consuming an adequate number of calories based on your body's needs is important to avoid excess weight or excessive weight loss, both of which can negatively affect inflammation and overall health.

Reduction of Inflammatory Foods: One aspect of nutritional balance in the anti-inflammatory diet is controlling the intake of foods known to promote inflammation. This includes reducing added sugars, saturated fats, highly processed foods, and foods with a high glycemic index.

Increase in Anti-Inflammatory Foods: At the same time, the nutritional balance promotes the increase in foods known for their anti-inflammatory properties, such as fruits, vegetables, fatty fish, nuts and seeds. These foods provide nutrients that can help reduce inflammation in the body.

Personalization: As mentioned above, the nutritional balance must be personalized based on individual nutritional needs and health conditions. Some people may need to adjust their intake of specific nutrients based on their needs.

Low Temperature Cooking Techniques

Low-temperature cooking techniques are particularly suitable for anti-inflammatory nutrition as they better preserve nutrients and reduce the formation of potentially harmful compounds during high-temperature cooking. Here are some of the most common low-temperature cooking techniques:

Sous Vide: This technique involves sous vide cooking foods in airtight bags at a constant temperature, often in a thermal tank. This method allows you to cook food slowly and evenly. It is particularly suitable for meat, fish and vegetables. Because the temperature is precise and constant, overheating and the loss of heat-sensitive nutrients can be avoided.

Steaming: Steaming is another low-temperature technique that retains most of the nutrients in foods. Food is placed on or in steam which gently cooks it. This technique is ideal for vegetables, fish and even eggs.

Slow Cooking: This technique involves cooking food over very low heat for a long period of time. For example, a slow cooker or slow cooker can be used to make soups, stews, or slow-cooked meats. This technique makes the meat tender and tasty and allows deep flavors to develop.

Low-temperature baking: This technique involves cooking food at a lower temperature than normal. For example, you can cook meat or fish at a temperature of 120-150°C instead of 180-220°C. This keeps the meat juicy and limits the formation of inflammatory substances such as acrylamide.

Steam oven: A steam oven uses water vapor to cook foods, which retains nutrients and prevents the formation of potentially harmful substances such as acrylamide. This type of oven is ideal for cooking vegetables, fish and even desserts.

Cold Marinating: Cold marinating involves soaking foods in a mixture of oil, vinegar, herbs and spices for a certain period of time before cooking them. This process can tenderize meats and add flavor without the use of high temperatures.

Low Temperature Dehydration: Dehydration is a technique that removes moisture from foods at low temperatures. This process is used to prepare healthy snacks such as fruit and vegetable chips.

Steaming in banana leaves: This traditional technique is used in some Asian cuisines. The food is wrapped in banana leaves and steamed, thus preserving the flavors and nutrients

Grilling the Healthy Way

Healthy grilling can be a delicious option for preparing anti-inflammatory meals, but it's important to do it right to minimize the formation of potentially harmful substances like acrylamide and to preserve the nutritional value of foods. Here are some guidelines for healthy grilling:

Use lean meat and fish: Choose lean cuts of meat such as skinless chicken breast, turkey breast or lean steak. Fish, such as salmon, trout or tuna, is a great choice rich in omega-3 fatty acids that can help reduce inflammation.

Marinate before grilling: Marinating meat or fish before grilling can add flavor and help reduce the formation of inflammatory compounds. Use marinades made with olive oil, herbs, garlic and spices such as turmeric or ginger.

Limit cooking time: Quick grilling over high heat is preferable to prolonged slow cooking. Cook the meat only until well done, avoiding burning it.

Avoid sugary marinades: Marinades high in sugar can burn easily on the grill, increasing acrylamide formation. Choose low-sugar or sugar-free marinades.

Use legumes and vegetables: Grilling vegetables such as peppers, courgettes, asparagus and mushrooms is a great alternative to meats. You can also grill tofu or tempeh for a source of plant-based protein.

Maintain a moderate temperature: Avoid cooking food at too high a temperature on the grill. A moderate temperature allows for even cooking without burning the outside of the food.

Use clean grills: Make sure your grill is clean before you start cooking. A dirty grill can contain residue from old cooking that can affect the flavor and quality of new foods.

Avoid direct contact with flames: If you are using a charcoal or wood-fired barbecue, avoid direct contact of food with flames. Place the meat or fish on a part of the grill where the heat is less intense.

Remove excess fat: Trim excess fat from meat before grilling. This helps reduce the formation of smoke and grease droplets that can cause flare-ups.

Add fresh herbs: After grilling, add fresh herbs like basil, parsley or rosemary to foods to enhance flavor without adding salt or sodium-rich seasonings.

Cooking Without Saturated Fats

Cooking without saturated fats is an important aspect of anti-inflammatory nutrition, as saturated fats can contribute to inflammation and increase the risk of chronic disease. Here are some cooking techniques you can promote in your book:

Steaming: Steaming is an excellent method for cooking food without adding saturated fat. You can steam vegetables, fish, chicken, and even grains like brown rice. This method keeps the nutrients and flavor of the food intact.

Baking in foil: Baking in foil is a fantastic way to prepare tasty dishes without saturated fat. Wrap the ingredients in aluminum foil or parchment and cook them in the oven or on the grill. You can add herbs, spices and citrus fruits to further flavor the food.

Oven cooking: The oven is a precious ally in cooking without saturated fats. You can roast vegetables, seafood, lean meats and even desserts without adding saturated fat. Use a nonstick or parchment-lined baking sheet to prevent food from sticking.

Low temperature cooking: Low temperature cooking is ideal for meat, fish and chicken. Slowly cooking foods at a low temperature can make them tender and flavorful without having to add oils or butter.

Cooking in broth or soup: Making soups and broths can be a delicious alternative to traditional cooking. Use low-fat vegetable or chicken broth as a base and add a variety of vegetables, lean proteins and spices for dishes that are full of flavor and nutrients.

Microwave steaming: If you're looking for a quick fix, microwave steaming is an option. Use special containers for steaming in the microwave and quickly cook vegetables and even fish.

Grilling without added oils: When you choose to grill meat, fish or vegetables, you can do it without adding oils or butter. Use spices, herbs, and yogurt- or citrus-based marinades to flavor your dishes.

Wok steaming: The wok is perfect for quickly and tasty cooking vegetables and proteins without the addition of saturated oils. Cooking occurs quickly, preserving the color and consistency of the ingredients.

Natural Flavors and Anti-inflammatory Spices

Turmeric: Turmeric is a powerful anti-inflammatory spice that can be used in many recipes. Add it to soups, stews, rice and even smoothies. You can also make a "golden milk" by mixing turmeric with non-dairy milk and a touch of black pepper to increase absorption.

Ginger: Fresh or powdered ginger is another natural anti-inflammatory. Add it to teas, juices, salads and meat or fish dishes for a health-boosting, spicy kick.

Cinnamon: Cinnamon is ideal for flavoring desserts, cereals, yogurt and even hot drinks. It is known for its potential benefit in helping regulate blood sugar levels.

Black Pepper: Black pepper contains piperine, which may improve the absorption of turmeric. Use a blend of turmeric and black pepper for maximum anti-inflammatory benefit.

Chili pepper: Chili pepper, or its powdered variant such as cayenne pepper, can give a spicy touch to your dishes and stimulate blood circulation.

Fresh herbs: Basil, parsley, thyme, rosemary and other fresh herbs can be used to add flavor to your dishes without adding salt or saturated fat.

Garlic and onion: These basic flavorings are rich in anti-inflammatory compounds. Add them to sofritos, gravies, salads or soups to enrich the flavor of your dishes.

Cardamom: Cardamom is an aromatic spice that pairs well with sweets, desserts and drinks. Add it to fruit-based foods, yogurt or even coffee.

Cloves: These aromatic spices are perfect for flavoring desserts and drinks. They can be used powdered or whole to add a touch of warmth.

Star anise: Star anise is a spice with a distinctive aroma that pairs well with meat, fish and soup dishes. It is also a common ingredient in some tea blends.

Sauces and Dressings Without Inflammation

Sauces and condiments can transform a dish, adding flavor and variety. In the anti-inflammatory diet, it is important to choose sauces and condiments that do not contribute to inflammation. Here are some inflammation-free options:

Extra virgin olive oil: Extra virgin olive oil is rich in heart-healthy monounsaturated fats and is an ideal choice for dressing salads or grilled vegetables. You can also use it to marinate lean meat or fish.

Balsamic vinegar: Balsamic vinegar adds a rich, sweet flavor to salads and vegetable dishes. Make sure you choose a high-quality variety with no added sugar.

Low Sodium Soy Sauce: Low sodium soy sauce is a flavorful condiment that can be used to add an Asian twist to your dishes. Check the label to make sure it contains less sodium.

Black Pepper Sauce: A sauce made with fresh black pepper, ginger, garlic, olive oil and lemon can add flavor to your lean protein or fish dishes without adding sugar or saturated fat.

Lemon and fresh herb sauce: By mixing fresh lemon juice with aromatic herbs such as parsley, basil and mint, you can create a light and fragrant sauce to flavor fish, chicken or vegetable dishes.

Low-sodium tomato sauce: No-sugar-added, low-sodium tomato sauce can be used to season whole-wheat pasta or as a base for meat or vegetable sauces.

Avocado Salsa: Avocado is rich in heart-healthy fats and can be blended with lime, garlic and pepper to create a creamy salsa to use on salads or as a topping for grilled chicken.

Hummus: This paste made from chickpeas, tahini, garlic and lemon is a versatile condiment that can be spread on whole-grain bread, used as a dip for vegetables or as a base for salads.

Basil Pesto: Basil pesto, made with fresh basil, pine nuts, parmesan and olive oil, is a flavor-packed condiment that can be mixed with whole-wheat pasta or used as a topping for fish.

Low-Sodium Peanut Sauce: This creamy sauce can be used to dress salads, grill vegetables, or make Asian dishes like chicken satay.

Chapter 14: Management of Food Allergies
How to adapt recipes for common food allergies
Recognize common food allergies

Recognizing common food allergies is a critical step in ensuring the safety and health of people with such allergies. This process requires a good understanding of the most common food allergies and associated symptoms. Here is an overview of common food allergies:

Gluten Allergy: This allergy is common among those who suffer from celiac disease or non-celiac gluten sensitivity. Gluten is a protein found in wheat, barley and rye. Symptoms may include gastrointestinal distress, skin rashes, fatigue and malnutrition.

Milk Allergy: Allergy to cow's milk proteins is frequent in children, but can persist into adulthood. Symptoms include skin rashes, bloating, abdominal cramps, and respiratory reactions.

Egg Allergy: Allergies to eggs, particularly egg white proteins, are more common in children and are often outgrown with age. Symptoms can range from mild to severe and include skin rashes, gastrointestinal upset, and respiratory reactions.

Nut Allergy: Allergies to nuts, such as common walnuts, pecans, Brazil nuts, and almonds, are often severe and can cause life-threatening anaphylactic reactions. Symptoms include itching, swelling, difficulty breathing and shock.

Fish Allergy: Allergies to fish, such as salmon, tuna and trout, are also notoriously serious and can cause anaphylactic reactions. Symptoms may be similar to those of nut allergies.

Shellfish Allergy: This category includes shrimp, lobsters and crabs. Shellfish allergies can be serious and cause anaphylactic reactions. The symptoms are similar to those of fish allergies.

Soy Allergy: Soy allergies are more common in children, but some people also suffer from them in adulthood. Symptoms may include gastrointestinal upset, skin rashes, and respiratory reactions.

Wheat Allergy: Wheat allergy is similar to celiac disease but involves an allergic reaction to wheat proteins, not an autoimmune reaction. Symptoms can vary and include gastrointestinal discomfort, skin rashes and itching.

Other food allergies: There are many other less common food allergies, such as allergy to strawberries, tomatoes, red meats, sesame seeds and more.

Safe ingredient substitutions

Safe ingredient substitutions are key to adapting recipes for people with common food allergies or intolerances. Here are some common and effective substitutions for allergenic ingredients:

Gluten Allergy:
Gluten-free flour (such as rice flour, almond flour, coconut flour) instead of wheat flour. Gluten-free pasta instead of wheat pasta. Gluten-free bread instead of wheat bread. Corn or rice bran instead of barley or rye cereals.

Milk Allergy:
Lactose-free milk or plant-based milk (such as almond milk, soy milk, coconut milk) instead of cow's milk. Vegan butter or margarine instead of traditional butter. Lactose-free yogurt or non-dairy yogurt instead of milk-based yogurt. Vegan cheese instead of traditional cheese.

Egg Allergy:
Banana or apple puree instead of eggs in sweet preparations (such as cakes and muffins).
Crumbled silken tofu instead of eggs in savory dishes (such as omelettes or quiche).
Vegan egg substitutes, commercially available, in many preparations.

Nut Allergy:
Chopped sunflower seeds, pumpkin seeds or chia seeds instead of nuts in salads and baking.
Sunflower seed butter or pumpkin seed butter instead of peanut butter.
Nut-free milk (such as oat milk) instead of almond or walnut milk.

Allergy to Fish or Shellfish:
Alternative fish or shellfish, such as oily fish, chicken or tofu, in fish or seafood recipes.
Vegetable fish substitutes, commercially available, for sushi-based dishes or fish salads.

Soy Allergy:
Soy-free plant-based milk (such as almond milk or coconut milk) instead of soy milk.
Sunflower seed butter or nut butter instead of soy butter.
Soy-free plant-based yogurt (such as coconut milk or almond milk) instead of soy yogurt.

Wheat Allergy:
Gluten-free flour or alternative flours (such as coconut flour, almond flour, or buckwheat flour) instead of wheat flour.
Gluten-free bread or bread made from alternative flours.
Gluten-free pasta or pasta made from legumes (such as lentil pasta) instead of wheat pasta.

Other food allergies:
There are several substitution options for specific ingredients, such as goat's milk in place of cow's milk for milk allergies, or corn flour in place of wheat flour for wheat allergies.

Food labels

Food labels are essential information found on the packaging of packaged foods and are critical for identifying and managing food allergies, intolerances or specific dietary preferences. Here are some key elements usually found on food labels:

List of Ingredients: Here are all the ingredients contained in the food, in descending order of quantity. Ingredients are often written in large print, making it easier to spot common allergens like wheat, milk, eggs, nuts and others.

Nutritional Information: This section provides information on the number of nutrients present in the food. It often includes calorie content, amounts of fat, carbohydrates, protein, fiber and sugar. This information is especially important for people following specific diets or monitoring their calorie and nutritional intake.

Declared Allergens: In the United States and many other jurisdictions, laws require that common food allergens, such as wheat, milk, eggs, peanuts, tree nuts, fish and shellfish, be clearly listed on the label. These allergens should be highlighted in bold or in different fonts.

Expiry Date or Preferential Consumption: This date indicates until when the food should be consumed to ensure maximum freshness and safety. It is important to follow these dates to avoid food spoilage.

Storage Instructions: This section provides guidance on how to store the food safely, such as whether it should be refrigerated, frozen or kept at room temperature.

Manufacturer Information: The label usually includes the name and address of the manufacturer or distributor of the food. This is useful for traceability purposes in case of food safety issues or requests for additional information.

Instructions for Use: Some food products, such as seasoning mixes or baking products, may provide instructions on how to use the product for best results.

Daily Percentage Values (VDG or DV%): These percentages indicate how much a single serving of food contributes to the recommended daily intake of nutrients, such as fats, carbohydrates, fiber, vitamins and minerals. They can be useful for assessing how much a food contributes to your overall diet.

Additional Ethical or Nutritional Information: Some labels may include claims about health, ethical sourcing of ingredients, or product features (for example, "GMO-free" or "organic").

Be careful at intersections

Attention to intersections is crucial for anyone who must cook for people with food allergies. Cross-contamination occurs when allergens or allergenic food particles come into contact with foods that should be safe for the allergic person. This can happen at various stages of the food preparation process, from shopping to cooking and serving the meal. That's why it's so important to take precautions to avoid cross-contamination:

1. Food separation: Keeping allergenic foods separate from safe foods is a fundamental rule. Use different surfaces and utensils to prepare allergenic and non-allergenic foods. For example, if you make peanut butter sandwiches for some family members, make sure none of it ends up in meals for allergy sufferers.

2. Proper Cleaning: Wash and clean surfaces, pots, pans and utensils between uses. This is especially important when working with common allergens like wheat, milk or eggs. Hands should also be washed thoroughly after handling allergenic foods.

3. Ingredient Awareness: Read food labels carefully to identify possible cross-contamination in products with allergens. Some foods may be manufactured in the same facility where allergens are processed. Also, check for labels "may contain traces of" or "processed in a facility that handles" specific allergens.

4. Clear Labeling: If you are cooking for someone with allergies, clearly label foods in your pantry or refrigerator to indicate whether they are safe or contain allergens. This helps avoid mistakes when preparing meals.

5. Choosing Safe Recipes: If you are cooking for someone with allergies, look for specific recipes that are safe for their needs. Avoid adapting recipes containing allergens unless you can guarantee total separation and cleanliness of the ingredients.

6. Clear Communication: If you are hosting or cooking for someone with allergies, communicate clearly with them to understand their specific dietary needs and allergies. Make sure you are aware of their needs before you start preparing meals.

Alternatives to common ingredients

When cooking for people with food allergies, it is important to know and use safe alternatives to common ingredients that could cause allergic reactions. Here are some alternatives to common ingredients often implicated in food allergies:

1. Milk: Plant-based milk (soy, almond, coconut, oat, rice), Plant-based yogurt, Vegan cheese.

2. Eggs: Commercial egg substitutes such as egg replacer, ripe banana puree, non-dairy yogurt.

3. Wheat: Rice flour, almond flour or coconut flour for gluten-free bread making, Gluten-free pasta such as rice or corn, Gluten-free bread.

4. Nuts (walnuts, almonds, etc.): Seeds such as sunflower seeds, pumpkin seeds or chia seeds, Health-safe dried fruits allergic person, sunflower seed butter or pumpkin seed butter.

5. Peanuts: Almond butter or nut butter, Roasted sunflower seeds as a snack, Sunflower seed butter.

6. Fish: Tofu or tempeh as alternatives in recipes, Heart of palm or banana heart to reproduce the consistency of fish. Plant-based fish substitutes.

7. Soy: Almond milk, oat milk or rice milk as alternatives in cereals or drinks, Tofu or tempeh to replace soy in recipes.

8. Celery: Parsley or basil to give flavor to soups and dishes, Black celery as a substitute for common celery.

9. Fresh and dried fruit: Choose fruit that is safe for the allergic person and use it to replace the risky one.

10. Foods with monosodium glutamate (MSG): - Use herbs and spices to flavor dishes without the use of MSG.

Chapter 15: Physical activity and stress reduction

Importance of physical activity in anti-inflammation

Weight control: Regular physical activity helps maintain a healthy body weight. Accumulation of excess body fat can contribute to chronic inflammation. Maintaining an ideal weight can reduce your risk of developing inflammation-related conditions such as obesity, type 2 diabetes and heart disease.

Improved insulin sensitivity: Exercise can increase your cells' sensitivity to insulin, which helps regulate blood sugar levels. This is especially important for those trying to manage inflammation related to type 2 diabetes.

Reduced Inflammation: Physical activity can directly help reduce inflammation in the body. Exercise promotes blood circulation, lymphatic flow and the release of beneficial hormones such as endorphins. These mechanisms can reduce systemic inflammation.

Boosting the Immune System: Moderate physical activity can improve the function of the immune system. A strong immune system can help the body fight inflammation and infections.

Improved joint health: For those who suffer from inflammatory joint conditions such as rheumatoid arthritis, regular exercise can help maintain flexibility, muscle strength and joint mobility.

Stress Reduction: Chronic stress is associated with inflammation. Physical activity is known for its beneficial effect on reducing stress through the release of endorphins and promoting psychological well-being.

Improved sleep: Quality sleep is essential for recovery and management of inflammation. Regular exercise can improve the quality of sleep, indirectly contributing to the reduction of inflammation.

Increased energy and vitality: Chronic inflammation can also cause tiredness and fatigue. Physical activity can increase energy and improve quality of life.

Stress management techniques for overall well-being

Meditation and Mindfulness: Reduce Stress and Promote Wellbeing

Meditation and mindfulness are age-old practices that involve mindful attention and concentration on breathing, thoughts and sensations without judgment. These techniques have become increasingly popular in managing stress and promoting overall health. Here are some significant things worth discussing:

Definition of meditation and mindfulness: Meditation involves focusing on a specific object or concept, while mindfulness focuses on being present in the current moment.

Health benefits: There are numerous health benefits associated with these practices, including the reduction of stress, anxiety and depression. Meditation and mindfulness can also improve concentration, sleep quality and emotional management.

Reduced inflammation: Meditation and mindfulness have been linked to reducing markers of inflammation in the body. This is especially relevant in an anti-inflammatory diet context.

Meditation Techniques: There is a varied overview of different meditation techniques, including guided meditation, transcendental meditation, and vipassana meditation.

Mindfulness in diet: The importance of mindfulness during meals is highlighted. Being aware of what you eat, the tastes and sensations during the meal can contribute to greater food satisfaction and better appetite regulation.

Practical Tips: Practical tips on how to integrate meditation and mindfulness into your daily life. These tips might involve creating a quiet space for practice, setting meditation goals, and pursuing consistency in your practice.

Chapter 16: Meal Planning and Maintenance

How to Plan Anti-Inflammatory Meals on a Budget

Guidelines for Correct Planning

Planning: Planning ahead can help you avoid waste and maximize efficiency in meal preparation.

Identifying Key Foods: Identify key anti-inflammatory foods to include in your diet. These might include fruits, dark green leafy vegetables, omega-3-rich fish, nuts, seeds, legumes and whole grains.

Grocery List: Create a grocery list based on what you need for your planned anti-inflammatory recipes. Stick to the list and avoid impulse purchases that can increase costs.

Buy in season: Buy fruits and vegetables in season, as they are often cheaper and of better quality. Consuming seasonal produce can also offer variety in your diet.

Packaged food vs. DIY: There are cost differences between packaged food and cooking from scratch. Cooking from scratch is often more convenient and allows you to control the ingredients.

Storage and freezing: Plan meals to avoid waste. For example, storing leftovers properly, freezing additional portions and using ingredients in multiple dishes to reduce waste.

Inexpensive Recipes: You can make inexpensive anti-inflammatory recipes that can be made with affordable ingredients. These recipes should be simple to follow and tasty.

Quantity and portions: Pay attention to portions to avoid food waste and save money. Plan your meals so you have leftovers that can be used for later meals.

Flexibility: Finally, use flexibility in meal planning. Adapting recipes based on ingredients on offer or promotions can help you stay on budget.

Monitor your progress and adjust your diet

Keep a food diary: Encourage readers to keep a food diary to record what they eat each day. This can help identify foods that may be triggering inflammatory reactions or digestive problems. Be sure to include spaces to note any symptoms or changes in well-being.

Evaluate Progress: Invite readers to regularly evaluate their progress and overall health. They might consider measures such as body weight, blood pressure, energy levels and sleep quality. Periodic evaluation can help see if the anti-inflammatory diet is producing benefits.

Consult a health professional: Suggest that readers consult a health professional, such as a nutritionist or dietician, to monitor their progress and receive personalized advice. This professional can also help you set specific health goals.

Controlled Experiments: Encourage readers to experiment with their diet in a controlled way. They can gradually introduce new foods and monitor how they affect their well-being. This approach can help identify specific food intolerances or sensitivities.

Listening to your body: Emphasizes the importance of listening to your body. Readers should be aware of how they feel after eating certain foods and make adjustments based on their body's responses. For example, if they notice symptoms of inflammation after consuming a certain food, they may consider eliminating it from their diet.

Flexibility in adjustment: Emphasize that the anti-inflammatory diet is not one size fits all. Each person has different food needs and tolerances. Encourage flexibility in adjusting nutrition based on individual needs.

Remember balance: Emphasize the importance of maintaining a balance in your diet. Anti-inflammatory nutrition should provide all the essential nutrients the body needs. Dietary extremism may not be sustainable in the long term.

Regularly Plan: Invite readers to plan their meals regularly to ensure they are eating a balanced, anti-inflammatory diet. Planning can help you avoid impulsive or unhealthy food choices.

Communicating with your health professional: If readers make significant changes to their diet, emphasize the importance of communicating with their health professional. This professional can evaluate the changes and provide further guidance.

Healthy lifestyle: In addition to diet, remind readers that a healthy lifestyle also includes regular exercise, stress management and quality sleep. All of these elements contribute to overall happiness.

Chapter 17: The Future of Anti-Inflammation

Future research and developments in anti-inflammation

Here are some examples of recent scientific research that highlights the crucial role of inflammation in disease:

Inflammation and cardiovascular disease: Numerous studies have confirmed the link between inflammation and cardiovascular diseases such as atherosclerosis. Chronic inflammation contributes to the formation of plaque in the arteries, increasing the risk of strokes and heart attacks. Research published in "Nature Reviews Cardiology" in 2019 delved into these links.

Inflammation and type 2 diabetes: The relationship between inflammation and type 2 diabetes is the subject of increasing attention. A study published in "Diabetes Care" in 2017 highlighted how chronic inflammation can interfere with insulin regulation and lead to insulin resistance.

Inflammation and cancer: Numerous studies have demonstrated the association between chronic inflammation and the risk of developing cancer. For example, a study published in "Cancer Research" in 2020 examined the role of inflammation in tumor metastasis, highlighting how it can facilitate the spread of tumor cells.

Inflammation and neurodegenerative diseases: Neuroinflammation has been linked to neurodegenerative diseases such as Alzheimer's and Parkinson's disease. Research published in "Nature Reviews Neuroscience" in 2021 delved into the role of inflammation in neuronal damage.

Inflammation and gastrointestinal disorders: Inflammation plays a key role in gastrointestinal disorders such as Crohn's disease and ulcerative colitis. Recent studies, such as those published in "Inflammatory Bowel Diseases" in 2022, seek to better understand the inflammatory mechanisms in these disorders.

Inflammation and obesity: Inflammation has been associated with obesity and its metabolic complications. Research continues to investigate the molecular pathways that link inflammation to body fat accumulation.

Inflammation and autoimmune diseases: Autoimmune diseases, such as lupus and multiple sclerosis, are characterized by inflammation and an abnormal immune response. Recent research is trying to better understand the mechanisms that trigger these inflammatory responses.

Inflammation and Aging: Aging studies have found that chronic inflammation can accelerate the cellular aging process. This research may help develop strategies to slow aging.

Role of inflammation on mental health

Depression and inflammation: A study published in "JAMA Psychiatry" in 2020 examined the links between depression and inflammatory markers. It highlighted that chronic inflammation may contribute to the development and severity of depression.

Neurodegenerative disorders and inflammation: Research continues to investigate the role of inflammation in the progression of neurodegenerative disorders such as Alzheimer's and Parkinson's disease, with studies published in journals such as "Nature Reviews Neuroscience."

Role of inflammation in aging

Cellular Aging and Inflammation: Recent research, such as a study published in "Cell Metabolism" in 2021, has highlighted the link between chronic inflammation and cellular aging. Inflammation can accelerate cell deterioration and contribute to aging processes.

Brain Aging and Inflammation: Studies on brain aging have revealed the importance of inflammation in cognitive degeneration. This is the subject of ongoing research, with publications in journals such as "Frontiers in Aging Neuroscience."

Role of inflammation in cancer types

Cancer and inflammation: Much research has confirmed the link between inflammation and the development of various types of cancer. For example, a study in "Cancer Research" in 2020 examined inflammation as a promoter of tumor metastasis.

Immunotherapy and cancer: Immunotherapy, an approach to fighting cancer that harnesses the immune system, has often been associated with inflammation. Scientists are trying to better understand how to manage inflammation to improve the effectiveness of these therapies.

Inflammatory inhibitors and anticancer therapies: Research published in "Cancer Cell" in 2021 examined the potential of anti-inflammatory drugs for the treatment of cancer, demonstrating that inflammation is an important therapeutic target.

The Role of Anti-Inflammation in Preventive Medicine

The preventative approach, in terms of anti-inflammatory diet, refers to a way of addressing health and well-being aimed at preventing the development of chronic diseases through proper nutrition and a healthy lifestyle. Its main role is to reduce or avoid chronic inflammation in the body, which is considered a key factor in the process of many diseases, including diabetes, heart disease, cancer, arthritis and other pathological conditions.

Here is a more detailed definition of these two components:

Preventive Approach: The preventive approach to health is based on the idea of preventing diseases from occurring rather than treating them after they have already occurred. This approach aims to identify and manage known risk factors and take steps to keep them under control. It includes a series of behaviors and lifestyle choices aimed at promoting well-being and preventing the development of pathological conditions. As part of anti-inflammatory nutrition, the preventative approach focuses on reducing chronic or excessive inflammation as a means of preventing or limiting the risk of chronic disease.

Role in the Anti-Inflammatory Diet: In the context of anti-inflammatory nutrition, the preventive approach manifests itself through a series of targeted food choices and a healthy lifestyle. This type of diet is based on foods known for their anti-inflammatory properties, such as fruits, vegetables, omega-3-rich fish, nuts, seeds and spices. The goal is to reduce consumption of foods known to promote inflammation, such as saturated fats, refined sugars and highly processed foods. At the same time, the anti-inflammatory diet encourages healthy lifestyle, including regular exercise, stress management, adequate sleep and maintaining a healthy body weight.

The role of the preventative approach in the anti-inflammatory diet is to provide individuals with tools and guidelines to adopt a way of life that is proactive in promoting health and preventing chronic diseases associated with inflammation. Additionally, it promotes awareness of how food choices and lifestyle directly influence the level of inflammation in the body and, consequently, long-term health.

Cooking Conversion Chart

Volume Equivalents (Liquid)

US STANDARD	US STANDARD (OUNCES)	METRIC (APPROXIMATE)
2 tablespoons	1 fl. oz.	30 mL
¼ cup	2 fl. oz.	60 mL
½ cup	4 fl. oz.	120 mL
1 cup	8 fl. oz.	240 mL
1½ cups	12 fl. oz.	355 mL
2 cups or 1 pint	16 fl. oz.	475 mL
4 cups or 1 quart	32 fl. oz.	1 L
1 gallon	128 fl. oz.	4 L

Volume Equivalents (Dry)

US STANDARD	METRIC (APPROXIMATE)
⅛ teaspoon	0.5 mL
¼ teaspoon	1 mL
½ teaspoon	2 mL
¾ teaspoon	4 mL
1 teaspoon	5 mL
1 tablespoon	15 mL
¼ cup	59 mL
⅓ cup	79 mL
½ cup	118 mL
⅔ cup	156 mL
¾ cup	177 mL
1 cup	235 mL
2 cups or 1 pint	475 mL
3 cups	700 mL
4 cups or 1 quart	1 L
½ gallon	2 L
1 gallon	4 L

Oven Temperatures

FAHRENHEIT (F)	CELSIUS (C) (APPROXIMATE)
250	120
300	150
325	165
350	180
375	190
400	200
425	220
450	230

Weight Equivalents

US STANDARD	METRIC (APPROXIMATE)
½ ounce	15 g
1 ounce	30 g
2 ounces	60 g
4 ounces	115 g
8 ounces	225 g
12 ounces	340 g
16 ounces or 1 pound	455 g

Concluding Message

Dear reader,

Let's conclude this journey together, a journey dedicated to health, well-being and the discovery of a food approach that can transform your life. I sincerely hope that you have found inspiration, knowledge and motivation to embrace anti-inflammatory nutrition and a lifestyle that can lead you to a healthier and more fulfilling future.

I want to thank you for choosing to take your time to explore these pages and invest in your health. Your dedication to improving your well-being is an act of love towards yourself and those around you.

Every small step you take towards a more balanced diet, a calmer mind and a more vibrant spirit will be an investment in your future. Remember that there is never a wrong time to start on a path to health, and every small change can make a significant difference.

I would also like to express my gratitude to all the experts, researchers and professionals who contributed their knowledge and experience to make this book possible. Your knowledge is a beacon in our pursuit of health and well-being.

Finally, I want to emphasize that your health is a precious and ongoing responsibility. Keep the flame of self-care alive, take care of your body and mind, and continue to explore the avenues of health through the anti-inflammatory diet.

I wish you a life in which well-being is your constant companion and your health is your greatest wealth.

With love,

Abbie Bates